Surgical Management of Spinal Cord Injury

Surgical Management of Spinal Cord Injury: Controversies and Consensus

Edited by

Arun Paul Amar, MD

Department of Neurosurgery
Stanford University School of Medicine
Stanford, CA

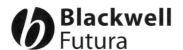

Blackwell Publishing, Inc., 350 Main Street, Malden, Massachusetts 02148-5020, USA
Blackwell Publishing Ltd, 9600 Garsington Road, Oxford OX4 2DQ, UK
Blackwell Science Asia Pty Ltd, 550 Swanston Street, Carlton, Victoria 3053, Australia

First published 2007

1 2007

ISBN: 978-1-4051-22061

Library of Congress Cataloging-in-Publication Data

Surgical management of spinal cord injury : controversies and consensus
/ edited by Arun Paul Amar
    p. ; cm.
  Includes bibliographical references and index.
  ISBN-13: 978-1-4051-2206-1 (hardcover : alk. paper)
  ISBN-10: 1-4051-2206-4 (hardcover : alk. paper)
  1. Spinal cord—Surgery. 2. Spinal cord—Wounds and injuries. I. Amar, Arun Paul.
  [DNLM: 1. Spinal Cord Injuries. 2. Spinal Cord Injuries—surgery. WL 400 S9615 2007]
RD594.3.S86 2007
617.4'82044—dc22   2006034606

A catalogue record for this title is available from the British Library

Acquisitions: Steve Korn & Gina Almond
Development: Lauren Brindley
Set by Charon Tec Ltd (A Macmillan Company), Chennai, India
Printed and bound in Singapore by C.O.S. Printers Pte Ltd

For further information on Blackwell Publishing, visit our website:
www.blackwellfutura.com

Contents

Contributors

Philipp R. Aldana, MD
Clinical Assistant Professor of Neurosurgery
Department of Neurosurgery
University of Florida-Jacksonville
and
Director of Clinical Services
Lucy Gooding Pediatric Neurosurgery Center
Jacksonville, FL

Arun Paul Amar, MD
Department of Neurosurgery
Stanford University School of Medicine
Stanford, CA

Edward C. Benzel, MD
Chairman
Cleveland Clinic Spine Institute
Cleveland, OH

Douglas L. Brockmeyer, MD
Professor
Division of Pediatric Neurosurgery
Primary Children's Medical Center
University of Utah
Salt Lake City, UT

Steven Casha, MD, PHD, FRCSC
Assistant Professor
University of Calgary
Clinical Neurosciences
Calgary, Alberta
Canada

Indro Chakrabarti, MD, MPH
Staff Neurosurgeon
Kaiser Permanente
Department of Neurosurgery
Sacramento, CA

Danny L. Chang, MD
Attending Emergency Physician
Sherman Oaks Hospital
Sherman Oaks, CA

Michael L. DiLuna, MD
Resident
Department of Neurosurgery
Yale University School of Medicine
New Haven, CT

Gordon L. Engler, MD
Professor Emeritus of Clinical Orthopaedic and
Neurological Surgery
University of Southern California
Los Angeles, CA

Richard G. Fessler, MD, PHD
John Harper Seeler Professor and Chief
Section of Neurosurgery
University of Chicago
Chicago, IL

Mark S. Gerber, MD
Resident Physician in Neurological Surgery
Barrow Neurological Institute
Phoenix, AZ

Steven L. Giannotta, MD
Chairman
Department of Neurological Surgery
USC Keck School of Medicine
Los Angeles, CA

Nestor R. Gonzalez, MD
Divisions of Neurosurgery and Interventional
Neuroradiology
David Geffen School of Medicine at UCLA
Los Angeles, CA

Barth A. Green, MD
Department of Neurological Surgery
University of Miami School of Medicine
Miami, FL

Mark N. Hadley, MD, FACS
Professor of Neurosurgery
Division of Neurosurgery
University of Alabama at Birmingham
Birmingham, AL

R. John Hurlbert, MD, PHD, FRCSC,
FACS
Associate Professor
Division of Neurosurgery
Department of Clinical Neurosciences
Calgary, Alberta
Canada

G. Alexander Jones, MD
Neurosurgery Resident
Cleveland Clinic Spine Institute
Cleveland, OH

Larry T. Khoo, MD
UCLA Comprehensive Spine Center
Santa Monica, CA

K. Anthony Kim, MD
Department of Neurological Surgery
Keck-USC Medical School
Los Angeles, CA

Jerry Larson, MA, D.ABNM
Clinical Instructor in Neurology
USC Keck Medical School
Neurology
LACUSC Medical Center
Los Angeles, CA

Michael L. Levy, MD, PhD
Professor and Head of Division of Pediatric
Neurosurgery
Children's Hospital of San Diego
San Diego, CA

Paul G. Matz, MD
Associate Professor of Surgery (Neurosurgery)
University of Alabama
Birmingham, AL

Eric P. Roger, MD, FRCS (C)
Surgical Spine Fellow
Department of Neurosurgery
Cleveland, OH

Joseph Silvaggio, MD
University of Calgary Spine Program and the
Department of Clinical Neurosciences
Foothills Hospital and Medical Centre
Calgary, Alberta
Canada

Volker K.H. Sonntag, MD, FACS
Vice Chairman, Division of Neurological Surgery
Director, Residency Program
Chairman, BNI Spine Section
Barrow Neurological Institute
and
Clinical Professor of Surgery (Neurosurgery)
University of Arizona
Tucson, AZ

**Stuart P. Swadron, MD, FRCPC,
FAAEM, FACEP**
Program Director
Residency in Emergency Medicine
Los Angeles County-University of Southern
California Medical Center
and
Assistant Professor
Keck School of Medicine of the University of
Southern California
Los Angeles, CA

Michael Y. Wang, MD
Assistant Professor and Spine Director
Department of Neurological Surgery
University of Southern California
Los Angeles, CA

Robert G. Watkins, MD
Center for Orthopedic Spinal Surgery
Los Angeles Spine Surgery Institute at St. Vincent
Medical Center
Los Angeles, CA

Brian R. Wilbur, MD, FACEP
Emergency Department
Lakewood Regional Medical Center
Lakewood, CA

Preface

The Edwin Smith papyrus, a surgical treatise drafted nearly 4000 years ago, recounted the devastation attendant to cervical spine injuries with quadriplegia and categorized them as "ailments not to be treated."[1] The nihilism implied by this proscription has remained the prevailing sentiment over the succeeding millennia. Indeed, relative to the triumphs achieved in some areas of modern medicine, spinal cord injury (SCI) has remained a debacle. It is estimated that traumatic SCI costs American society between 6 and 40 billion dollars annually.[2] As staggering as this economic impact appears, it is overshadowed by the emotional toll and personal tragedy that attend such disabling injuries.

The acute management of the SCI patient begins at the scene of an accident the moment that such an insult is suspected and progresses until the time of discharge to a rehabilitation facility. At each stage along this continuum, the goals of treatment remain identical:[3,4]

1 To maximize neurological recovery.
2 To restore normal alignment and correct deformity.
3 To promote spinal stability and/or fusion.
4 To minimize pain, both acutely and chronically.
5 To facilitate early mobilization and rehabilitation.
6 To minimize hospitalization and cost.
7 To prevent secondary complications of disability.

Although these tasks can only be accomplished by the concerted efforts of a multidisciplinary team of doctors, therapists, and nurses, the surgeon's role remains preeminent. However, *in vitro* studies, animal models, and clinical outcome analyses have all failed to yield incontrovertible guidelines that define the role of surgery in SCI. As a result, there is no consensus regarding the necessity, timing, nature, or approach of surgical intervention. Intuitive hunches and anecdotal accounts have not been corroborated by scientific studies, and individual or institutional preferences abound. Because of numerous methodological limitations, including ethical concerns about withholding potentially beneficial treatments to victims of SCI, it has not been feasible to subject such theories to prospective, randomized, controlled trials. Thus, the majority of the extant literature consists of retrospective analyses, unrandomized case series, and experimental models that may fail to simulate human SCI.[5-7]

This book reviews the controversies pertaining to the emergency, diagnostic, medical, and surgical management of SCI and summarizes the foundations of rational treatment paradigms. Scrutiny of the scientific data has yielded objective truths, though there remains some latitude for subjectivity and personal experience. Collectively, the insights disclosed within these pages justify a sense of optimism and compel the practicing surgeon to refute the archaic, defeatist notions of the past. In 2007, SCI is an ailment to be treated.

References

1 Wilkins RH (ed.). *Neurosurgical Classics*. American Association of Neurological Surgeons, Chicago, 1992, pp. 1–5.
2 Berkowitz M. Assessing the socioeconomic impact of improved treatment of head and spinal cord injuries. *J Emerg Med* 1993;11:63–67.
3 Fessler RG, Masson RL. Management of thoracic fractures. In Menezes AH and Sonntag VKH (eds): *Principles of Spinal Surgery*. McGraw-Hill, New York, 1996, pp 899–918.
4 Wilberger J. Acute spinal cord injury. In Menezes AH and Sonntag VKH (eds): *Principles of Spinal Surgery*. McGraw-Hill, New York, 1996, pp. 753–768.
5 Amar AP, Levy ML. Surgical controversies in the management of spinal cord injury. *J Am Coll Surg* 1999;188:550–566.
6 Amar AP, Levy ML. Pathogenesis and pharmacological strategies for mitigating secondary damage in acute spinal cord injury. *Neurosurgery* 1999;44:1027–1040.
7 American Association of Neurological Surgeons and Congress of Neurological Surgeons Section on Disorders of the Spine and Peripheral Nerves. Guidelines for the management of acute cervical spine and spinal cord injuries. *Neurosurgery* 2002;50(suppl):S1–S199.

Foreword by Charles H. Tator

In the last two decades the management of spinal cord injuries has changed dramatically, and major improvements have occurred in both the diagnosis and surgical treatment of spinal cord injury. Furthermore, these accomplishments have been underpinned by major advances in the basic science of both spinal injury and spinal cord injury. We now have a much greater understanding of the mechanisms of these injuries, especially improved knowledge of the pathophysiological processes in the acute, subacute, and chronic stages of traumatic spinal cord injury.

As well, it is now apparent that there should be regionalization and specialization in the management of all phases of spinal cord injury, and that all patients with acute injury should reach a specialized unit for definitive management within about two hours of injury. Certainly, this goal can be achieved in most centers in North America, except those in very remote regions. Early triage is essential for improved patient outcomes because we now know that the spinal cord suffers from major vascular impairments that worsen over time, and that best practice guidelines include careful and judicial management of hemodynamic factors as soon as possible after injury in order to prevent progressive posttraumatic infarction of the spinal cord.

Also, it has become apparent that a multidisciplinary approach to the management of spinal cord injury is the best way to ensure optimal outcome in terms of enhancement of neurological recovery, achievement of a stable, pain-free spine, and social and psychological rehabilitation. This team approach in the acute stage must be followed by a similar team approach in the rehabilitation and chronic stages in order to maximize recovery and minimize complications. The tragic passing of Christopher Reeve emphasizes the importance of management of the whole individual to prevent the potential fatal complications of spinal cord injury.

Surgical treatment has been marvelously improved, and one of the major reasons for the improvement is the accuracy with which the diagnosis of both the spinal and spinal cord injuries can be made. The importance of obtaining early complete definition of both the spinal and spinal cord injuries must be stressed: all patients with spinal cord injuries must have unimpeded access to early and expert imaging with both computerized tomography (CT) and magnetic resonance imaging (MRI). Both modalities are essential for accurate diagnosis and management, and serial imaging is essential for determining the reasons for any early deterioration. It is important to keep in mind that a significant percentage of patients deteriorate within the first few days of injury, and that the causes can often be detected by serial neurological examination and serial imaging.

The spinal cord injury field has benefited greatly from the efforts to standardize and improve the grading and scoring neurological function. Indeed, careful monitoring of clinical neurological status is just as important today as it was 50 years ago when CTs and MRIs were not available. In contrast, neurophysiologic monitoring, although useful intraoperatively, has been somewhat disappointing because it has proven to be less accurate than careful, serial, clinical neurological examinations. Thus, all practitioners in spinal cord injury must continue to remain expert in performing the clinical neurological examination. Furthermore, this examination should be based on the American Spinal Injury Association (ASIA) system because it is the best available for accurate, serial monitoring. Although it is important for surgeons to teach the neurological examination to other members of the team, especially to nurses, and physical and occupational therapists, it is essential for surgeons to continue to be skilled in this aspect of care.

The advances in our ability to repair the injured vertebral column have been staggering, and it is wonderful to behold the array of surgical approaches, strategies, and devices that are now available for patients with spinal injuries. Furthermore, it is heartening to see the cooperation between the spinal neurosurgeons and the spinal orthopedic surgeons, and the convergence of expertise toward the goal of training spinal surgeons from both training streams. The emphasis must be on training for this difficult and complicated field.

Unfortunately, the medical and surgical treatments available for reconstructing the injured spinal cord have lagged behind those available for the spinal column, and there have been no "breakthroughs" in the past 50 years. We can be proud of the many high-quality clinical trials that have occurred including the nine randomized prospective clinical trials (RPCTs) for neuroprotection, although only one RPCT for the surgical management of spinal cord injury. The lack of these "gold standard" RPCTs for surgical treatment of spinal cord injury is disappointing, and some of the blame must rest with the national funding agencies including the National Institutes of Health that have chosen to deny funds for these trials since the last National Acute Spinal Cord Injury Study (NASCIS) trial ended in approximately 1990. Hopefully, this will be rectified in the future because it is essential to conduct RPCTs of important issues such as the timing and effectiveness of acute surgical decompression of the spinal cord. In my view, almost every patient with an acute spinal cord injury should be entered into a formal clinical trial. If we do not do this, individuals writing Forewords to books such as this, 50 years from now will continue to be faced with a lack of knowledge of important issues in this field. For example, the efforts of the Surgical Treatment for Acute Spinal Cord Injury Study (STASCIS) group that I founded several years ago should be supported.

Arun Amar has performed a real service to the practitioners involved in the surgical management of spinal injuries by putting together this excellent group of chapters, and I am optimistic that the knowledge transfer will result in improved patient outcomes.

Charles H. Tator, CM, MD, PhD, FRCSC, FACS
Professor and Robert Campeau Family Foundation Chair,
Division of Neurosurgery, University of Toronto,
Toronto Western Hospital

Foreword by Michael L. J. Apuzzo

Unraveling a Gordian Knot

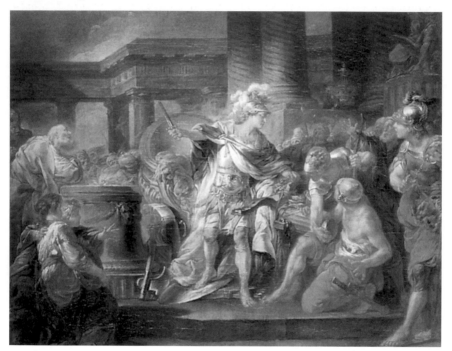

Jean-Simon Berthélemy: Alexander durchschlägt den gordischen Knoten (Alexander cuts the Gordian Knot)

The surgical discipline of neurosurgery is replete with challenges, many of which have seemed insurmountable in spite of the dramatic progress in neuroscience and clinically meaningful therapies over the past generation of effort. This collection of disorders will be the focus of intense scrutiny over the next generation. They include, among others, the glia tumor spectrum, cerebral vasospasm, and neural injury, which includes those of the spinal cord.

Functional restoration and capability for neural repair remains a "holy grail" for the investigators of the 21st century.[1] However, during our time, we can appreciate remarkable improvement in the general management of these problematical injuries through refinements in initial and more sustained stabilization techniques as well as the development of probes that offer apertures to understanding that which will eventually allow the unraveling of the Gordian knot of neural injury.

It would seem that issues attendant to comprehending the application of molecular and cellular biology will fuel a true evolution of the concept of cellular and molecular neurosurgery in these matters. Nanotechnology, although now a half-century-old concept, is only in its infancy regarding potential application in matters of injury that involve spinal column and neuronal elements.[2–4]

For the time being, we will be required to provide what is considered an optimum milieu for recovery and the creation of the setting for what might be termed, "natural restoration."[5]

Arun Amar has edited a succinct, but substantive presentation of practical issues attendant to this problem, while providing a review of the promising "seminal" concepts that will allow progress to reach the resolution of the central problem – neural injury.

The content of this volume is essential material for all clinical neuroscientists and an important presentation for all those seeking to develop a grasp of modernity of concept and practical action relating to this problem.

Michael L. J. Apuzzo, M.D.
Edwin M. Tood/Trent H. Wells,
Jr. Professor of Neurological Surgery and
Professor of Radiation Oncology, Biology, and Physics,
University of Southern California Keck School of Medicine,
Los Angeles, CA
Editor, Neurosurgery, Neurosurgery-Online,
and Operative Neurosurgery

References

1 Apuzzo MLJ. Editor's letter. *Neurosurgery* 2001;48:1.
2 Leary SP, Liu CY, Apuzzo ML. Toward the emergence of nanoneurosurgery: Part I. Progress in nanoscience, nanotechnology, and the comprehension of events in the mesoscale realm. *Neurosurgery* 2005;57:606–634.
3 Leary SP, Liu CY, Apuzzo ML. Toward the emergence of nanoneurosurgery: Part II. Nanomedicine: Diagnostics and imaging at the nanoscale level. *Neurosurgery* 2006;58:805–823.
4 Leary SP, Liu CY, Apuzzo ML. Toward the emergence of nanoneurosurgery: Part III. Nanomedicine: Targeted nanotherapy, nanosurgery and progress toward the realization of nanoneurosurgery. *Neurosurgery* 2006;58:1009–1026.
5 Hadley MH, Walters BC, Grabb PA, Oyesiku NM, Przybylski GJ, Resnick DK, Ryken TC. Section on disorders of the spine and peripheral nerves of the American Association of Neurological Surgeons and the Congress of Neurological Surgeons. Guidelines for the management of acute cervical spine and spinal cord injuries. *Neurosurgery* 2002;50 (March Suppl):S1–S199.

CHAPTER 1

Pathogenesis of acute spinal cord injury and theoretical bases of neurological recovery

Arun Paul Amar

Introduction

Experimental models and clinical observations of spinal cord injury (SCI) support the concepts of primary and secondary injury, in which the initial mechanical insult is succeeded by a series of deleterious events that promote progressive tissue damage and ischemia. Whereas the primary injury is fated by the circumstances of the trauma, the outcome of the secondary injury may be amenable to therapeutic modulation. This chapter, derived from a more detailed analysis,[1] reviews the pathogenetic determinants of these two phases of injury and summarizes the bases for interventions that may restore neurological function following SCI.

Pathogenesis

Models of SCI

Several experimental systems have been employed to investigate the pathophysiology of SCI and to test the effects of neuroprotective agents in the laboratory. Interest in such models dates as far back as the 2nd century AD, when Galen sectioned the spinal cord of monkeys and other animals in order to conduct studies on differential spinal lesions.[2] Current experimental paradigms involve neuronal cell cultures or anatomically intact segments of spinal cord subjected to various mechanical or ischemic insults such as weight drop, focal or circumferential extradural balloon compression, clip pressure, photochemical or thermal injury, distractional forces, or piston trauma.[3–10] The resultant injury can be assessed by histological examination (e.g. light or electron microscopy, special staining, and tracing methods), electrophysiological outcome measures (e.g. evoked potentials), or behavioral assessments (e.g. open field locomotion or postural stability on an inclined plane).[6,8,9,11]

Such studies are susceptible to a number of inherent flaws in experimental design that impair their ability to simulate human SCI. For instance, the weight drop method only mimics the trauma of initial impact and omits the force of persistent compression. Whereas most humans suffer anterior or circumferential cord compression from fracture dislocations of a closed vertebral system, most animal models create posterior compression through an open laminectomy.[2] Animal models may not account for neurogenic shock or concomitant injuries that produce systemic hypoxia and hypotension, factors which are known to aggravate the extent of injury resulting from any given mechanical stress.[12] Also, these models often fail to analyze the effects of repetitive mechanical trauma to the spinal cord from an unstable fracture.[6] Furthermore, few animal studies examine the same range of injury severity that is encountered in human trials, in which patients with both complete and incomplete deficits are often randomized to the same treatment group.

Because of differences in drug metabolism, results in animal models often fail confirmation in human trials. Other variations in experimental methodology, such as the type of species being studied, may also play a role. Unlike human trials, animal studies all require the use of anesthesia, which may affect the response to the substance being tested. Conversely, in the clinical setting, humans receive myriad drugs besides the one being studied, and adverse pharmacological interactions may antagonize the efficacy of the agent in question. Furthermore, neuroprotective therapies are often administered in the laboratory more promptly after injury than may be feasible in clinical practice.

As a result of these discrepancies in drug kinetics, the inability to extrapolate the results of animal models to the human condition does not necessarily invalidate the potential utility of the agent being tested. However, these factors contribute to conflicting or irreproducible results in the literature and hinder attempts at constructing a unified theory of pathogenesis and treatment in SCI.[13]

Despite these limitations, laboratory models have proven relevant to human SCI. Developments in the fields of basic neuroscience, including studies of the cerebral cortex and spinal cord, support the theory that the central nervous system (CNS) responds to injury in an archetypal fashion, whether the inciting insult represents trauma, hypoxia, hypoglycemia, epilepsy, various toxins, neurodegenerative disorders, or other pathophysiological processes.[14–20] The concepts of primary and secondary injuries, first advanced over 80 years ago, have emerged as an explanation for this phenomenon of a rehearsed mechanism of neuronal death. According to this paradigm, the initial mechanical insult in SCI is succeeded by a series of deleterious events that promote progressive tissue damage, largely mediated by ischemia and aberrant calcium influx into neurons. While the primary injury is fated by the circumstances of the trauma, the outcome of the secondary injury may be amenable to therapeutic modulation.

Determinants of primary injury

SCI may follow many types of trauma to the cord itself or to the surrounding vertebral column, and the extent of subsequent damage depends on several biomechanical factors that may be unrelated to the degree of bony fracturing.[21,22] Distractional forces associated with flexion, extension, dislocation, or rotation can all result in stretching or shearing of the neural elements themselves or spinal cord vasculature, and damage to either substrate could incur clinical deficit.[3,21,22] Other possible mechanical stresses include compression and contusion from bone fragments, ligaments, and hematoma within the spinal canal. These mechanisms may be responsible for cord injury even when the bony alignment appears normal at the time of admission. For instance, momentary dislocation may occur from ligamentous disruption, resulting in transitory cord compression or distraction. These distortions are substantially greater than what is depicted by initial radiographs, since soft tissue elasticity and postural influences tend to initiate spontaneous recoil, and muscle spasm tends to maintain the reduction by the time such radiographs are taken.

These forces may be operant not only acutely, at the moment of injury, but also chronically, secondary to persistent deformity. Mechanical instability can lead to further structural deformations, such as posttraumatic kyphosis or subluxation, which add additional compressive or distractive forces and result in worsening neurological deficit. Kyphosis, for instance, has been shown to cause tension within axonal tracts and constriction of intramedullary blood vessels.[3,21]

For any force applied to the neural elements, the extent of subsequent injury also depends on the relative dimensions of the spinal canal at that level. Whereas larger canals might provide a buffer for any given mechanical stress, stenotic canals lack such reserve. Thus, 53% of fractures of thoracic spine result in neurological injury compared with only 39–47% in the cervical region.[1,23] Similarly, one study revealed a much higher likelihood of complete injury resulting from lesions of the thoracic region (77.5%) than the cervical (60.4%) or thoracolumbar junction (64.7%) regions.[22] This discrepancy probably relates to the narrower canal of the thoracic spine, such that the degree of cord compression tends to be more severe for any given encroachment, as well as the relative paucity of blood flow to the thoracic cord.[21–23] Likewise, Eismont measured the midsagittal canal diameter in patients with fracture dislocations of the cervical spine and found that those with smaller canals were prone to more significant neurological injury, while larger canal diameters afforded a protective effect.[24] Other studies have shown that the relative stenosis incurred by cervical spondylitic disease predisposes to SCI following minor trauma, even in the absence of detectable bony injury.[3,22]

The anatomic location of injury in relation to the conus medullaris also seems to have some prognostic significance. Cauda equina injuries have a better prognosis for neurological recovery than comparable injuries to the spinal cord itself, since lower motor neurons are inherently more resistant to trauma, with fewer mechanisms of secondary injury and greater regenerative capacity than upper motor neurons and their tracts.

Determinants of secondary injury

In addition to local forces that potentially compromise spinal cord function, systemic pulmonary and cardiac factors that determine tissue oxygenation and perfusion can profoundly modulate the extent of injury resulting from any given mechanical stress.[12] Taken together, these considerations of local and systemic influences imply that ischemia underlies much of the mechanism of posttraumatic SCI. While other pathological processes such as edema, intramedullary hemorrhage, axonal degeneration, or demyelination may also play a role, these all have an integral relationship with impaired cord perfusion and bioenergetic failure at the cellular level. Experimental models employing the basic mechanisms of both compression and distraction have confirmed that SCI is associated with long-lasting ischemia that parallels the force of the experimental insult and the severity of the clinical deficit.[3,9,10,25,26] The ischemia is worse in the gray matter and may extend focally for considerable distances rostral and caudal to the injured segment.[3,8,9,12,25,26] The impaired perfusion may be followed by a phase of "hyperemia" or "luxury perfusion" due to the reduction of perivascular pH from accumulation of acid metabolites such as lactate.[26] This tissue reperfusion may increase cellular damage by promoting the influx of free radicals and other toxic byproducts.[18]

The intrinsic mechanisms occurring during SCI have been well documented and are schematically diagrammed in Figure 1.1.[1] In the initial phase, petechial hemorrhages develop within the spinal cord substance due to rupture of postcapillary venules or sulcal arterioles, either from mechanical disruption by the inciting force itself or from intravascular coagulation due to fibrin and platelet thrombi leading to venous stasis and distension.[8,10,12,21,27] Leakage of proteinaceous fluid from the intrinsic vessels of the cord then leads to edema at the injury site and surrounding tissues.[8,26] Because the spinal cord is contained within a relatively inelastic pial membrane, edema produces increased interstitial pressure that may diminish local spinal cord blood flow.[2] Vasoactive substances released by injured cells, including endothelin released from damaged capillaries, and other mechanical, biochemical, or neurogenic mechanisms may also play a role in impairing cord perfusion.[8,12,26–28] Focal narrowing, disruption, aneurysmal dilation, or occlusion of sulcal arterioles and intramedullary capillaries have all been demonstrated with the use of microangiographic techniques and three-dimensional vascular corrosion casts.[27,28] These changes may represent the morphological correlates of microvascular spasm, thrombosis, and rupture that underlie regional impairments in spinal cord perfusion. This focal ischemia is compounded by hypotension or hypoxia, since autoregulation is lost in SCI and spinal cord blood flow passively follows alterations in systemic hemodynamics.[8,9,12,21,26]

Ischemia initiates a cascade of secondary pathogenetic mechanisms collectively known as excitotoxicity because of their dependence on endogenous excitatory amino acid (EAA).[15,20] Ischemia depletes the supply of adenosine triphosphate (ATP), leading to dysfunction of energy-dependent processes such as the sodium–potassium pump that preserves cellular homeostasis. Ionic species then move passively across the cell membrane according to concentration gradients previously maintained between the intracellular and extracellular spaces, leading to a net efflux of potassium and a large influx of sodium, chloride, and calcium into the cell. Acute cellular swelling results. Furthermore,

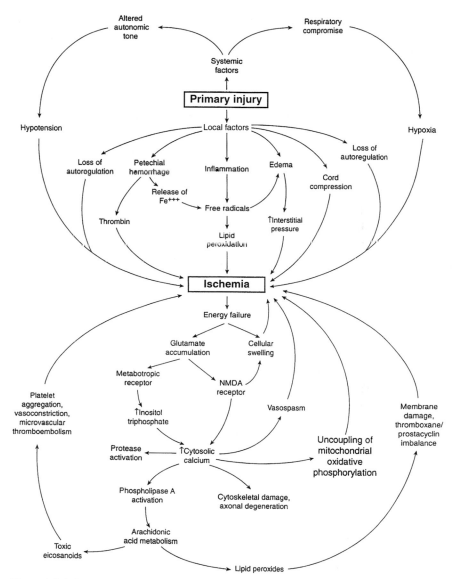

Figure 1.1 Schematic representation of key mechanisms, molecular species, and interrelationships underlying the pathogenesis of acute SCI. Principal pathways of secondary injury that converge upon ischemia are emphasized, while others have been omitted for simplicity. These pathogenetic determinants represent the logical targets for therapeutic modulation (reprinted with permission from Ref. [1]).

the altered composition of the extracellular and intracellular spaces leads to changes in membrane polarization that promote the release of EAA neurotransmitters such as glutamate and aspartate from synaptic vesicles. This release is compounded by impaired cellular uptake mechanisms in neurons and glia, which depend on the presence of high-energy phosphates and are inactivated by the ATP depletion accompanying hypoxia.[14,29,30] As a result of these two mechanisms, the local concentration of glutamate in the extracellular space can increase by a factor of eight following an ischemic insult.[14,30]

Extracellular accumulation of glutamate may also occur through non-ischemic mechanisms. The intracellular glutamate concentration in brain tissue is approximately 10 mmol/l, while its extracellular concentration is normally only 0.6 μmol/l.[18] Excitotoxic damage to neurons can occur when the latter concentration reaches 2–5 μmol/l.[18] Thus, ambient glutamate concentrations are precariously close to those that can destroy neurons, and the injury of even a single cell from direct traumatic mechanisms could produce a local accumulation of glutamate that places neighboring cells at risk for excitotoxic damage.[18] Although the glutamate concentrations within the spinal cord are less well documented, they may approximate those found in the brain. Glutamate receptors have been demonstrated in both the dorsal and ventral horns, and many pathways mediating locomotion and nociception, including the corticospinal and rubrospinal tracts, appear to rely on EAA neurotransmitters.[31] Extracellular EAA concentrations within the spinal cord have been shown to reach toxic levels 15 min after experimental SCI.[31]

Glutamate may act upon several families of receptors, each with distinct pharmacological and electrophysiological properties.[18,20,29] These receptor classes are named for the agonist compounds that selectively activate them. Some of these receptors, such as the N-methyl-D-aspartate (NMDA), α-amino-3-hydroxy-5-methyl-4-isoxazole-propionic acid (AMPA), and kainate receptors, are collectively termed "ionotropic" because they comprise ligand-gated ion channels. Others are termed "metabotropic" and comprise transmembrane proteins coupled with changes in the concentration of intracellular second messengers such as cyclic nucleotides or phosphoinositol through GTP-binding proteins.

Although activation of the AMPA and kainate receptors results primarily in the influx of sodium from the extracellular space, some subtypes may be permeable to calcium as well. In contrast, the NMDA receptor principally mediates calcium entry. The NMDA receptor contains a binding site for glycine, which acts as an obligate co-agonist. Furthermore, at resting membrane potential, inward current through the NMDA receptor is prevented by voltage-dependent blockade of its ion channel by magnesium, even if the glutamate and glycine sites are occupied. However, the degree of this magnesium blockade is reduced as the neuron becomes depolarized. Thus, any process which impairs the neuron's ability to maintain its normal membrane potential, such as bioenergetic defects or simultaneous activation of the AMPA receptor, can lead to electrophysiological decoupling that causes additional calcium influx through the NMDA receptor, even in the face of ambient glutamate concentrations. Membrane depolarization also promotes calcium entry through activation of voltage-dependent calcium channels. Finally, glutamate can trigger the accumulation of intracellular calcium through activation of metabotropic receptors, leading to the metabolism of inositol phospholipids and mobilization of intracellular calcium stores as well as inactivation of energy-dependent calcium transporters that pump cytosolic calcium across the cell membrane or sequester it within intracellular compartments such as the mitochondria and endoplasmic reticulum.[14,18–20,29]

These aberrant calcium fluxes trigger a myriad of calcium-dependent processes, such as activation of phospholipase A2, mobilization of free fatty acids, synthesis of toxic eicosanoids, generation of free radicals, further depletion of energy reserves through activation of calcium-dependent ATPase, covalent modification of receptor proteins, modification of the microtubular and neurofilament components of the cytoskeleton, impairment of mitochondrial oxidative phosphorylation, axonal degeneration, and activation of lytic enzymes such as proteases, phosphatases, and endonucleases.[14,18–20,25] This sustained elevation of cytosolic calcium concentration is postulated to be the final common pathway mediating cell death in many tissue types.[14–16,18–20]

Potentiating factors in this sequence of events include increased phospholipase activity, either from direct mechanical stimulation or from mobilization of calcium, resulting in the liberation of free arachidonic acid from membrane phospholipids.[25,32] This substrate is rapidly metabolized by cyclo-oxygenase to prostanoids such as thromboxane and prostacyclin. Thromboxane stimulates platelet adherence to endothelium, intravascular platelet aggregation, microvascular occlusion, vascular stasis, microvascular thromboembolism, and vasoconstriction; prostacyclin has the opposite effects on the microcirculation. Other byproducts of the cyclo-oxygenase pathway include free radicals such as lipid peroxides. These latter molecules selectively inhibit prostacyclin production, and the resultant thromboxane–prostacyclin imbalance contributes to an environment favoring thromboembolism and a tendency toward further ischemia.[25,32]

In addition to altering the ratio between thromboxane and prostacyclin production, lipid peroxides interact with polyunsaturated fatty acid components of the cell membrane to cause a chain reaction of phospholipid peroxidation that compromises the structural and functional integrity of the cell membrane and, ultimately, produces cell death.[25,33] Free radicals may also directly damage the nervous tissue's vascular integrity, cellular proteins, and nucleic acids. Besides cyclo-oxygenase, other enzymatic sources of free radicals include xanthine oxidase, which catalyzes production of the superoxide anion and hydrogen peroxide in response to CNS ischemia.[34] Because this enzyme is located primarily in the endothelial cells, the oxygen-derived free radicals induced by the xanthine oxidase system act primarily at the capillary level, altering vascular permeability and worsening posttraumatic edema.[34] Reactive iron species contained within the hemoglobin of extravasated blood may also act as a catalyst of free radical formation and lipid peroxidation reactions.[2] The subsequent release of these substances into the local environment as the cellular and vascular barriers disintegrate can impair neighboring cells and result in progression of deficit.

One limitation of this paradigm is that the excitotoxic model cannot directly account for injury to the white matter and glial elements of the CNS. Although ischemic damage is commonly observed in this tissue, most studies have failed to demonstrate that axons, myelin, astrocytes, and oligodendrocytes are endowed with NMDA receptors or are vulnerable to glutamate administration.[29] However, the concept of a "bad neighborhood" resulting from the local accumulation of lytic enzymes, free radicals, and other toxic factors derived from glutamate-mediated injury in adjacent neuronal tissue may explain the pervasive effects of focal CNS ischemia.[15,25] Furthermore, some studies suggest that periaxonal astrocytes may express certain subtypes of the AMPA and kainate receptors on their surface, thus implicating these cells in glutaminergic white matter injury.[35]

In the ensuing phases of SCI, inflammation and demyelination prevail. Two waves of peripheral leukocytic influx occur. In the early peak, neutrophils predominate, and their lytic enzymes may further damage vascular, neuronal, and glial cell populations.[2] Later, macrophages participate in the phagocytosis of hemorrhagic and necrotic tissue. Both phases of inflammation have been implicated in the demyelination of spared axons, which starts within the first 24 h after injury and increases over the next several days.[2] Well-demarcated areas of cavitation within the gray and white matter, extensive Wallerian degeneration, and scarring represent the final stages of histopathological evolution.[2] Although this scar is predominantly comprised of astroctyes and other glia, fibroblasts also make a significant contribution.

Theoretical bases of neurological recovery

Although the propensity for neurological improvement following both complete and incomplete SCI has been verified by experimental models and clinical observations, the biological basis of such recovery remains enigmatic. As Tator has suggested, functional restoration probably involves a combination of several different processes acting upon numerous anatomical substrates, including nerve roots at the level of injury, gray and white matter, and spinal cord vasculature.[11] Neural regeneration, the regrowth of lesioned neural elements with the restoration of functional synaptic connections, may account for late recovery occurring months to years after injury.

Root recovery
Several studies have confirmed that the peripheral nervous system is more resistant to injury and has a greater capacity for repair than the CNS.[2,11] This resilience is manifested by the frequency with which improved nerve root function is detected among patients with acute SCI. Re-establishment of segmental function at the site of injury, reflecting recovery in one or more nerve roots at that level, may restore innervation to particular muscle groups, organs or dermatomes, although motor roots generally have increased vulnerability to injury and decreased capacity for recovery than sensory roots.[11] Root recovery is expected in both complete and incomplete lesions in 66–90% of patients.[36] However, the greatest proportion of total neurological recovery occurs caudal

to the level of injury, reflecting improvements in the function of long spinal tracts themselves.

Resolution of cord ischemia

Surrounding the zone of irreparable ischemic damage is a penumbra of hypoxic tissue, whose cells may remain viable, even while lacking the capacity to maintain normal neuronal function. This tissue may be marginally supported by collateral circulation. If the ischemia exceeds a critical level, or persists beyond a certain threshold of time, irreversible damage will ensue and the zone of infarction will extend. If, however, blood flow can be restored before the onset of permanent injury, normal physiological function may be re-established.

Salvage of the ischemic penumbra can result from both medical and surgical interventions. Autopsy reports have shown that in most cases of SCI, including complete injuries, the cord remains anatomically intact.[2,9] Furthermore, animal studies of SCI suggest that preservation of a small proportion of spinal axons can support neurological recovery.[2,10,37] In a rat model, for instance, persistence of only 12% of the normal number of axons following clip compression injury conferred substantial maintenance of inclined plane performance and open field walking.[5] Thus, any manipulation that increases the fraction of functional axons traversing the injury site above this threshold, or that enhances the response of lower motor neurons to the attenuated input from those axons, can have a significant impact on neurological recovery.[10,37] Alternatively, since injured vasculature of the CNS tends to lose its autoregulatory response to hypertension, spinal cord blood flow could be increased passively by improving systemic hemodynamic parameters or selective infusion of CNS vasodilators.[8,12,26]

The central gray matter of the spinal cord is inherently more susceptible to trauma because it has higher metabolic activity and because it contains neuronal bodies whose machinery for biomolecular repair may be directly damaged. In contrast, the circumferential white matter tracts at the site of injury have a lower metabolic rate and have intact cell bodies that are distant from the locus of injury.[37] Thus, delayed pharmacological and physiological interventions are more likely to restore function to the white matter elements of the cord. Metabolic factors may also underlie the fact that motor tracts have increased vulnerability to injury and decreased propensity for recovery than sensory ones.[11]

Resolution of other injury events

Abnormalities of membrane polarization and excitability may accompany acute SCI. These changes in ionic equilibrium could result from the leakage of potassium into the interstitial fluid or from alterations in sodium permeability across the axolemma.[38,39] Such electrolyte shifts might underlie the early neuronal dysfunction associated with spinal shock and may account for the immediate inability to conduct action potentials across the injury segment.[38,39]

With time, however, restoration of the normal sodium and potassium gradients may re-establish impulse conduction in the long tracts and produce features of clinical recovery.[11] Spontaneous resolution of other processes, such as intramedullary hemorrhage, edema, and inflammation, are also likely to improve neurological outcome.[11]

Neural plasticity

Neural regeneration, the regrowth of lesioned neural elements with restoration of functional synaptic connections, has been the topic of intense experimentation over the past decade. Although the inability of injured CNS tissue to regenerate was traditionally considered an inviolable "law of nature," it now appears that many therapeutic interventions can promote the crucial aspects of neurite outgrowth, guidance, target recognition, and synaptic stabilization.[2] Current knowledge concerning the theoretical foundations of inducing regeneration following SCI and the practical limitations to its implementation have been reviewed elsewhere.[2,11] The reparative process depends on a complex interplay of cellular elements, extracellular matrix (ECM) components, paracrine hormones, and other factors.

Cellular elements

Following SCI, Schwann cells of peripheral nerve origin can migrate along the dorsal and ventral spinal roots and invade the cord parenchyma.[2,40,41] There, they may proliferate and foster many mechanisms of neuronal regeneration, including remyelination of CNS axons, which has been shown to restore action potential conduction through lesioned central pathways.[2,11,35,40–43] In addition, they may produce various neurotrophic factors such as nerve growth factor (NGF), brain-derived neurotrophic factor (BDNF), and ciliary neurotrophic factor.[43] Finally, they play an important role in axonal guidance.[44] The versatility of these salutary properties forms the rationale for various attempts at transplanting Schwann cell populations into sites of CNS injury. In 1911, fibers of the cerebral cortex were found to grow along the denervated Schwann cell bands of peripheral nerve grafts.[2] More recently, transplantation of peripheral nerve segments into the injured spinal cord have provided bridges along which CNS axons can extend for up to several centimeters.[45,46] Purified Schwann cell implants, injected as suspensions or as guidance channels supported by a semipermeable membrane, have served as similar substrates for regenerating CNS fibers following spinal cord transection.[2,44]

The proliferative, migratory, and regenerative capacities of ependymal cells have also been recognized. These properties underlie much of the spontaneous repair following traumatic SCI in lower animals.[11] In the newt, for instance, ependymal cells proliferate in the stump of an amputated tail and form a scaffold that directs the growth of regenerating central fibers while in the rat, invagination of proliferating sheets of ependymal cells by growing axons after spinal cord transection provides morphological evidence for a similar neurotrophic role in mammals.[41,47] Recently, a self-renewing population of mitotically active, multipotent neural stem cells has been recovered from the central canal of the adult mammalian spinal cord.[48] While such progenitors may impede regenerative attempts by contributing to the glial scar, Tator and others have speculated about their therapeutic potential as well, either through stem cell transplantation or application of exogenous growth factors that promote neuronal differentiation.[11,48,49]

Although the proliferative potential of oligodendrocytes remains uncertain, it is clear that surviving cells extend new cytoplasmic processes that can remyelinate adjacent axons.[40] Because this process is typically incomplete, future strategies that enhance recruitment, expansion, and migration of the quiescent oligodendroglial population may play a significant role in therapeutic attempts at inducing neural regeneration.[2]

The lesion scar representing the final stage of histopathological evolution following SCI has historically been regarded as an impermeable barrier to neurite outgrowth. More recent evidence suggests that astrocytes, which comprise the predominant cellular elements of this scar, may engender aspects of regeneration as well.[2,44] Membrane proteins, ECM components, and soluble factors expressed by the astrocyte all contribute to the complexity of these growth-promoting and growth-inhibitory effects, and the biochemical composition of the lesion scar awaits further characterization. In general, attempts at manipulating the lesion scar, such as the injection of pyrogens or collagenase or the use of spinal cord irradiation to reduce scar formation, have only achieved limited success in enhancing neural regeneration.[2]

ECM components

Several molecules normally found in the ECM contribute to a local microenvironment favoring neurite elongation and guidance. Fibroblasts, Schwann cells, and macrophages that migrate to sites of cord injury, as well as astrocytes residing within the glial scar, can all deposit various components of the ECM.[2] Schwann cells, for instance, synthesize and secrete laminin, which is known to modulate neurite outgrowth, as well as heparan sulfate proteoglycans, type IV collagen, and other components of the basal lamina associated with the peripheral axon–myelin unit.[43,44] This cell's ability to ensheathe and myelinate axons is entirely dependent on deposition of the basal lamina, and if the latter process is interrupted by conditions preventing the formation of ECM components (e.g. ascorbic acid deficiency, which impairs collagen production), myelination will not occur.[43] Conversely, neural regeneration could theoretically be enhanced by interventions which induce the formation of these crucial ECM proteins.

Paracrine and humoral factors

In newborn rats, rubrospinal and corticospinal neurons undergo massive cell death following axotomy, but injections of BDNF or neurotrophin-3 (NT-3) can largely counteract this event.[2] Similarly, the collateral sprouting response of transected corticospinal tract fibers in adult rats can be significantly enhanced by soluble factors elaborated by embryonic spinal cord grafts or local application of NT-3.[2,50] Likewise, topical administration of NGF to corticospinal tract axons following spinal cord transection in adult rats partially restores the pattern of regenerative behavior typical of newborn animals, characterized by the induction of axonal sprouting and elongation.[51]

These experiments provide compelling evidence for the existence of endogenous trophic factors that can promote neurite regeneration. In addition, much attention has been focused toward identifying the nonpermissive factors that ordinarily impede this process. It appears that CNS myelin and oligodendrocytes are associated with a number of potent growth-inhibitory factors, including membrane-bound proteins, glycolipids such as galactocerebroside, and glycosaminoglycans.[2] Monoclonal antibodies directed against some of these molecules can neutralize the inhibitory effects and facilitate the elongation and sprouting of transected axons which otherwise would not regenerate.[2,50]

The complementary actions of these two treatment approaches suggest that future therapeutic strategies may combine the use of neurotrophic factors with antibodies against CNS myelin-associated neurite growth inhibitors.[50,51] However, these high molecular weight proteins are unlikely to cross the blood–CNS barrier after systemic administration. Furthermore, they may only demonstrate efficacy after prolonged administration.[11] For these reasons, intrathecal delivery or direct parenchymal injection is typically required.[11] A phase 1 clinical trial was undertaken to study the pharmacokinetics of intrathecal ciliary neurotrophic factor in four patients suffering from amyotrophic lateral sclerosis. Although a therapeutic benefit could not be demonstrated, the study confirmed the feasibility of chronic intrathecal administration of recombinant neurotrophic factors through the use of a drug pump, suggesting potential applicability for future SCI therapies as well.[52]

Rationale for therapeutic intervention

Comprehension of the pathogenetic determinants of SCI, the theoretical bases of neurological recovery, and the principles of neural regeneration establish the foundation for rational therapy. Emerging concepts of the CNS response to injury have engendered much interest in the potential for mitigating secondary damage and restoring neurological function through both pharmacological and surgical interventions.[1]

Pharmacological strategies

The molecular events outlined above that represent logical targets for pharmacological modulation include glutamate accumulation, aberrant calcium fluxes, free radical formation, lipid peroxidation, and generation of arachidonic acid metabolites. Because of the complexity of these processes, numerous strategies have been devised. Although many therapeutic agents show promise in animal models, only methylprednisolone has been proven in large, randomized, double-blinded human studies to enhance the functional recovery of neural elements following acute SCI.[1]

It has been demonstrated that pharmacological agents must be given within a narrow window of opportunity in order to be effective. In fact, it has been proposed that paramedical personnel administers a bolus of methylprednisolone to suspected SCI victims in the field, but the clinical utility of this practice remains unproven.

The cascade of events that lead to impaired spinal cord perfusion is complex, and the diversity of molecular species that converge upon cord ischemia suggests that future therapies must consist of various combinations of these agents, each directed toward counteracting a different aspect of pathogenesis. Detailed preclinical studies must precede such therapy, because of potential drug interactions that may undermine the efficacy of already proven strategies. For instance, gangliosides have been shown to block some of the neuroprotective effects of methylprednisolone; similarly, the combination of naloxone and methylprednisolone increased mortality in some spinal-injured animals.[53,54]

The effects of glucocorticoids, lazeroids, gangliosides, opiate antagonists, calcium channel blockers, glutamate receptor antagonists, antioxidants, free radical scavengers, and other pharmacological agents in both animal models and human trials are summarized in the next chapter and elsewhere.[1]

Operative strategies

In vitro studies, animal models, and clinical outcome analyses of SCI have all failed to yield incontrovertible guidelines that define the role of surgery in the comprehensive management of the cord-injured patient. As a result, there is no consensus regarding the necessity, timing, nature, or approach of operative intervention. Intuitive hunches and anecdotal accounts have not been consistently corroborated by scientific studies, and individual or institutional preferences abound. Because of numerous methodological limitations, including ethical concerns about withholding potentially beneficial treatments to victims of SCI, it has not been feasible to subject such theories to prospective, randomized, controlled trials. Thus, the majority of the extant literature consists of retrospective analyses of unrandomized case series. The benefits of surgical intervention as opposed to natural history are difficult to discern from these papers.[55]

Historically, neurosurgical treatment of SCI has been confined to the mechanical elements of decompressing or stabilizing the vertebral column that surrounds the damaged cord. The controversies pertaining to these interventions are scrutinized in subsequent chapters of this book.

Recent advances in molecular and cell biology, however, suggest possible roles for surgical manipulation of the cord itself. For instance, neural transplantation has been employed as a strategy to modulate the milieu of the injured cord and enhance its endogenous reparative potential. Tissue sources for transplantation have included peripheral nerve grafts, dorsal root ganglia,

Schwann cells, olfactory ensheathing cells, adrenal tissue, and fetal spinal cord tissue.[56–58]

The exact mechanisms by which transplanted tissue may induce functional recovery remain unknown. Neural grafts may act as a bridge or scaffold for the passage of host axons that regrow and find appropriate targets caudal to the lesion. Alternatively, transplanted neurons may integrate into the host spinal cord and establish new synaptic connections, thereby restoring intraspinal circuitry or acting as a relay between supraspinal pathways and intrinsic central pattern generators within the caudal stump. Remyelination of anatomically intact, but functionally disrupted axons may enhance action potential conduction across the lesion. Lastly, the graft may elaborate neuroprotective factors that mitigate against axonal retraction and promote the survival or regeneration of host neuronal tissue.

Conclusions

The concepts of primary and secondary injury are well established and have broad implications for the treatment of acute SCI. The notion of SCI as a momentary, irreversible event has been supplanted by that of a dynamic and complex process amenable to therapeutic manipulation at each stage. Whereas the optimal timing of surgical interventions such as decompression remains a matter of debate, it appears that the pharmacological strategies aimed at mitigating secondary injury must be implemented within a narrow window of opportunity after trauma. The theoretical efficacy of these therapies warrants cautious optimism about the prognosis of acute SCI, and it is no longer tenable to consider it an ailment "not to be treated (see preface)".

References

1 Amar AP, Levy ML. Pathogenesis and pharmacological strategies for mitigating secondary damage in acute spinal cord injury. *Neurosurgery* 1999;44:1027–1040.

2 Schwab ME, Bartholdi D. Degeneration and regeneration of axons in the lesioned spinal cord. *Physiol Rev* 1996;76:319–370.

3 Dolan EJ, Transfeldt EE, Tator CH, *et al.* The effect of spinal distraction on regional spinal cord blood flow in cats. *J Neurosurg* 1980;53:756–764.

4 Faden AI. Pharmacotherapy in spinal cord injury: a critical review of recent developments. *Clin Neuropharmacol* 1987;10:193–204.

5 Fehlings MG, Tator CH. The relationships among the severity of spinal cord injury, residual neurological function, axon counts, and counts of retrogradely labeled neurons after experimental spinal cord injury. *Exp Neurol* 1995;132:220–228.

6 Geisler FH. Neuroprotection and regeneration of the spinal cord. In Menezes AH and Sonntag VKH (eds): *Principles of Spinal Surgery.* McGraw-Hill, New York, 1996, pp. 769–784.

7 Janssen L, Hansebout RR. Pathogenesis of spinal cord injury and newer treatments: a review. *Spine* 1989;14:23–32.

8 Sandler AN, Tator CH. Effect of acute spinal cord compression injury on regional spinal cord blood flow in primates. *J Neurosurg* 1976;45:660–676.

 9 Tator CH, Fehlings MG. Review of the secondary injury theory of acute spinal cord trauma with emphasis on vascular mechanisms. *J Neurosurg* 1991;75:15–26.

10 Young W. Secondary injury mechanisms in acute spinal cord injury. *J Emerg Med* 1993;11:13–22.

11 Tator CH. Biology on neurological recovery and functional restoration after spinal cord injury. *Neurosurgery* 1998;42:696–708.

12 Dolan EJ, Tator CH. The effect of blood transfusion, dopamine, and gamma hydroxybutyrate on posttraumatic ischemia of the spinal cord. *J Neurosurg* 1982;56:350–358.

13 Faden AI, Salzman S. Pharmacological strategies in CNS trauma. *Trends Pharmacol Sci* 1992;13:29–35.

14 Choi DW. Calcium-mediated neurotoxicity: relationship to specific channel types and role in ischemic damage. *Trends Neurosci* 1988;11:465–468.

15 Choi DW. The role of glutamate neurotoxicity in hypoxic-ischemic neuronal death. *Annu Rev Neurosci* 1990;13:171–182.

16 Choi DW, Koh J, Peters. Pharmacology of glutamate neurotoxicity in cortical cell culture: attenuation by NMDA antagonists. *J Neurosci* 1988;8:185–196.

17 Faden AI, Demediuk P, Panter SS, et al. The role of excitatory amino acids and NMDA receptors in traumatic brain injury. *Science* 1989;244:798–800.

18 Lipton SA, Rosenberg PA. Excitatory amino acids as a final common pathway for neurologic disorders. *New Engl J Med* 1994;330:613–622.

19 Siesjo BK. Historical overview: calcium, ischemia, and death of brain cells. *Ann NY Acad Sci* 1988;522:638–661.

20 Tymianski M, Tator CH. Normal and abnormal calcium homeostasis in neurons: a basis for the pathophysiology of traumatic and ischemic central nervous system injury. *Neurosurgery* 1996;38:1176–1195.

21 Chapman JR, Anderson PA. Thoracolumbar spine fractures with neurologic deficit. *Orthop Clin North Am* 1994;25:595–612.

22 Tator CH. Spine–spinal cord relationships in spinal cord trauma. *Clin Neurosurg* 1983;30:479–494.

23 Fessler RG, Masson RL. Management of thoracic fractures. In Menezes AH and Sonntag VKH (eds): *Principles of Spinal Surgery*. McGraw-Hill, New York, 1996, pp. 899–918.

24 Eismont FJ, Clifford S, Goldberg M, et al. Cervical sagittal spinal canal size in spine injury. *Spine* 1984;9:663–666.

25 Hall ED, Wolf DL. A pharmacological analysis of the pathophysiological mechanisms of posttraumatic spinal cord ischemia. *J Neurosurg* 1986;64:951–961.

26 Sandler AN, Tator CH. Review of the effect of spinal cord trauma on the vessels and blood flow in the spinal cord. *J Neurosurg* 1976;45:638–646.

27 Tator CH, Koyanagi I. Vascular mechanisms in the pathophysiology of human spinal cord injury. *J Neurosurg* 1997;86:483–492.

28 Koyanagi I, Tator CH, Lea PJ. Three-dimensional analysis of the vascular system in the rat spinal cord with scanning electron microscopy of vascular corrosion casts. Part 2: Acute spinal cord injury. *Neurosurgery* 1993;33:285–291.

29 Greenamyre JT, Porter RH. Anatomy and physiology of glutamate in the CNS. *Neurology* 1994;44(Suppl 8):S7–S13.

30 Rothman SM, Olney JW. Glutamate and the pathophysiology of hypoxic-ischemic brain damage. *Ann Neurol* 1986;19:105–111.

31 Wrathall JR, Teng YD, Choiniere D. Amelioration of functional deficits from spinal cord trauma with systemically administered NBQX, an antagonist of non-*N*-methyl-D-aspartate receptors. *Exp Neurol* 1996;137:119–126.

32 Hsu CY, Halushka PV, Hogan EL, *et al.* Alteration of thromboxane and prostacyclin levels in experimental spinal cord injury. *Neurology* 1985;35:1003–1009.

33 Hall ED. The role of oxygen radicals in traumatic injury: clinical implications. *J Emerg Med* 1993;11:31–36.

34 Kinuta Y, Kimura M, Itokawa Y, *et al.* Changes in xanthine oxidase in ischemic rat brain. *J Neurosurgery* 1989;71:417–420.

35 Agrawal SK, Fehlings MG. Role of NMDA and non-NMDA ionotropic glutamate receptors in traumatic spinal cord axonal injury. *J Neurosci* 1997;17:1055–1063.

36 Stauffer ES. Neurological recovery following injuries to the cervical spinal cord and nerve roots. *Spine* 1984;9:532–534.

37 Geisler FH, Dorsey FC, Coleman WP. Recovery of motor function after spinal-cord injury – a randomized placebo-controlled trial with GM-1 ganglioside. *New Engl J Med* 1991;324:1829–1838.

38 Eidelberg E, Sullivan J, Brigham A. Immediate consequences of spinal cord injury: possible role of potassium in axonal conduction block. *Surg Neurol* 1975;3:317–321.

39 Kobrine AI. The neuronal theory of experimental traumatic spinal cord dysfunction. *Surg Neurol* 1975;3:261–264.

40 Hughes TJ. Regeneration in the human spinal cord: a review of the response to injury of the various constituents of the human spinal cord. *Paraplegia* 1984;22:131–137.

41 Wallace MC, Tator CH, Lewis AJ. Chronic regenerative changes in the spinal cord after cord compression injury in rats. *Surg Neurol* 1987;27:209–219.

42 Blight AR, Young W. Central axons in injured cat spinal cord recover electrophysiological function following remyelination by Schwann cells. *J Neurol Sci* 1989; 91:15–34.

43 Bunge RP. Expanding roles for the Schwann cell: ensheathment, myelination, trophism and regeneration. *Curr Opin Neurobiol* 1993;3:805–809.

44 Xu XM, Guenard V, Kleitman N, *et al.* Axonal regeneration into Schwann cell-seeded guidance channels grafted into transected adult rat spinal cord. *J Comp Neurol* 1995; 351:145–160.

45 Cheng H, Cao Y, Olson L. Spinal cord repair in adult paraplegic rats: partial restoration of hind limb function. *Science* 1996;273:510–513.

46 Richardson PM, McGuinness UM, Aguayo AJ. Axons from CNS neurones regenerate into PNS grafts. *Nature* 1980;284:264–265.

47 Simpson SB. Morphology of the regenerated spinal cord in the lizard, *Anolis carolinensis.* *J Comp Neurol* 1968;134:193–210.

48 Weiss S, Dunne C, Hewson J, *et al.* Multipotent CNS stem cells are present in the adult mammalian spinal cord and ventricular neuroaxis. *J Neurosci* 1996;16:7599–7609.

49 Frisen J, Johansson CB, Torok C, *et al.* Rapid, widespread, and longlasting induction of nestin contributes to the generation of glial scar tissue after CNS injury. *J Cell Biol* 1995; 131:453–464.

50 Schnell L, Schneider R, Kolbeck R, *et al.* Neurotrophin-3 enhances sprouting of corticospinal tract during development and after adult spinal cord lesion. *Nature* 1994; 367:170–173.

51 Fernandez E, Pallini R, Lauretti L, *et al.* Spinal cord transection in adult rats: effects of local infusion of nerve growth factor on the corticospinal tract axons. *Neurosurgery* 1993; 33:889–893.

52 Penn RD, Kroin JS, York MM, *et al.* Intrathecal ciliary neurotrophic factor delivery for treatment of amyotrophic lateral sclerosis (phase 1 trial). *Neurosurgery* 1997;40:94–100.

53 Constantini S, Young W. The effects of methylprednisolone and the ganglioside GM1 on acute spinal cord injury in rats. *J Neurosurg* 1994;80:97–111.

54 Young W, DeCescito V, Flamm ES, *et al.* Pharmacological therapy of acute spinal cord injury: studies of high dose methylprednisolone and naloxone. *Clin Neurosurg* 1988;36:675–697.

55 Amar AP, Levy ML. Surgical controversies in the management of spinal cord injury. *J Am Coll Surg* 1999;188:550–566.

56 Christie SD, Mendez I. Neural transplantation in spinal cord injury. *Can J Neurol Sci* 2001;28:6–15.

57 Bartolomei JC, Greer CA. Olfactory ensheathing cells: bridging the gap in spinal cord injury. *Neurosurgery* 2000;47:1057–1069.

58 Barami K, Diaz FG. Cellular transplantation and spinal cord injury. *Neurosurgery* 2000; 47:691–700.

CHAPTER 2

Pharmacotherapy for spinal cord injury

Steven Casha, Joseph Silvaggio and R. John Hurlbert

Introduction

The pharmacological management of acute spinal cord injury (ASCI) remains the source of significant controversy. Optimism that a greater understanding of the pathogenesis of ASCI would lead to effective pharmacological treatment strategies, aimed at mitigating secondary injury, has been met with disappointment in the clinical arena. In March 2002, the American Association of Neurological Surgeons/Congress of Neurological Surgeons Joint Section on Disorders of the Spine and Peripheral Nerves, with the collaboration of the Joint Section on Trauma, published the *Guidelines for the Management of Acute Cervical Spine and Spinal Cord Injury*. The document, representing enormous effort and collaboration, was generally well accepted and praised. Clearly, the most controversial section dealt with pharmacological therapy after acute cervical SCI. The editor's comment advising readers to "carefully review the available data and comments ... [and] to establish their own perspective on this evolving matter" demonstrates the controversial and politically sensitive nature of the topic. In this chapter the various pharmacological agents that have been investigated in the treatment of human ASCI are reviewed, focusing on available medical evidence. The wealth of animal studies that have not reached clinical investigation are beyond the scope of this discussion. Treatment strategies aimed at neuro-augmentation and neuro-regeneration, applicable to the spinal cord injured patient later in their management, are the focus of Chapter 1.

Methylprednisolone

Steroids have been anecdotally administered to patients with ASCI for many years and in various forms and dosages. However, following publication and popularization of the National Acute Spinal Cord Injury Study (NASCIS) II results a degree of scientific credibility became associated with methylprednisolone administration that very quickly led many centers to adopt it as a standard of care, almost overnight. Whether this change in practice was fueled by media attention, by misguided interpretation of the results, or by both remains a source of considerable debate. Nonetheless, independent re-evaluation of the published NASCIS results consistently suggests that this reputation was not

Table 2.1 Level of evidence for clinical studies using steroids for SCI.

Author	Year	Design	Level	Agent	Result*
Bracken *et al.* (NASCIS I)	1984	Prospective, randomized, double-blind	I	Methylprednisolone	Negative
Bracken *et al.* (NASCIS II)	1990 and 1992	Prospective, randomized, double-blind	I	Methylprednisolone	Positive
Bracken *et al.* (NASCIS III)	1997 and 1998	Prospective, randomized, double-blind	I	Methylprednisolone/ Tirilizad	Positive
Otani *et al.*	1994	Prospective, randomized, no blinding	I	Methylprednisolone	Positive
Pointillart *et al.*	2000	Prospective, randomized, blinded	I	Methylprednisolone/ nimodipine	Negative
Kiwerski	1993	Retrospective, concurrent case control	II-2	Dexamethasone	Positive
Poynton *et al.*	1997	Retrospective, concurrent case control	II-2	Methylprednisolone	Negative
George *et al.*	1995	Retrospective, historical case control	II-3	Methylprednisolone	Negative
Gerhart *et al.*	1995	Retrospective, historical case control	II-3	Methylprednisolone	Negative
Prendergast *et al.*	1994	Retrospective, historical case control	II-3	Methylprednisolone	Negative

*As reported by the authors.

deserved.[1–4] Indeed, a recent survey of Canadian Spinal Surgeons confirms that only 17% prescribe methylprednisolone because they believe it works while 83% prescribe it because of peer pressure or for fear of litigation.[5]

Several studies besides the NASICS trials have been published that attempt to define the usefulness of steroids in ASCI. They can be summarized in tabular form ranked by level of evidence (Tables 2.1 and 2.2). Briefly Level I evidence is gained through prospective randomized trials. Level II evidence arises from prospective non-randomized trials or retrospective studies that make use of concurrent or historical case controls. Level III evidence is gained from descriptive uncontrolled studies or through expert opinion.[6] Level I evidence is generally required to establish a treatment as a "standard of care", while Level II evidence defines a treatment as "recommended", and Level III

Table 2.2 Level of evidence for clinical studies using non-steroid medications for SCI.

Author	Year	Design	Level	Agent	Result*
Geisler *et al.*	1991	Prospective, randomized, double-blind	I	GM-1 Gangliocyde	Positive
Geisler *et al.*	2001	Prospective, randomized, double-blind	I	GM-1 Gangliocyde	Negative
Bracken *et al.* (NASCIS II)	1990 and 1992	Prospective, randomized, double-blind	I	Naloxone	Negative
Flamm *et al.*	1985	Prospective feasibility/ safety study	III	Naloxone	N/A
Pitts *et al.*	1995	Prospective, randomized, double-blind	I	Thyrotropin-releasing hormone	Positive
Tadie *et al.* (abstract only)	1999	Prospective, randomized, double-blind	**	Gacyclidine	Negative
Pointillart *et al.*	2000	Prospective, randomized, blinded	I	Nimodipine	Negative

*As reported by the authors.
**To our knowledge this study has not been published in the peer-reviewed literature and has only been presented in abstract form. Therefore level of evidence is not assigned.

evidence supports the treatment as a therapeutic "option". However, despite the rigorous structure of this classification, proper weighting can become problematic because of flaws in data harvesting, reporting, and/or analyses that are independent of trial design.[3]

NASCIS II and III

Results of NASCIS II and III form the highest level of evidence arguing for the use of methylprednisolone in ASCI.[7–10] The 6-month data was released initially for each study, followed by publication of the 12-month data under separate cover. Both trials were well designed and executed. Patient follow-up was meticulous. Without dispute, the primary analyses looking for a steroid treatment effect were negative in both studies. Only *post-hoc* analyses revealed potential and admittedly minor treatment effects on motor scores at 1 year when 24-h therapy was initiated within 8 h (NASCIS II) and when 48-h therapy initiated within 3–8 h (NASCIS III) (Figure 2.1). In NASCIS III motor scores were reported significantly improved in patients treated with steroids for 48 h compared to the original 24-h administration, when started between 3 and 8 h after injury ($P = 0.053$). However, the chance of death from respiratory compromise in the 48-h group was six times that of the 24-h group ($P = 0.056$). Interestingly the authors concluded that 48-h steroid administration should be given to patients with ASCI treated between 3 and 8 h, yet interpreted the

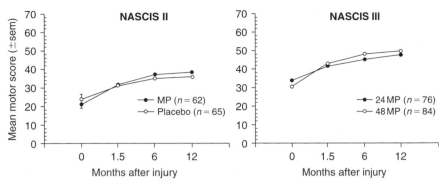

Figure 2.1 Summary of positive *post-hoc* results reported in the NASCIS II and III trials. No differences were observed in any primary outcome measures. *Post-hoc* sensory scores were no different amongst treatment groups. Only relative improvement in motor score was reported significantly improved in 24-h methylprednisolone (MP) patients (NASCIS II) and 48-h MP patients (NASCIS III) at 12 months. Although reported as statistically significant, the actual differences observed between treatment and control groups are not compelling.

increased mortality rate from 48-h therapy as irrelevant. None of the sensory scores were different between treatment groups at 1 year in either study, even in the *post-hoc* analyses.

Several questions remain unanswered about the *post-hoc* comparisons performed in NASCIS II and III, casting serious doubt that even a small benefit might be provided to SCI patients by methylprednisolone administration. The left-sided motor scores were never published but reported as "similar". Only right-sided scores were reported representing half the available data. No attempt was made to correct for multiple statistical comparisons. Over 65 *t*-tests were performed in NASCIS II and over 100 *t*-tests in NASCIS III (ignoring Naloxone and Tirilizad comparisons). Hence, the likelihood of encountering statistical significance through random chance alone was high. The rationale behind an 8-h sub-analysis in NASCIS II is uncertain. It has been claimed that the *post-hoc* 8-h therapeutic window for steroid administration was based on median time-to-treatment. Analysis of a true median time-to-treatment (8.5 h) should assign 50% of patients (244 of 487) before cut-off and 50% after. However, within the 8-h window only 38% of patients (183 of 487) were included in the *post-hoc* analysis, thereby excluding well over half the randomized patients. Similarly the justification of a 3–8 h window in NASCIS III is obscure. Improvement in function meaningful to the patient was not documented in either study.

Other steroid studies

In 1994 Otani *et al.* published a prospective trial investigating methylprednisolone administration using the NASCIS II dosing regimen.[11] Although patients were randomized, the investigators were not blinded to treatment.

In addition the control group was allowed to receive alternate steroids at the physicians' discretion. Of 158 patients entered 117 were analyzed. American Spinal Injury Association (ASIA) motor and sensory scores, the primary outcome measures, were not different between treatment groups. *Post-hoc* analyses suggested that more patients improved on the NASCIS II steroid regimen compared to controls. However, these analyses ignored the fact that in order for a greater number of steroid treated patients to improve, the small number of control patients who also improved must have demonstrated a larger magnitude of recovery (since overall ASIA motor and sensory score were no different between groups). Thus on closer inspection, conclusions based on such *post-hoc* analyses become nonsensical and meaningless.

The only other study claiming to demonstrate a benefit to steroid administration was a retrospective study with concurrent case controls from Poland published in 1993.[12] The dose of dexamethasone was left up to the discretion of the attending physician. Treatment was instituted within 24 h of injury. Length of follow-up was not specified. A novel but unvalidated neurological grading system was utilized for assessment. The author reported the percentage of patients improved to be significantly higher in the steroid treated group compared to controls. However, closer examination of the data demonstrated much higher mortality rates within the control groups, suggesting these patients to be more severely injured (Figure 2.2). A systematic selection bias such as this would reasonably allow the healthier patients (those tending to receiving methylprednisolone) to have better outcomes. The overall magnitude of the mortality rates in all reported patients causes concern about the ability to generalize the results.

In summary there exists no Class I evidence to suggest that methylprednisolone or any other steroid is beneficial in the treatment of ASCI. Weak *post-hoc* analyses are proposed to show a small effect on motor function in the

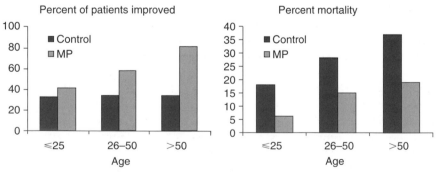

Figure 2.2 Graphical representation of Kiwerski[12] data demonstrating that more patients in the steroid treated group improved neurologically compared to controls. However, when one examines mortality data, approximately twice as many patients in the control group died. The results suggest that the control group was more seriously injured than the steroid treated group. In addition, the high mortality rates observed overall suggests that the study population may not be representative and the results not generalizable.

three Class I trials. However, all of these analyses contain serious flaws rendering conclusions of efficacy no better than speculative. Furthermore, there exists no compelling Class II or III evidence to further support the role of methylprednisolone in ASCI. These observations have led two national organizations to classify methylprednisolone administration as a treatment option rather than as a standard of care or even as recommended treatment.[13,14] Forty-eight hour methylprednisolone administration should be avoided as the evidence of death holds approximately the same weight as the evidence of slight motor improvement.

Gangliosides

Gangliosides are sialic acid-containing glycophosphingolipids which are found in high concentration in the outer cell membranes of central nervous system cells, especially in the vicinity of synapses. Although their exact function is unknown, they appear to play a role in neural development and plasticity. The proposed mechanisms of action of exogenously administered gangliosides include anti-excitotoxic activities, apoptosis prevention, augmentation of neurite outgrowth, and induction of regeneration and sprouting of neurons.[15–18]

GM-1 ganglioside has been evaluated in both animal and human studies of ASCI. In 1991, the first of two prospective randomized placebo-controlled trials studying the efficacy of GM-1 ganglioside in the treatment of ASCI was published.[19] Of the 37 patients enrolled, 1-year follow-up was available on 34. All patients received a 250 mg bolus of methylprednisolone followed by 125 mg every 6 h for 72 h. Patients were administered 100 mg of GM-1 ganglioside or placebo intravenously per day for 18–32 days, with the first dose given within 72 h of injury. Neurological recovery was assessed using the Frankel scale and the ASIA motor score. The authors reported a significant difference between groups in improvement of Frankel grades from baseline at 1-year ($P = 0.034$). The GM-1 treated patients also had a significantly greater mean improvement in ASIA motor score from baseline to the 1-year follow-up than the placebo treated patients ($P = 0.047$). When recovery of individual muscles was analyzed, the increased recovery in the GM-1 treated group was attributed to recovery of useful strength in initially paralyzed muscle groups, rather than to strengthening of paretic muscles. There were no reported adverse effects attributed to the administration of the study drug. The authors concluded that their small study provided evidence that GM-1 enhances recovery of neurological function 1 year following ASCI in humans. They recommended a larger study examining the safety and efficacy of GM-1 in ASCI.

In 1992, a larger GM-1 ganglioside ASCI study was initiated.[20] The study was designed as a prospective, multicenter, double-blind, randomized trial. When the study was concluded in 1997, 797 patients had been enrolled. All patients received methylprednisolone according to NASCIS II protocol. Patients were randomized into three groups: placebo, low-dose GM-1 (300 mg loading dose then 100 mg/day for 56 days), and high-dose GM-1 (600 mg loading dose then 200 mg/day for 56 days). Study medication, placebo or GM-1, was initiated at the completion of the 23-h methylprednisolone infusion. Clinical outcomes were assessed using the modified Benzel Classification and the ASIA motor and sensory examinations at 4, 8, 16, 26, and 52 weeks after injury. The primary efficacy assessment was the proportion of patients who demonstrated improvement of at least two grades (modified Benzel score) from baseline, at week 26 of the study. Secondary outcomes included timing of recovery, the ASIA motor score and the ASIA sensory evaluations, relative and absolute sensory levels of impairment, and assessments of bladder and bowel function. A planned interim evaluation after the first 180 patients resulted in discontinuation of the high-dose treatment strategy because of an early trend toward higher mortality. At the conclusion of the study, 760 patients remained for primary efficacy analysis. The results of the trial were published in 2001.[20] The authors found no significant difference in mortality between the groups. The GM-1 treated group did not have a significantly higher proportion of patients with marked recovery at 26 weeks when compared to placebo treated patients. The time course of recovery suggested earlier attainment of marked recovery in GM-1 treated patients, regardless of baseline severity. The authors also reported that there was a large, consistent and, at some points, significant effect in the primary outcome in the sub-group of non-operated patients through week 26. The ASIA motor, light touch and pinprick scores showed a consistent trend in favor of GM-1, as did bladder function, bowel function sacral sensation, and anal contraction. Less significantly injured patients appeared to have greater beneficial drug effect; however this was not statistically significant. The authors concluded that despite the lack of statistical significance in the primary analysis, numerous positive secondary analyses indicate that GM-1 ganglioside may be a useful drug in the management of severe ASCI. Of interest, the authors could not confirm the previous NASCIS II findings in their group of methylprednisolone treated "placebo" patients.

In summary, the available evidence does not support a significant, lasting, clinical benefit from the administration of GM-1 ganglioside in the treatment of patients after ASCI. Two North American randomized-controlled trials have been completed.[19,20] Improvement in neurological recovery with the administration of GM-1 ganglioside following ASCI has been suggested but not convincingly proven.

Opiate antagonists

Shock and microcirculatory collapse are thought to negatively influence SCI by adding an ischemic insult to the spinal cord (Chapter 1). Hypovolemic and spinal shock syndromes in the poly-trauma patient as well as microcirculatory collapse contribute to this phenomenon. Opiate receptor antagonists and physiological opiate antagonists improve blood pressure and survival following traumatic shock.[21] Furthermore, animal studies have demonstrated release of endogenous opiod peptides after ASCI.[22,23] Dynorphin, through the kappa opioid receptor decreases microcirculatory bloodflow in the spinal cord and may contribute directly to neurotoxicity possibly through the N-methyl-D-aspartate (NMDA) receptor.[24–26] These observations have led to exploration of the role of opiod antagonists in neuroprotection after ASCI. Three agents have shown neuroprotective effects in animal models: Naloxone, Nalmefene, and Thyrotropin-releasing hormone (TRH).[22,27–37] Conversely however, some studies of Naloxone have failed to shown neuroprotection.[38–41]

In human studies, Naloxone was included as one of the treatment arms in NASCIS II.[7] The 154 patient Naloxone group was given a 5.4 mg/kg bolus followed by a 23 h, 4.0 mg/kg/h infusion and compared to the 171 patient placebo group. Motor and sensory functions were assessed by systematic neurological examination on admission and 6 weeks and 6 months after injury. This study failed to demonstrate a therapeutic benefit.[7,8] Subsequent *post-hoc* reanalysis did reveal that while there was no effect on neurological recovery at the level of the lesion there was an effect on long tract recovery when Naloxone was administered within 8 h of injury, suggesting that this effect may warrant further study.[42]

Flamm *et al.* conducted a phase 1 study of Naloxone in ASCI prior to the NASCIS II investigation.[43] Two groups were included in the study. A group of 20 patients received a low dose of Naloxone (0.14–1.43 mg/kg loading followed by 20% of loading 47 h infusion), while the other group of nine patients received a high dose (2.7–5.4 mg/kg loading dose followed by 75% of loading 23 h infusion). The study was designed with an escalating dosage as patients were enrolled so as to explore safety and feasibility of the medication over a dose range. The high- and low-dose groups also differed in that more patients in the low-dose group had complete injuries (85% versus 44%) and initiated their treatment later (average 12.9 h versus 6.6 h). The low-dose group showed no improvement in neurological examination or somatosensory evoked potentials (SSEPs). In the high-dose group a small number of patients demonstrated neurological improvement and improvement in SSEPs that was sustained and progressive months later. This study was designed as a phase 1 study and as such did not have the appropriate placebo group or statistical power to examine drug efficacy. The observed improvements were encouraging but not statistically validated. The authors were able to show that the high doses of Naloxone indicated by animal studies of ASCI would be tolerated clinically with minimal side effects.

TRH has been the subject of one human study in which 20 ASCI patients sub-classified as complete and incomplete injured were administered TRH (0.2 mg/kg bolus followed by 0.2 mg/kg/h 6 h infusion) or placebo within 12 h of injury.[44] No discernible treatment effect was found in patients with complete injuries (six patients), while at 4 months, in the incomplete injury sub-group (11 patients), TRH treatment was associated with significantly higher motor and sensory recovery, and Sunnybrook Cord Injury Scale scores. The small sample size in this study led the authors to recommend caution in interpreting their statistical evaluation and they were unwilling to confidently dismiss the null hypothesis.

In summary, to date opioid receptor antagonism has shown experimental promise but the limited human trials do not support there role in the current management of ASCI. Three human studies have been conducted which have produced preliminary evidence supporting further study of this matter. Some animal studies have suggested a bell-shaped efficacy curve for Naloxone necessitating further determination of optimal dosing prior to definitive human-randomized placebo control studies.[31]

Excitatory amino acid receptor antagonists

Excitotoxicity has been a key biochemical process implicated in secondary injury following ASCI (Chapter 1). Animal evidence points to an increase in extracellular glutamate and aspartate after injury,[45,46] leading to toxicity of both neurons and glia through ligand gated ionotropic receptors as well as G-protein coupled metabotropic receptors.[47–51] Inhibition of these mechanisms in rodents has resulted in improved behavioral and histological outcome.[47,52,53] However, the application of these observations to clinical studies has been difficult. Glutamate is a ubiquitous excitatory neurotransmitter in the central nervous system and as such its inhibition is fraught with adverse reactions. Furthermore, the rise in excitatory amino acids seen after injury occurs early and is transient (likely complete within 2 h) suggesting that the therapeutic window is small.[45]

To date one clinical study of the compound Gacyclidine, an inhibitor of NMDA type ionotropic glutamate receptors, failed to show efficacy.[54,55] This study succeeded in enrolling 280 ASCI patients within 2 h of injury. Patients received 0.005 mg/kg, 0.01 mg/kg, or 0.02 mg/kg Gacyclidine or placebo at randomization and 4 h later. While the 1-month data showed a non-significant trend to better outcome in the high-dose group this effect was not sustained at 1 year;[54(abstract)] 72% of the patients suffered complete injuries. There was a suggestion in the data of a more promising effect in the incomplete injured group.

Thus, amino acid excitotoxicity has long been established as a key secondary injury mechanism following neurotrauma. The animal data suggests that inhibitors are likely to be efficacious in the treatment of ASCI. A single human study has been completed, which did not show efficacy. These agents likely deserve further development and study.

Calcium channel blockers

Dysregulation of calcium homeostasis and in particular rise in cytoplasmic calcium is thought to be an event common to many pathways leading to cell death.[56] Calcium is frequently employed by the cell for intracellular signaling and enzyme regulation. As such a host of calcium dependant proteases, nucleases, and lipases have been identified, which together with other less directly calcium regulated cellular events (e.g. increased free radical production) contribute to cellular demise after injury.[56] In the setting of neurotrauma, calcium channel blockers may have a direct effect in ameliorating these calcium fluxes and thus decreasing cell death. In addition they may also be effective through vascular smooth muscle and decrease injury induced vasospasm. This potentially advantageous effect on spinal cord perfusion must be balanced with the potential hypotensive effect caused by peripheral vascular dilation seen with these drugs. In animal models calcium channel blockade has been neuroprotective[57–60] and has been shown to increase post-traumatic spinal blood flow.[61,62]

In human SCI a single randomized placebo-controlled trial of the calcium channel blocked nimodipine has been published.[63,64] In this study, 106 ASCI patients were administered methylprednisolone (NASCIS II protocol), nimodipine (0.015 mg/kg/h for 2 h followed by 0.03 mg/kg/h for 7 days), both agents, or placebo. No difference in blinded neurological recovery (ASIA score) was found among these groups at 1 year.

Thus to date, cellular calcium fluxes are thought to be a key event in secondary injury after neurotrauma and remain a popular topic in the scientific literature. However, the application of calcium channel antagonists to human SCI has been limited to a single study which did not show efficacy.

Antioxidants and free radical scavengers

After neurotrauma several conditions promote formation of free radicals. Increased cytosolic calcium induces several free radical producing pathways including xanthine oxidase, nitrous oxide synthetase, and the phospholipase A2 – cyclooxygenase pathway.[65] Free radicals (superoxide) are also produced through the Fe^{2+} dependent Fenton and Haber-Weiss reactions.[65] Alterations in the inner mitochondrial membrane proteins (removal, release, or inactivation) may reduce the efficiency of the electron transport chain leading to increased production of superoxide radical.[65,66] Activated inflammatory cells yield reactive oxygen species.[65] The resultant increased production of free radicals overwhelms the cell's free radical scavenging systems (e.g. superoxide dysmutases – catalyases, glutathione, ascorbic acid) leading to oxidation of lipid proteins and nucleic acids. This in turn may lead to cell death.[67]

Several animal studies provide good evidence for the involvement of free radicals and peroxidation reactions in the pathophysiology of ASCI specifically. Studies have demonstrated increases in specific free radicals,[68–71] evidence of increased macromolecular oxidation after SCI,[69,72–74] and evidence that free radical scavenging compounds, decreased free radical production and increased free radical scavenging are neuroprotective.[69,75–79]

In human studies, the mechanism of action of methylprednisolone, which was the subject of the NASCIS studies, likely includes inhibition of peroxidation reactions. As discussed above, these studies have not shown conclusively that this agent is useful in the treatment of ASCI. Tirilizad mesylate is believed to inhibit iron-dependent lipid peroxidation in central nervous system tissue and was also included in the NASCIS III investigation.[80] One hundred and sixty-six patients in the Tirilizad group received a 2.5 mg/kg bolus infusion every 6h for 48h after their 30 mg/kg methylprednisolone bolus (administered before randomization). When compared to the control group in this study, which received methylprednisolone 5.4 mg/kg/h for 24h, no difference in motor recovery was found.[9,10] This study indicates that Tirilizad mesylate is equally effective to methylprednisolone in the treatment of ASCI. Given the lack of conclusion regarding the role of methylprednisolone (as discussed above), the role of both these agents in the treatment of ASCI will require further scrutiny.

In summary, while macromolecular peroxidation likely contributes to cell death and neurological dysfunction as supported by animal studies in ASCI, the human data to date on methylprednisolone and Tirilizad mesylate, which are believed to decrease peroxidation, do not support conclusively their use in the treatment of ASCI.[81–85]

Conclusions

From the generally accepted injury model of SCI stems the hypothesis that amelioration of either primary or secondary injury mechanisms will decrease tissue damage in the spinal cord and lead to improved neurological outcome. Animal studies addressing the large array of secondary injury mechanisms have significantly improved our understanding of these phenomena and have yielded encouraging behavioral and histological results. Some of this basic science research has been successfully translated into human clinical trials through admirably complex protocols in multiple centers. Unfortunately the results of these studies to date, while encouraging, have not yielded any clearly effective therapies for the treatment of ASCI. Furthermore, a number of publications have generated considerable controversy by the way in which their data were reported.

It is reasonable to expect that manipulation of a single pathway in the large milieu of secondary injury mechanisms will have only a small overall effect in a system as complex as the central nervous system. Ultimately a treatment strategy of multiple agents with broad specificity will likely evolve from our present efforts. The task of proving efficacy in human ASCI is made more difficult by the reality that the injury is heterogeneous, unlike the uniform injury of animal models used in the laboratory. Interventions shown efficacious in animals may produce similar effects in human tissue, but perhaps on a scale too small to measure with the crude clinical tools presently at our disposal. Nonetheless, the encouraging results and broad scope of activities in animal models combined with a now well-established track record in the execution of complex clinical trials secures an exciting arena in which the goal of effective pharmacological strategies in ASCI will ultimately be achieved. Until that time, maintenance of airway and support of tissue oxygenation through ventilatory and circulatory augmentation where necessary remain the principles of care for acutely spinal cord injured patients.

References

1 Nesathurai S. Steroids and spinal cord injury: revisiting the NASCIS 2 and NASCIS 3 trials. *J Trauma* 1998;45:1088–1093.

2 Coleman WP, Benzel E, Cahill DW, *et al.* A critical appraisal of the reporting of the National Acute Spinal Cord Injury Studies (II and III) of methylprednisolone in acute spinal cord injury. *J Spinal Disord* 2000;13:185–199.

3 Hurlbert RJ. Methylprednisolone for acute spinal cord injury: an inappropriate standard of care. *J Neurosurg* 2000;93:1–7.

4 Short DJ, El Masry WS, Jones PW. High dose methylprednisolone in the management of acute spinal cord injury – a systematic review from a clinical perspective. *Spinal Cord* 2000;38:273–286.

5 Hurlbert RJ, Moulton R. Why do you prescribe methylprednisolone for acute spinal cord injury? A Canadian perspective and a position statement. *Can J Neurol Sci* 2002;29: 236–239.

6 Woolf SH, Battista RN, Anderson GM, *et al.* Assessing the clinical effectiveness of preventive maneuvers: analytic principles and systematic methods in reviewing evidence and developing clinical practice recommendations. A report by the Canadian Task Force on the Periodic Health Examination. *J Clin Epidemiol* 1990;43:891–905.

7 Bracken MB, Shepard MJ, Collins WF, *et al.* A randomized, controlled trial of methylprednisolone or naloxone in the treatment of acute spinal-cord injury. Results of the Second National Acute Spinal Cord Injury Study. *New Engl J Med* 1990;322:1405–1411.

8 Bracken MB, Shepard MJ, Collins WF, *et al.* Methylprednisolone or naloxone treatment after acute spinal cord injury: 1-year follow-up data. Results of the Second National Acute Spinal Cord Injury Study. *J Neurosurg* 1992;76:23–31.

9 Bracken MB, Shepard MJ, Holford TR, *et al.* Administration of methylprednisolone for 24 or 48 hours or tirilazad mesylate for 48 hours in the treatment of acute spinal cord injury. Results of the Third National Acute Spinal Cord Injury Randomized Controlled Trial. National Acute Spinal Cord Injury Study. *JAMA* 1997;277:1597–1604.

10 Bracken MB, Shepard MJ, Holford TR, *et al.* Methylprednisolone or tirilazad mesylate administration after acute spinal cord injury: 1-year follow up. Results of the Third National Acute Spinal Cord Injury Randomized Controlled Trial. *J Neurosurg* 1998; 8:699–706.

11 Otani K, Abe H, Kadoya S. Beneficial effect of methylprednisolone sodium succinate in the treatment of acute spinal cord injury. *Sekitsui Sekizui J* 1994;7:633–647.

12 Kiwerski JE. Application of dexamethasone in the treatment of acute spinal cord injury. *Injury* 1993;24:457–460.

13 Hugenholtz HM, Cass DE, Dvorak MF, *et al.* High-dose methylprednisolone for acute closed spinal cord injury – only a treatment option. *Can J Neurol Sci* 202;29:227–235.

14 Hadley MN, Walters BC, Grabb PA, *et al.* Guidelines for the management of acute cervical spine and spinal cord injuries – pharmacological therapy after acute cervical spinal cord injury. *Neurosurgery* 2002;50:S63–S72.

15 Zeller CB, Marchase RB. Gangliosides as modulators of cell function. *Am J Physiol* 1992;262:C1341–C1355.

16 Rahmann H. Brain gangliosides and memory formation. *Behav Brain Res* 1995;66:105–116.

17 Sabel BA, Stein DG. Pharmacological treatment of central nervous system injury. *Nature* 1986;323:493.

18 Gorio A. Gangliosides as a possible treatment affecting neuronal repair processes. *Adv Neurol* 1988;47:523–530.

19 Geisler FH, Dorsey FC, Coleman WP. Recovery of motor function after spinal-cord injury – a randomized, placebo-controlled trial with GM-1 ganglioside. *New Engl J Med* 1991; 324:1829–1838.

20 Geisler FH, Coleman WP, Grieco G, *et al.* The Sygen multicenter acute spinal cord injury study. *Spine* 2001;26:S87–S98.

21 McIntosh TK, Faden AI. Opiate antagonist in traumatic shock. *Ann Emerg Med* 1986; 15:1462–1465.

22 Faden AI, Jacobs TP, Mougey E, *et al.* Endorphins in experimental spinal injury: therapeutic effect of naloxone. *Ann Neurol* 1981;10:326–332.

23 Faden AI, Holaday JW. A role for endorphins in the pathophysiology of spinal cord injury. *Adv Biochem Psychopharmacol* 1981;28:435–446.

24 Winkler T, Sharma HS, Ghord T, *et al.* Topical application of dynorphin A (1–17) antiserum attenuates trauma induced alterations in spinal cord evoked potentials, microvascular permeability disturbances, edema formation and cell injury. An experimental study in the rat using electrophysiological and morphological approaches. *Amino Acids* 2002; 23:273–281.

25 Hauser KF, Knapp PE, Turbek CS. Structure-activity analysis of dynorphin A toxicity in spinal cord neurons: intrinsic neurotoxicity of dynorphin A and its carboxyl-terminal, nonopioid metabolites. *Exp Neurol* 2001;168:78–87.

26 Hu WH, Lee FC, Wan XS, *et al.* Dynorphin neurotoxicity induced nitric oxide synthase expression in ventral horn cells of rat spinal cord. *Neurosci Lett* 1996;203:13–16.

27 Behrmann DL, Bresnahan JC, Beattie MS. A comparison of YM-14673, U-50488H, and nalmefene after spinal cord injury in the rat. *Exp Neurol* 1993;119:258–267.

28 Benzel EC, Khare V, Fowler MR. Effects of naloxone and nalmefene in rat spinal cord injury induced by the ventral compression technique. *J Spinal Disord* 1992;5:75–77.

29 Akdemir H, Pasaoglu A, Ozturk F, *et al.* Histopathology of experimental spinal cord trauma. Comparison of treatment with TRH, naloxone, and dexamethasone. *Res Exp Med (Berl)* 1992;192:177–183.

30 Hashimoto T, Fukuda N. Effect of thyrotropin-releasing hormone on the neurologic impairment in rats with spinal cord injury: treatment starting 24 h and 7 days after injury. *Eur J Pharmacol* 1991;203:25–32.

31 Benzel EC, Hoffpauir GM, Thomas MM, *et al.* Dose-dependent effects of naloxone and methylprednisolone in the ventral compression model of spinal cord injury. *J Spinal Disord* 1990;3:339–344.

32 Faden AI, Sacksen I, Noble LJ. Opiate-receptor antagonist nalmefene improves neurological recovery after traumatic spinal cord injury in rats through a central mechanism. *J Pharmacol Exp Ther* 1988;245:742–748.

33 Arias MJ. Treatment of experimental spinal cord injury with TRH, naloxone, and dexamethasone. *Surg Neurol* 1987;28:335–338.

34 Arias MJ. Effect of naloxone on functional recovery after experimental spinal cord injury in the rat. *Surg Neurol* 1985;23:440–442.

35 Flamm ES, Young W, Demopoulos HB, *et al.* Experimental spinal cord injury: treatment with naloxone. *Neurosurgery* 1982;10:227–231.

36 Faden AI, Jacobs TP, Holaday JW. Opiate antagonist improves neurologic recovery after spinal injury. *Science* 1981;211:493–494.

37 Faden AI, Jacobs TP, Holaday JW. Thyrotropin-releasing hormone improves neurologic recovery after spinal trauma in cats. *New Engl J Med* 1981;305:1063–1067.

38 Black P, Markowitz RS, Gillespie JA, *et al.* Naloxone and experimental spinal cord injury: effect of varying dose and intensity of injury. *J Neurotrauma* 1991;8:157–171.

39 Black P, Markowitz RS, Keller S, *et al*. Naloxone and experimental spinal cord injury: Part 2. Megadose treatment in a dynamic load injury model. *Neurosurgery* 1986;19:909–913.

40 Black P, Markowitz RS, Keller S, *et al*. Naloxone and experimental spinal cord injury: Part 1. High dose administration in a static load compression model. *Neurosurgery* 1986;19:905–908.

41 Wallace MC, Tator CH. Failure of blood transfusion or naloxone to improve clinical recovery after experimental spinal cord injury. *Neurosurgery* 1986;19:489–494.

42 Bracken MB, Holford TR. Effects of timing of methylprednisolone or naloxone administration on recovery of segmental and long-tract neurological function in NASCIS 2. *J Neurosurg* 1993;79:500–507.

43 Flamm ES, Young W, Collins WF, *et al*. A phase I trial of naloxone treatment in acute spinal cord injury. *J Neurosurg* 1985;63:390–397.

44 Pitts LH, Ross A, Chase GA, *et al*. Treatment with thyrotropin-releasing hormone (TRH) in patients with traumatic spinal cord injuries. *J Neurotrauma* 1995;12:235–243.

45 Farooque M, Hillered L, Holtz A, *et al*. Changes of extracellular levels of amino acids after graded compression trauma to the spinal cord: an experimental study in the rat using microdialysis. *J Neurotrauma* 1996;13:537–548.

46 Panter SS, Yum SW, Faden AI. Alteration in extracellular amino acids after traumatic spinal cord injury. *Ann Neurol* 1990;27:96–99.

47 Mills CD, Johnson KM, Hulsebosch CE. Group I metabotropic glutamate receptors in spinal cord injury: roles in neuroprotection and the development of chronic central pain. *J Neurotrauma* 2002;19:23–42.

48 Liu D, Xu GY, Pan E, *et al*. Neurotoxicity of glutamate at the concentration released upon spinal cord injury. *Neuroscience* 1999;93:1383–1389.

49 Liu D. An experimental model combining microdialysis with electrophysiology, histology, and neurochemistry for studying excitotoxicity in spinal cord injury. Effect of NMDA and kainate. *Mol Chem Neuropathol* 1994;23:77–92.

50 Agrawal SK, Fehlings MG. Role of NMDA and non-NMDA ionotropic glutamate receptors in traumatic spinal cord axonal injury. *J Neurosci* 1997;17:1055–1063.

51 Agrawal SK, Theriault E, Fehlings MG. Role of group I metabotropic glutamate receptors in traumatic spinal cord white matter injury. *J Neurotrauma* 1998;15:929–941.

52 Lang-Lazdunski L, Heurteaux C, Vaillant N, *et al*. Riluzole prevents ischemic spinal cord injury caused by aortic crossclamping. *J Thorac Cardiovasc Surg* 1999;117:881–889.

53 Wrathall JR, Choiniere D, Teng YD. Dose-dependent reduction of tissue loss and functional impairment after spinal cord trauma with the AMPA/kainate antagonist NBQX. *J Neurosci* 1994;14:6598–6607.

54 Tadie M. Acute spinal cord injury: early care and treatment in a multicenter study with Gacyclidine. Abstract 444.2 in Soc Neurosci Abstr. Miami: Society for Neuroscience 1090 (1999).

55 Mitha AP, Maynard KI. Gacyclidine (Beaufour-Ipsen). *Curr Opin Investig Drug* 2001; 2:814–819.

56 Tymianski M, Tator CH. Normal and abnormal calcium homeostasis in neurons: a basis for the pathophysiology of traumatic and ischemic central nervous system injury. *Neurosurgery* 1996;38:1176–1195.

57 Ross IB, Tator CH, Theriault E. Effect of nimodipine or methylprednisolone on recovery from acute experimental spinal cord injury in rats. *Surg Neurol* 1993;40:461–470.

58 Agrawal SK, Nashmi R, Fehlings MG. Role of L- and N-type calcium channels in the pathophysiology of traumatic spinal cord white matter injury. *Neuroscience* 2000; 99:179–188.

59 Pointillart V, Gense D, Gross C, *et al.* Effects of nimodipine on posttraumatic spinal cord ischemia in baboons. *J Neurotrauma* 1993;10:201–213.

60 De Ley G, Leybaert L. Effect of flunarizine and methylprednisolone on functional recovery after experimental spinal injury. *J Neurotrauma* 1993;10:25–35.

61 Ross IB, Tator CH. Spinal cord blood flow and evoked potential responses after treatment with nimodipine or methylprednisolone in spinal cord-injured rats. *Neurosurgery* 1993;33:470–476.

62 Guha A, Tator CH, Piper I. Effect of a calcium channel blocker on posttraumatic spinal cord blood flow. *J Neurosurg* 1987;66:423–430.

63 Pointillart V, Petitjean ME, Wiart L, *et al.* Pharmacological therapy of spinal cord injury during the acute phase. *Spinal Cord* 2000;38:71–76.

64 Petitjean ME, Pointillart V, Dixmerias F, *et al.* Medical treatment of spinal cord injury in the acute stage. *Ann Fr Anesth Reanim* 1998;17:114–122.

65 Lewen A, Matz P, Chan PH. Free radical pathways in CNS injury. *J Neurotrauma* 2000; 17:871–890.

66 Kowaltowski AJ, Castilho RF, Vercesi AE. Ca(2+)-induced mitochondrial membrane permeabilization: role of coenzyme Q redox state. *Am J Physiol* 1995;269:C141–C147.

67 Gardner AM, Xu FH, Fady C, *et al.* Apoptotic vs. nonapoptotic cytotoxicity induced by hydrogen peroxide. *Free Radic Biol Med* 1997;22:73–83.

68 Liu D, Ling X, Wen J, *et al.* The role of reactive nitrogen species in secondary spinal cord injury: formation of nitric oxide, peroxynitrite, and nitrated protein. *J Neurochem* 2000;75:2144–2154.

69 Liu D, Li L, Augustus L. Prostaglandin release by spinal cord injury mediates production of hydroxyl radical, malondialdehyde and cell death: a site of the neuroprotective action of methylprednisolone. *J Neurochem* 2001;77:1036–1047.

70 Liu D, Liu J, Wen J. Elevation of hydrogen peroxide after spinal cord injury detected by using the Fenton reaction. *Free Radic Biol Med* 1999;27:478–482.

71 Liu D, Sybert TE, Qian H, *et al.* Superoxide production after spinal injury detected by microperfusion of cytochrome c. *Free Radic Biol Med* 1998;25:298–304.

72 Leski ML, Bao F, Wu L, *et al.* Protein and DNA oxidation in spinal injury: neurofilaments – an oxidation target. *Free Radic Biol Med* 2001;30:613–624.

73 Springer JE, Azbill RD, Mark RJ, *et al.* 4-hydroxynonenal, a lipid peroxidation product, rapidly accumulates following traumatic spinal cord injury and inhibits glutamate uptake. *J Neurochem* 1997;68:2469–2476.

74 Barut S, Canbolat A, Bilge T, *et al.* Lipid peroxidation in experimental spinal cord injury: time-level relationship. *Neurosurg Rev* 1993;16:53–59.

75 Kaptanoglu E, Sens S, Beskonakli E, *et al.* Antioxidant actions and early ultrastructural findings of thiopental and propofol in experimental spinal cord injury. *J Neurosurg Anesthesiol* 2002;14:114–122.

76 Farooque M, Isaksson J, Olsson Y. Improved recovery after spinal cord injury in neuronal nitric oxide synthase-deficient mice but not in TNF-alpha-deficient mice. *J Neurotrauma* 2001;18:105–114.

77 Fujimoto T, Nakamura T, Ikeda T, *et al.* Effects of EPC-K1 on lipid peroxidation in experimental spinal cord injury. *Spine* 2000;25:24–29.

78 Katoh D, Ikata T, Katoh S, *et al.* Effect of dietary vitamin C on compression injury of the spinal cord in a rat mutant unable to synthesize ascorbic acid and its correlation with that of vitamin E. *Spinal Cord* 1996;34:234–238.

79 Naftchi NE. Treatment of mammalian spinal cord injury with antioxidants. *Int J Dev Neurosci* 1991;9:113–126.

80 Kavanagh RJ, Kam PC. Lazaroids: efficacy and mechanism of action of the 21-aminosteroids in neuroprotection. *Br J Anaesth* 2001;86:11011–11019.

81 Gerhart KA, Johnson RL, Menconi J, *et al.* Utilization and effectiveness of methylprednisolone in a population-based sample of spinal cord injured persons. *Paraplegia* 1995;33:316–321.

82 George ER, Scholten DJ, Buechler CM, *et al.* Failure of methylprednisolone to improve the outcome of spinal cord injuries. *Am Surg* 1995;61:659–663.

83 Poynton AR, *et al.* An evaluation of the factors affecting neurological recovery following spinal cord injury. *Injury* 1997;28:545–548.

84 Prendergast MR, Saxe JM, Ledgerwood AM, *et al.* Massive steroids do not reduce the zone of injury after penetrating spinal cord injury. *J Trauma* 1994;37:576–579.

85 Bracken MB, Collins WF, Freeman DF, *et al.* Efficacy of methylprednisolone in acute spinal cord injury. *JAMA* 1984;251:45–52.

CHAPTER 3

Prehospital and emergency department management of spinal cord injury

Stuart P. Swadron, Danny L. Chang and Brian Wilbur

Introduction

The first minutes and hours after injury are disproportionately important in the management of trauma. This is true in both patients with isolated spinal cord injury (SCI) as well as those with concomitant injuries. Multiple factors in the prehospital and emergency department (ED) phases of management influence the outcome of patients with SCI. In these early phases, optimal outcomes are achieved primarily by avoiding secondary injury until more definitive management can occur.

Over the past several decades, the fields of emergency medicine and trauma surgery have grown substantially and management protocols have evolved. In some these protocols are supported by evidence from SCI trials, but in most cases "general," practice continues to be based on a consensus of expert opinion.

Prehospital care

There exist two relatively distinct models of prehospital care in the developed world. The Franco-German model involves the dispatch of physicians to the accident scene. In this model, important components of the initial resuscitation are carried out at the scene itself. Attempts at stabilization in the field may include advanced airway management, aggressive fluid resuscitation, the full spectrum of emergency parenteral drugs, and emergency surgical interventions. In the Anglo-American model, resuscitation is initiated in the field, but a heavy emphasis is placed on timely transport of patients to the hospital, where it is believed that a more optimal resuscitation can be performed. This is the model utilized by the vast majority of emergency medical systems throughout North America.

Despite the different emphases of these two models of prehospital care, both involve the institution of spinal precautions at the scene of injury. The institution of spinal precautions prior to transport necessarily increases scene time and delays transport to the hospital. In addition, there is surprisingly little evidence for the effectiveness of our current practice of spinal precautions for transport, which were developed largely on the basis of anecdotal reports and descriptive studies.[1] Poor outcomes in patients with SCI have been attributed to improper positioning and handling of the patient in transport and during initial resuscitation. The causal effect of such mishandling may appear clear in an individual case, such as when a patient becomes suddenly quadriplegic after manipulation of the neck during airway intervention. However, a lack of controlled data makes it difficult to be precise about the extent and degree to which current immobilization protocols improve outcomes in patients with SCI on the whole.[2,3] Although ethical and legal concerns will limit the availability of data to prove the benefit of spinal precautions, it may be possible to identify subgroups of patients where the use of spinal precautions is unnecessary or for whom the risks of an adverse outcome from delayed transport outweigh its benefits.

Because of the potentially devastating effects of worsening a spinal injury, criteria for the application of spinal immobilization in the field should be as sensitive as possible. Thus, every patient with a clinically unstable injury must be immobilized, even at the expense of the unnecessary immobilization of many other patients without spinal injury. Attempts have been made to apply clinical decision rules to the prehospital phase similar to those used by emergency physicians to clear the cervical spine in the hospital. Domeier *et al.*[4] and Stroh *et al.*[5] both report large series of patients where the application of such decision rules results in the appropriate immobilization of the vast majority of patients with SCI. However, in both studies, their decision rules yield lower sensitivities for the detection of SCI than is found in the more rigorously controlled trials performed in the ED. The sensitivity of any prehospital screening for SCI must be at least as sensitive as the screening that takes place in the ED, otherwise some patients with injury will be transported without precautions. In addition, other research shows that the interrater reliability for cervical spine clearance rules differs significantly between physicians and non-physician providers such as nurses and emergency medical technicians.[6] Thus, until a prehospital rule for spinal clearance with nearly 100% sensitivity is prospectively validated in the field, spinal precautions should be applied very liberally in the prehospital phase to any patient with a mechanism that may possibly result in spinal trauma.[7]

There is a paucity of evidence to support any particular method for applying cervical spine precautions. In addition, research on the efficacy of various methods invariably uses normal volunteers – not patients with unstable spinal injuries.[8–10] Nonetheless, current practice is guided by the best available evidence and is consistent across most emergency medical systems. The application of cervical spine immobilization begins before the patient is extricated from a vehicle or other enclosed space during their initial rescue. In this scenario, a rigid cervical collar is typically placed before further efforts at extrication are made. In addition to the rigid collar, a short backboard placed behind the patient may also be employed for additional stability during the extrication. If the patient is conscious, he or she should be asked to actively move their neck to the neutral position. The neutral position has been defined by one author as the "normal anatomic position of the head and torso that one assumes when standing and looking ahead."[11] If active movement of the neck to the neutral position is not possible, gentle passive movement can be attempted, however, this should be abandoned if there is any pain, resistance, or neurological deterioration during the procedure. In these cases, the neck should be immobilized in the position in which it lies. If the patient is wearing a helmet, it may remain as part of the immobilization apparatus.

In order to achieve a neutral position on a backboard, most patients will require the placement of padding under the occiput, although the amount varies greatly from patient to patient. After the patient in a rigid collar is placed on the backboard, the head is further stabilized by the placement of side head supports, consisting of sandbags or proprietary foam blocks. The two side head supports are then connected together over the patients forehead via adhesive tape or Velco straps. Lastly, the entire patient must be secured to the backboard by straps or tape. Care should be taken to include straps at the level of the shoulders and at the pelvis because rotation at these areas results in movement of the spine. The balance of evidence suggests that better immobilization is achieved when all of these techniques are employed together; the rigid collar is used in combination with a backboard and secured side head supports, with the whole body completely secured to the backboard.[12]

Aside from prolonging time spent at the accident scene, the application of spinal immobilization raises additional concerns, even with short-term application. Patients are at increased risk of aspiration, and should be rolled together with the backboard toward their side at the first signs of vomiting. Aggressive suctioning of the airway should also occur in the event of vomiting. Because immobilizing the entire body involves straps around the thorax and abdomen, a patient's respiratory excursion is often compromised. In an otherwise healthy patient with a high cervical SCI or severe chest injury, or those with diminished pulmonary reserve, this may prove detrimental. Lastly, prolonged maintenance of prehospital spinal precautions results in pain and discomfort, complicating the emergency phase of treatment by causing back pain that may not have existed had a backboard not been used. After several hours, the patient strapped to a backboard may ultimately develop pressure sores, which in turn may result in sepsis and even death. It is for this reason that the backboard devices placed in the field be removed as soon as possible after the patient arrives in the ED.

Prehospital care providers and emergency physicians consider the immobilization of the cervical spine simultaneously with the management of the airway. In the multiply injured patient, the use of high-flow oxygen is recommended, principally to avoid hypoxia and to prevent tissue ischemia. When a patient is unable to oxygenate or ventilate adequately, immediate active airway management becomes necessary. The specific management depends on the degree of training and scope of practice of the prehospital personnel. In the United States, emergency medical technicians are trained to maintain spinal precautions while assisting ventilation with a bag-valve-mask device. Paramedics are trained in endotracheal intubation and maintain in-line stabilization of the cervical spine during this procedure. In most systems, the use of paralytic agents to facilitate intubation is not within the scope of practice of paramedics, although they are used in some systems, more commonly, particularly in those utilizing aeromedical transport.

Because of the concern of untoward movement in the patient with spinal injury, paramedics are less likely to attempt endotracheal intubation when an injured patient continues to breathe, even if it appears likely that intubation may soon be required. Endotracheal intubation, whether through the oral or nasal route, presents significant risks in this uncontrolled environment, particularly in patients with cervical spine injuries without paralytic and without the assistance of paralytic agents. If paramedics can temporize by successfully assisting ventilations with a bag-valve-mask device, they will frequently do so rather than attempt intubation, especially when transport times are short. A recent large-scale study of head injured patients in San Diego County examined the use of paralytic agents to facilitate intubation in the field. Patients intubated using a newly implemented paralytic protocol were compared to a group of historical controls treated before the implementation of paralytic agents. The investigators found that the rate of mortality was higher in the group that received paralytics, leading to an early termination of the project.[13] An analysis of data from field instruments revealed a possible explanation – patients receiving paralytics experienced sustained episodes of hypoxia and hypercarbia in the prehospital phase.[14] This highlights the differences between the prehospital environment, which is often chaotic, and the more controlled environment of the ED. Although the San Diego study examined head injured patients, not those with SCI, it clearly raises concerns about the prehospital use of paralytic agents in SCI patients as well.

The practice of using the Trendelenberg position (head lower than feet) in the management of hemorrhagic shock has fallen out of favor in recent years. A lack of evidence for its benefit, coupled with concerns about the restriction of cerebral venous drainage in the head injured patient are responsible for this trend.[15] In fact, patients with high cervical SCI, who have impaired control of the diaphragm may benefit from the reverse Trendelenberg position, to offload the pressure of the abdominal contents from the flaccid diaphragm, improving ventilation.

Some controversy has surrounded the use of intravenous fluids in the field for hypotensive trauma patients. In particular, "permissive hypotension" for victims of penetrating thoracoabdominal trauma has been proposed after a landmark study showing improved survival when fluids to such patients were held during their prehospital phase.[16] These results were achieved in victims of penetrating trauma in an urban emergency medical services (EMS) system with short transit times; the external validity of these findings to other populations of trauma victims is likely limited.[17] Untreated hypotension in patients with known or presumed SCI is likely to be deleterious and should be avoided in the prehospital phase. The administration of boluses of crystalloid, such as normal saline, while in transit to hospital, should thus be used to restore systemic blood pressure to pre-traumatic levels in patients with SCI.

Although there are descriptive studies of a specialized prehospital system to triage patients with SCI directly to specialized SCI centers, the majority of patients with SCI receive care in unspecialized centers that are designated to receive victims of trauma.[18] In fact, because the likelihood of SCI increases with the severity of mechanism, patients with SCI are frequently only known as "multiply injured" or "head injured" until after their evaluation in hospital.

There is some evidence that prolonged transport time to a facility where definitive neurosurgical care is available is associated with poorer outcomes. Nonetheless, the actual mode of transport of the patient with SCI is usually determined by other factors, such as the distance to the nearest trauma center and the extent and nature of other injuries.[19] For example, an SCI patient with concomitant airway extremis may be taken by ground ambulance to the closest facility hospital, whereas a hypotensive patient with a seat belt sign across the abdomen may be brought taken by air ambulance to a trauma center if ground transport time is considered to be unacceptably long.

Indirect evidence points to an improvement in outcomes of patients with SCI in the prehospital phase over the past several decades.[20] Between the 1970s and 1980s, the percentage of patients presenting to hospital with complete cord lesions decreased from 55% to 39%.[21-23] Although some have attributed this to improved immobilization techniques, the cause is more likely to be multifactorial, also related to advances in other elements of prehospital care, such as improved airway, ventilation, and fluid management.[24]

Emergency department resuscitation

The majority of patients with SCI have major concomitant injuries of the head, chest, abdomen, pelvis, and extremities – only approximately 40% sustain isolated SCI.[25,26] The initial stages in trauma resuscitation proceed in the same fashion regardless of whether a SCI is present: these begin with a primary survey, a resuscitative phase and a secondary survey. These steps in resuscitation were formally outlined by the American College of Surgeons in their Advanced Trauma Life Support (ATLS) courses that began in 1980.[27]

The primary survey

The primary survey consists of assessment of the airway with attention to spinal protection, breathing, circulation, neurological disability, and exposure of the entire patient for signs of injury. In the primary survey, intervention occurs concurrently with assessment, and the nature of intervention can be tailored to the specific circumstances of each resuscitation. Neurological disability appears later in the primary survey than the cardiopulmonary assessment, because the most direct threat to neurological outcome is secondary injury from exacerbation of the ischemic insult. This can be avoided by prompt stabilization of concomitant life-threatening injuries.

Airway

Airway management in trauma has undergone a substantial evolution in recent decades. The most notable change has been the widespread availability of paralytic medications in EDs. Rapid sequence intubation (RSI) is now standard curriculum in American emergency medicine residency programs and it is employed routinely by emergency physicians. In the trauma patient who is unable to protect their airway or unable to maintain adequate oxygenation and ventilation, the need for immediate endotracheal intubation is readily apparent. However, there are many other instances when the decision to intubate is based on subtler data. In these more elective intubations the risks should be weighed carefully against the potential benefits. Examples include, the patient with multiple injuries in severe pain and those who require prolonged diagnostic or painful surgical procedures. Although the potential for worsening a cord injury during RSI exists, intubation can be achieved safely and effectively. In addition, in the agitated patient with altered mental status, controlling the airway with RSI and sedating the patient prevents secondary injury from uncontrolled movement.

Careful attention to the patient's rate and pattern of breathing and the presence of paradoxical or abdominal breathing will assist in the airway management decisions in patients with SCI. It should be noted, however, that for patients with high cervical SCI, delayed intubation may result in further morbidity.[28] In one series from our institution, of 31 patients with SCI but no overt signs of respiratory compromise on admission, 13 patients (42%) required intubation within the first 53 h. Six of the thirteen patients were intubated in emergency situations after a precipitous failure of oxygenation and developed pulmonary complications as a result.[29] It is difficult to provide guidelines on the basis of such descriptive data, however, it is clear that endotracheal intubation should be considered early in patients with SCI. The potential morbidity associated with RSI under controlled conditions is likely far less than that associated with leaving the airway unsecured.

RSI involves the use of a paralytic agent in combination with agent(s) to render the patient unconscious to facilitate endotracheal intubation. If possible, intubation is achieved without the need for bag-valve-mask ventilation, which increases the risk of vomiting and aspiration. The procedure begins by providing preoxygenation to the patient through a tight-fitting non-rebreather mask. This maximizes the time available for achieving intubation after the paralytic is administered. Pretreatment with certain medications such as fentanyl prior to the administration of the paralytic agent may result in hypotension, and should be undertaken with caution, if at all. A simple regimen of a paralytic such as succinylcholine or rocuronium in combination with an induction agent such as etomidate is ideal, as it does not significantly alter the patient's hemodynamic status and central nervous system perfusion. Once the paralytic and induction agent are administered, gentle downward pressure to the cricoid cartilage to prevent passive aspiration should be provided (the Sellick maneuver). The collar is temporarily removed, and an assistant

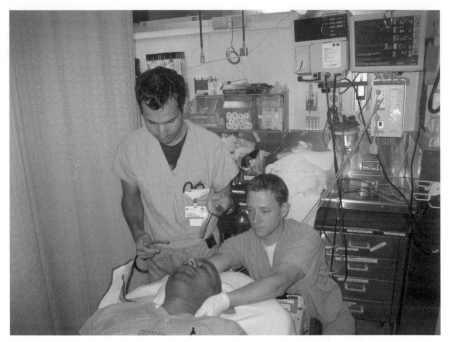

Figure 3.1 Technique of in-line cervical spine stabilization during rapid sequence endotracheal intubation. The Sellick maneuver (gentle cricoid cartilage pressure to prevent passive regurgitation and pulmonary aspiration) would require a third person (not shown).

provides in-line stabilization of the cervical spine while the trachea is intubated orally by a dedicated operator (see Figure 3.1). After the tube is placed, confirmation of placement must be verified. This is ideally achieved with waveform capnography, but may also consist of a combination of less definitive techniques such as auscultation, quantitative end-tidal CO_2 detection, and syringe aspiration.

Nasotracheal intubation, once recommended in the ATLS course for breathing patients with suspected SCI, has fallen out of practice. RSI with orotracheal intubation and in-line stabilization is thought to be more consistently successful and ultimately result in less movement of the cervical spine. Some evidence supports this transformation in practice, and there is consensus across disciplines that it is safer, although no data exist from controlled trials.[30,31] Cricothyroidotomy has also become less common. This is mostly due to the success of RSI techniques and the increasing use of adjunctive airway techniques and devices that help the emergency physician achieve a definitive airway when traditional laryngoscopy is unsuccessful. These devices include the intubating laryngeal mask airway, lighted stylet, and elastic bougie devices among many others. Endoscopic techniques of intubation that do not require laryngoscopy are becoming more common, and may eventually replace the traditional techniques, especially when neck movement is to be avoided.

Breathing

Hyperventilation ("overbagging") of a newly intubated patient is very frequent, especially during the charged environment of a critical trauma resuscitation. Care must be taken to avoid this. Not only does excessive hyperventilation have the potential to exacerbate traumatic brain injury, but overzealous bag-valve-mask ventilation prevents venous return and has deleterious effects on systemic blood pressure. Once the patient is attached to a ventilator, a determination of blood gases should be made after several minutes to ensure adequate oxygenation and ventilation. Hypoxia and hypercarbia are both deleterious to the injured spinal cord.

Circulation

Although data from controlled studies in humans may never be available, hypotension exacerbates injury in experimental models of SCI (see Chapter 1). Data are also available to point to the deleterious effects of hypotension in those patients with concomitant brain injury. The consensus of expert opinion is that hypotension should be avoided in the resuscitation of patients with SCI. In addition, there is some evidence that augmentation of blood pressure in the first week after SCI through aggressive volume expansion and the use of pressor agents may improve outcome.[32–34] Although some authorities go as far as to propose minimum values for mean arterial pressure, it is more likely that the optimal pressures vary from patient to patient and circumstance to circumstance. All authors recommend that systolic blood pressures in adults should be kept >90 mmHg at all times during the emergency phase of management.[35]

Shock states are common in patients presenting with SCI. Although the physical examination may provide clues to the underlying cause of shock, the assumption during the prehospital and emergency phases of care must be that a component of hypovolemic shock causing ongoing hemorrhage is present. This assumption is made not only because hemorrhage is the most common form of shock in the trauma patient, but it requires aggressive and systematic treatment with crystalloid, blood products, and surgical hemostasis. The initial stages of hypovolemic shock are not characterized by hypotension, but rather by more subtle signs such as a narrowing of the pulse pressure. Recognizing these signs and anticipating hypotension before it is allowed to occur is an important goal for the resuscitation team.

Neurogenic shock, which occurs to varying degrees in patients with SCI, is the result of decreased sympathetic outflow through the sympathetic chain in the cervical and high thoracic region. In neurogenic shock, the loss of sympathetic tone results in peripheral vasodilation and a lower than expected heart rate. The classic picture of a paralyzed, hypotensive patient with warm, dry, hyperemic extremities, and bradycardia contrasts sharply with the patient with cool, pale, clammy extremities, and tachycardia more typical of hypovolemic or cardiogenic shock. Nonetheless, shock states may be mixed and present atypically; aggressive efforts to eliminate the possibility of ongoing hemorrhage are essential before a conclusion is made that hypotension is due to a neurogenic shock. Fortunately, the initial treatment of both neurogenic shock and hypovolemic shock is with volume expansion. Further treatment with inotropic agents and pressors is often required in patients with neurogenic shock to prevent systemic hypotension. In addition to neurogenic shock, other causes of relative bradycardia in the face of hypotension also must be considered by the emergency physician, including cardiogenic shock from cardiac contusion or coronary artery disease and the action of negative chronotropic medications, such as beta blockers and calcium channel blockers.

Disability

When the decision has been made to intubate the patient during the airway, breathing, and circulation steps of the primary survey, a rapid neurological assessment should be made prior to the administration of paralytic agents. This consists of checking the pupils for size and reactivity, an assessment of level of consciousness, and a gross measure of movement of the extremities. It also ideally includes an assessment of rectal tone as another indicator of spinal function. In critically injured patients, when more detailed examination is not feasible, these steps in the primary survey must be considered a minimum.

Exposure

During the exposure component of the primary survey, the patient is typically "logrolled" to examine the back and the entire length of the spine for signs of trauma. Although some prehospital studies have proposed that other techniques for moving a patient on or off a backboard may result in less motion of the spine, such techniques do not necessarily allow for visualization of the back.[36] Careful logrolling, with one caregiver maintaining cervical spine stabilization while others rotate the body at the shoulders and pelvis, remains the standard practice in the ED.

Whether or not SCI is present, the backboard used for patient transport must be removed – the remaining elements of immobilization used for transport remain or may be replaced by better fitting and comfortable devices. This may occur after the primary survey, or if the backboard remains briefly to facilitate movement of the patient for imaging studies, immediately thereafter. Patients who have not yet been evaluated for injuries of the thoracic, lumbar, or sacral spine should remain lying flat and restricted to their bed, until such evaluation has occurred.[37]

The resuscitation phase and secondary survey

Resuscitation is begun upon first contact with the patient in the prehospital setting and continues throughout the primary survey. The resuscitation phase of the ATLS protocol involves a continuation and reassessment of the interventions begun in the primary survey, obtaining historical details about the patient and the circumstances surrounding the injury, diagnostic imaging and other studies, as well as the insertion of nasogastric and urinary catheters.

For the most seriously injured patients, the ED phase often ends here, as the venue for further resuscitation changes to the operating room, interventional angiography suite, or intensive care unit. In these patients, the likelihood of SCI increases from approximately 2–3% in the unselected trauma patient to around 10%.[7,38] In the face of other immediate life-threatening injuries, no further ED evaluation of the spine and spinal cord may be possible. A more complete physical examination and radiological evaluation of the spine may be deferred temporarily with the understanding that the patient must be handled as if they have a spinal injury until proved otherwise.

The secondary survey: neurological examination

For less critically injured patients and those patients that remain in the ED, the secondary survey can proceed. The secondary survey, which examines all systems from head-to-toe more thoroughly, includes a complete neurological examination. The presence of a spinal injury is first suspected based on the chief complaint(s), mechanism of injury, and physical examination findings. If the patient is communicative and complains of localized pain in the neck or back, this directs a careful physical examination and imaging to that location. The entire spine should be inspected for tenderness, step-off deformities, edema, and ecchymoses. It must be remembered, however, that extra-spinal injuries, such as long bone fractures or even moderately severe soft tissue injuries, may serve to distract the patient and mask the symptoms and signs of SCI. Such painful, distracting injuries are present in approximately half of all patients with SCI.[7]

If the patient is communicative and interactive, the neurological examination should be performed quickly and thoroughly, especially in the face of possible clinical deterioration or the need for sedation, paralysis, and intubation. The initial neurological examination helps to localize the level of injury, predicts the type of injury by recognition of various spinal cord syndromes, and serves as a baseline examination for the rest of the hospital stay, against which improvement or deterioration can be compared.

Following the cursory assessment in the primary survey, a complete neurological examination includes testing of bilateral motor, sensory, and reflex function. The use of standardized scoring instruments for SCI has not yet become routine or even common among emergency physicians. This is due, in part, to the many different scoring systems that have been developed and abandoned over the past decades. Many of these scoring systems did not have good interrater reliability and many were cumbersome to utilize. The latest instrument from the American Spinal Injury Association (ASIA) is relatively straightforward and has demonstrated good interrater reliability.[39]

In the ASIA system, the sensory evaluation includes bilateral testing of sensation in 28 dermatomes to light touch and pinprick, and are scored as being absent, impaired, normal, or not testable. The motor evaluation includes bilateral testing of motor strength on a standard 6 point scale in 10 key muscles. Finally, voluntary anal sphincter contraction and anal sensation are evaluated, with any intact function indicating an incomplete spinal cord lesion.[40] Dorsal column function should also be evaluated, particularly in the setting of anterior cord syndrome. The standardization of this evaluation allows for reproducible serial examinations, even by different examiners. However, this examination is only useful in the cooperative patient. If the patient presents with an altered level of consciousness, the neurological examination may be less complete but it is nonetheless critically important to do as thorough an examination as possible.

Although the determination of whether SCI is complete or incomplete may be made in the ED, this information should not be used by the emergency physician to guide management. Because a complete lesion may eliminate potential therapies and has important prognostic implications, it is safest for the emergency physician to assume the presence of an incomplete lesion until the patient has been fully evaluated by a neurosurgeon. The determination of the status of the lesion may be confounded by the presence of spinal shock. Spinal shock is the transient condition during which all neurological function below the level of SCI is absent, usually in conjunction with severe SCI. The motor and sensory components of spinal shock may take up until an hour or more to resolve. Return of spinal reflexes such as the anal wink and bulbocavernosus reflex heralds the end of spinal shock, after which time any remaining motor or sensory impairment cannot be attributed to spinal shock. The deficits seen at 24 h after a complete cord injury have <3% chance of recovery of any meaningful function, and this falls to essentially 0% at 48 h after injury.[41,42]

Incomplete cord injuries are those in which some sensory and/or motor function remains below the level of cord injury, and these have a better prognosis for recovery. There are several types of incomplete SCIs that are recognizable as discrete syndromes that may be predicted based on the mechanism of injury and may also direct the clinicians to other possible associated injuries. The *anterior cord syndrome* is characterized by compromise of the anterior two-thirds of the spinal cord, affecting the corticospinal and spinothalamic tracts and resulting in bilateral weakness and decreased sensation to pain and temperature below the level of the lesion. The anterior cord syndrome may occur in the setting of direct compression of the anterior spinal cord by bony or cartilaginous structures in hyperflexion injuries, or by compromise of the anterior spinal artery. The anterior cord syndrome has the worst prognosis of all incomplete spinal cord syndromes. The *central cord syndrome* has been classically described to result from compression of the cervical spinal cord in hyperflexion or hyperextension injuries between degenerative osteophytic protuberances anteriorly and buckling of a calcified ligamentum flavum into the central cord posteriorly. The syndrome is characterized by weakness in the upper more than lower extremities and variable sensory and bowel and bladder symptoms. The *Brown–Sequard syndrome* is characterized by the loss of ipsilateral proprioception and fine touch, ipsilateral weakness, and contralateral loss of pain and temperature below the level of a hemi-transection of the spinal cord. This syndrome usually occurs in the setting of penetrating trauma to the spinal cord. The *conus medullaris syndrome* can present with bilateral lower extremity motor and sensory deficits, in addition to bowel and bladder symptoms. This syndrome is similar to the *cauda equina syndrome*, but the former usually is associated with little or no radicular pain, unlike the latter. In addition, as a peripheral injury as opposed to a true SCI, the cauda equina syndrome has a better prognosis for recovery of function.

The secondary survey: other systems

The mechanism of trauma should be used by the emergency physician as a guide in the search for associated injuries in the patient with SCI. Depending on the nature of the SCI, the physical examination of the spinal-injured patient in the secondary survey may be unreliable, and advanced imaging is often necessary. Important associations in patients with SCI are as follows.

Head

In the setting of severe head trauma and a comatose, non-interactive patient, cervical SCI should be an immediate concern. In severely head-injured patients there is a >5% incidence of associated SCI,[44] and in spinal-injured patients there is a 25–50% incidence of associated head injury.[43,44] In a large study at our institution, there was a directly inverse relationship between Glasgow Coma Scale (GCS) on presentation and the incidence of SCI.[29] Associated head injury may alter the order of emergency interventions in a patient with SCI, but also underscores the importance of maintaining optimal perfusion and metabolic status of the central nervous system during the emergency phase of management.

Chest

Chest injuries are common in the multiply injured patient. Respiratory compromise may occur by any number of mechanisms. Direct injury to the chest wall, rib fractures, pulmonary contusions, hemothoraces, and pneumothoraces may be immediately apparent upon the primary survey and with portable chest radiography. The patient's respiratory rhythm and rate, chest wall expansion, oxygen saturation, and if available, end-tidal CO_2 should be carefully monitored. While high cervical cord injury may cause immediate respiratory failure due to loss of control of the diaphragm via the phrenic nerve, slower respiratory deterioration may occur in the setting of upper thoracic SCI due to loss of control of the intercostal musculature. Underlying medical conditions such as chronic pulmonary or cardiac disease should lower the threshold for intubation of the patient with an upper SCI, as the patient has little pulmonary reserve. Early placement of a nasogastric or orogastric tube may help prevent aspiration and to relieve abdominal distention that compromises chest expansion. Of the many possible causes of chest pain in the victim of a rapid deceleration injury, traumatic aortic injury and thoracic spine fracture are critically important ones and should be considered early on. Both of these may exhibit a widened mediastinum on plain chest radiography.

Abdomen

If an SCI compromises sensation of the abdominal viscera and peritoneum, a traumatic intra-abdominal process may not be detectable by clinical examination. Continuous monitoring of the patient's vital signs looking for evidence of shock, serial checks of the patient's hemoglobin, and serial use of bedside ultrasonography all aid in the rapid detection of intra-abdominal hemorrhage in the ED. Computerized tomography (CT) imaging of the abdomen and pelvis is routinely employed in these patients when they are considered sufficiently stable to leave the resuscitation area. Chance fractures are horizontal vertebral fractures due to hyperflexion injuries that occur most often in the setting of lap seat-belted passengers involved in motor vehicle crashes. The incidence of intestinal and mesenteric injuries in patients with Chance fractures is reported to be as high as 63%.[45,46] Because these injuries may not be well visualized on CT, it is important to serially assess these patients by other means as well (physical examination, laboratory studies) and to continue to watch for signs of evolving abdominal emergencies well after the patient has left the ED.

Pelvis

In the setting of possible SCI and particularly with lower lumbar vertebral injuries, pelvic fractures must be considered. Pelvic fractures can be devastating, with both a high incidence of morbidity and mortality. The genitourinary examination is performed, checking for pelvic instability, blood at the urethral meatus, bladder distention, perianal sensation, sphincter tone, a superiorly displaced prostate gland, and priapism, which reflects autonomic dysfunction associated with SCI. In the multiply injured patient, a pelvic X-ray to look for fractures and dislocations is considered a routine part of the initial resuscitation. Pelvic fractures are associated with significant blood loss and are one of the most common sites of injury accounting for seemingly occult hemorrhage. In the patient with a spinal injury and pelvic fracture who has urinary retention, SCI cannot be assumed to be the cause of urinary retention without consideration of possible urethral transection, bladder rupture, or pelvic fracture causing compromise of the sacral nerve plexus.

Extremities

Orthopedic injuries can easily be missed as attention is given to more obvious or severe injuries. Careful assessment of the extremities for tenderness, bruising, edema, lacerations, crepitus, and joint range of motion should be performed, and imaging should be used liberally to search for fractures and dislocations, especially in the non-interactive patient.

Imaging studies in the ED

Although the imaging of patients with SCI is discussed in detail in Chapter 5, it should be noted that large, well-controlled trials studying the use of screening radiography for cervical spine injury have been conducted in the ED setting. Two validated clinical decision rules exist to clinically clear the cervical spine and obviate the need for radiographic evaluation. The NEXUS (National Emergency X-ray Utilization Study) criteria are somewhat easier to apply and have a sensitivity of 99.6% for the detection of cervical spine injury, with an even higher sensitivity for the detection of potentially unstable injuries[7] (see

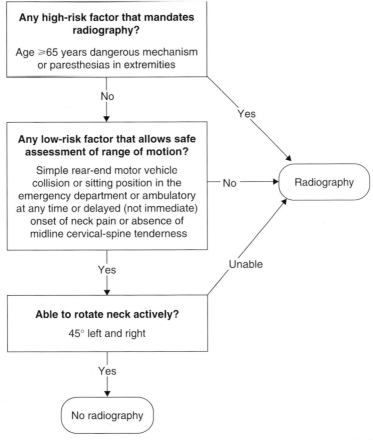

Figure 3.2 Canadian C-spine decision rule. For patients with trauma who are alert (as indicated by a score of 15 on the Glasgow Coma Scale) and in stable condition and in whom cervical-spine injury is a concern, the determination of risk factors guides the use of cervical-spine radiography. A dangerous mechanism is considered to be a fall from an elevation ⩾3 ft or 5 stairs; an axial load to the head (e.g. diving); a motor vehicle collision at high speed (>100 km/h) or with rollover or ejection; a collision involving a motorized recreational vehicle; or a bicycle collision. A simple rear-end motor vehicle collision excludes being pushed into oncoming traffic, being hit by a bus or a large truck, a rollover, and being hit by a high-speed vehicle. *Source*: Steill *et al. New Engl J Med* 2003;349:2510–2518. Reproduced with permission.

box below). The Canadian C-Spine Rule, although somewhat more detailed, is equally sensitive and also effective at safely reducing the overall use of X-ray studies in the ED.[47] These clinical decision rules are provided in Figure 3.2.

Clinical decision rules for clearance of the cervical spine: the NEXUS low-risk criteria

Cervical-spine radiography is indicated for patients with trauma unless they meet all of the following criteria:

No posterior midline cervical-spine tenderness

No evidence of intoxication

A normal level of alertness

No focal neurologic deficit

No painful distracting injuries

Once the decision to perform imaging is made, there is no consensus on what constitutes radiographic clearance. CT scanning is becoming increasing common to image the spine, and for the patient who is going to the CT scanner for other studies, there is general agreement that CT of the cervical spine should be done in the place of plain films, provided that either scout films or lateral reconstruction views are also provided to assess alignment.[48–50] For patients who do not need any other CT studies, plain films are still considered an acceptable screening tool, although they may rarely miss clinically significant injuries.[51]

Once an abnormality is seen on plain films, a CT should be performed of the entire cervical spine rather than a more limited study that just focuses on the suspicious area. This assertion is based on the finding that patients with multiple clinically significant injuries on CT often only have a single area of abnormality identified on plain films. Because one spinal column injury predicts a 6–16% chance of another non-contiguous column injury, the entire spine should be imaged once a spinal injury is identified.[52–54]

Magnetic resonance imaging (MRI) can be obtained from an increasing number of EDs and is indicated as soon as possible in patients with neurological deficits.

Disposition

Although only weak evidence exists to point to improved outcomes when patients with SCI are monitored in intensive care settings after admission, disposition to such settings is nonetheless recommended.[20,33–34,55,56] SCI is a major systemic insult which evolves over time – many patients who appear to be compensating well in the initial hour after injury deteriorate precipitously – neurologically and systemically.[57–59] In addition, it appears that even brief periods of suboptimal perfusion may be disproportionately deleterious to patients with SCI. In a monitored unit, it is more likely that subtle changes in hemodynamic and respiratory status will be noted earlier, so that immediate corrective action can be taken.

Conclusions

SCI occurs most commonly in the setting of other traumatic injuries. Even when it appears isolated, the initial evaluation of patients with SCI still must reflect a vigilant search for associated injuries because they are often masked by the SCI itself or an associated head injury. Moreover, the outcome of SCI will be linked to the identification and management of concomitant injuries. In each phase of emergency care, from the initial extrication of the patient from the accident scene to the point of discharge from the ED, the focus in the care of patients with SCI is to prevent further neurological injury and create an optimal environment for more definitive and specific therapy.

References

1 Joint Section on Disorders of the Spine and Peripheral Nerves of the American Association of Neurological Surgeons and the Congress of Neurological Surgeons. *Neurosurgery* 2002;50(Suppl 3):S18–S20.

2 Hauswald M, *et al.* Out-of-hospital spinal immobilization: its effect on neurologic injury. *Acad Emerg Med* 1998;5(3):214–219.

3 Hoffman JR, Mower WR. Out-of-hospital cervical spine immobilization: making policy in the absence of definitive information. *Ann Emerg Med* 2001;37(6):632–634.

4 Domeier RM, *et al.* Multicenter prospective validation of prehospital clinical spinal clearance criteria. *J Trauma* 2002;53(4):744–750.

5 Stroh G, Braude D. Can an out-of-hospital cervical spine clearance protocol identify all patients with injuries? An argument for selective immobilization. *Ann Emerg Med* 2001; 37(6):609–615.

6 Hoffman JR, *et al.* Validity of a set of clinical criteria to rule out injury to the cervical spine in patients with blunt trauma. National Emergency X-Radiography Utilization Study Group. *New Engl J Med* 2000;343(2):94–99.

7 Meldon SW, *et al.* Out-of-hospital cervical spine clearance: agreement between emergency medical technicians and emergency physicians. *J Trauma* 1998;45(6):1058–1061.

8 Podolsky S, *et al.* Efficacy of cervical spine immobilization methods. *J Trauma* 1983; 23(6):461–465.

9 Mazolewski P, Manix TH. The effectiveness of strapping techniques in spinal immobilization. *Ann Emerg Med* 1994;23(6):1290–1295.

10 De Lorenzo RA, *et al.* Optimal positioning for cervical immobilization. *Ann Emerg Med* 1996;28(3):301–308.

11 Schriger DL. Immobilizing the cervical spine in trauma: should we seek an optimal position or an adequate one? *Ann Emerg Med* 1996;28(3):351–353.

12 De Lorenzo RA. A review of spinal immobilization techniques. *J Emerg Med* 1996; 14(5):603–613.

13 Davis DP, *et al.* The effect of paramedic rapid sequence intubation on outcome in patients with severe traumatic brain injury. *J Trauma* 2003;54(3):444–453.

14 Davis DP, *et al*. The impact of hypoxia and hyperventilation on outcome after paramedic rapid sequence intubation of severely head-injured patients. *J Trauma* 2004;57(1):1–8; discussion 8–10.

15 Bridges N, Jarquin-Valdivia AA. Use of the trendelenburg position as the resuscitation position: to T or not to T? *Am J Crit Care* 2005;14(5):364–368.

16 Bickell WH, *et al*. Immediate versus delayed fluid resuscitation for hypotensive patients with penetrating torso injuries. *New Engl J Med* 1994;331(17):1105–1109.

17 Pepe PE, Eckstein M. Reappraising the prehospital care of the patient with major trauma. *Emerg Med Clin North Am* 1998;16(1):1–15.

18 Tator CH, *et al*. Management of acute spinal cord injuries. *Can J Surg* 1984;27(3):289–293, 296.

19 Burney RE, Waggoner R, Maynard FM. Stabilization of spinal injury for early transfer. *J Trauma* 1989;29(11):1497–1499.

20 Tator CH, *et al*. Neurological recovery, mortality and length of stay after acute spinal cord injury associated with changes in management. *Paraplegia* 1995;33(5):254–262.

21 DeVivo MJ, *et al*. Trends in spinal cord injury demographics and treatment outcomes between 1973 and 1986. *Arch Phys Med Rehabil* 1992;73(5):424–430.

22 Gunby P. From "regeneration" to prostheses: research on spinal cord injury. *JAMA* 1981;245(13):1293–1297, 1301.

23 Tator CH, *et al*. Changes in epidemiology of acute spinal cord injury from 1947 to 1981. *Surg Neurol* 1993;40(3):207–215.

24 Deane SA, Ramenofsky ML. Advanced trauma life support in the 1980s: a decade of improvement in trauma care. *Aust N Z J Surg* 1991;61(11):809–813.

25 Reiss SJ, *et al*. Cervical spine fractures with major associated trauma. *Neurosurgery* 1986;18(3):327–330.

26 Saboe LA, *et al*. Spine trauma and associated injuries. *J Trauma* 1991;31(1):43–48.

27 Collicott PE. Advanced Trauma Life Support (ATLS): past, present, future – 16th Stone Lecture, American Trauma Society. *J Trauma* 1992;33(5):749–753.

28 Velmahos GC, *et al*. Intubation after cervical spinal cord injury: to be done selectively or routinely? *Am Surg* 2003;69(10):891–894.

29 Demetriades D, *et al*. Nonskeletal cervical spine injuries: epidemiology and diagnostic pitfalls. *J Trauma* 2000;48(4):724–727.

30 McCrory C, Blunnie WP, Moriarty DC. Elective tracheal intubation in cervical spine injuries. *Ir Med J* 1997;90(6):234–235.

31 Rhee KJ, *et al*. Oral intubation in the multiply injured patient: the risk of exacerbating spinal cord damage. *Ann Emerg Med* 1990;19(5):511–514.

32 Zach GA, Seiler W, Dollfus P. Treatment results of spinal cord injuries in the Swiss Parplegic Centre of Basle. *Paraplegia* 1976;14(1):58–65.

33 Vale FL, *et al*. Combined medical and surgical treatment after acute spinal cord injury: results of a prospective pilot study to assess the merits of aggressive medical resuscitation and blood pressure management. *J Neurosurg* 1997;87(2):239–246.

34 Levi L, Wolf A, Belzberg H. Hemodynamic parameters in patients with acute cervical cord trauma: description, intervention, and prediction of outcome. *Neurosurgery* 1993;33(6):1007–16; discussion 1016–1017.

35 Amar AP, Levy ML. Surgical controversies in the management of spinal cord injury. *J Am Coll Surg* 1999;188(5):550–566.

36 McGuire RA, *et al*. Spinal instability and the log-rolling maneuver. *J Trauma* 1987; 27(5):525–531.

37 Savitsky E, Votey S. Emergency department approach to acute thoracolumbar spine injury. *J Emerg Med* 1997;15(1):49–60.

38 Wright SW, Robinson II GG, Wright MB. Cervical spine injuries in blunt trauma patients requiring emergent endotracheal intubation. *Am J Emerg Med* 1992;10(2):104–109.

39 Association ASI. *International Standards for the Neurological Classification of Spinal Cord Injury (Revised 2002).* 2002.

40 Schrader SC, Sloan TB, Toleikis JR. Detection of sacral sparing in acute spinal cord injury. *Spine* 1987;12(6):533–535.

41 Chapman JR, Anderson PA. Thoracolumbar spine fractures with neurologic deficit. *Orthop Clin North Am* 1994;25(4):595–612.

42 Stauffer ES. Neurologic recovery following injuries to the cervical spinal cord and nerve roots. *Spine* 1984;9(5):532–534.

43 Chiles III BW, Cooper PR. Acute spinal injury. *New Engl J Med* 1996;334(8):514–520.

44 Widder S, *et al.* Prospective evaluation of computed tomographic scanning for the spinal clearance of obtunded trauma patients: preliminary results. *J Trauma* 2004;56(6):1179–1184.

45 Anderson PA, *et al.* The epidemiology of seatbelt-associated injuries. *J Trauma* 1991; 31(1):60–67.

46 Anderson PA, *et al.* Flexion distraction and chance injuries to the thoracolumbar spine. *J Orthop Trauma* 1991;5(2):153–160.

47 Stiell IG, *et al.* The Canadian C-spine rule for radiography in alert and stable trauma patients. *JAMA* 2001;286(15):1841–1848.

48 Barba CA, *et al.* A new cervical spine clearance protocol using computed tomography. *J Trauma* 2001;51(4):652–656; discussion 656–657.

49 Schenarts PJ, *et al.* Prospective comparison of admission computed tomographic scan and plain films of the upper cervical spine in trauma patients with altered mental status. *J Trauma* 2001;51(4):663–668; discussion 668–669.

50 Thomas M, Teece S. Towards evidence based emergency medicine: best BETs from Manchester Royal Infirmary. Computed tomography and the exclusion of upper cervical spine injury in trauma patients with altered mental state. *Emerg Med J* 2002;19(6):551–552.

51 Mower WR, *et al.* Use of plain radiography to screen for cervical spine injuries. *Ann Emerg Med* 2001;38(1):1–7.

52 Vaccaro AR, *et al.* Noncontiguous injuries of the spine. *J Spinal Disord* 1992;5(3):320–329.

53 Keenen TL, Antony J, Benson DR. Non-contiguous spinal fractures. *J Trauma* 1990; 30(4):489–491.

54 Barrett TW, *et al.* Injuries missed by limited computed tomographic imaging of patients with cervical spine injuries. *Ann Emerg Med* 2006;47(2):129–133.

55 Hachen HJ. Idealized care of the acutely injured spinal cord in Switzerland. *J Trauma* 1977;17(12):931–936.

56 McMichan JC, Michel L, Westbrook PR. Pulmonary dysfunction following traumatic quadriplegia. Recognition, prevention, and treatment. *JAMA* 1980;243(6):528–531.

57 Lu K, *et al.* Delayed apnea in patients with mid- to lower cervical spinal cord injury. *Spine* 2000;25(11):1332–1338.

58 Lehmann KG, *et al.* Cardiovascular abnormalities accompanying acute spinal cord injury in humans: incidence, time course and severity. *J Am Coll Cardiol* 1987;10(1):46–52.

59 Reines HD, Harris RC. Pulmonary complications of acute spinal cord injuries. *Neurosurgery* 1987;21(2):193–196.

CHAPTER 4

Radiographic workup of spinal cord injury

Nestor R. Gonzalez, Larry T. Khoo and Richard G. Fessler

Introduction

The diagnosis and therapeutic planning of spine and spinal cord injuries (SCIs) frequently require the utilization of imaging examinations such as plain films, computerized tomography (CT), or magnetic resonance imaging (MRI). Each of these studies provides valuable information regarding the type of injury, the structural stability, and the mechanism that could cause the trauma. In addition, these imaging techniques are key factors in determining the surgical approach that would better benefit the patient, details of the anatomy of the spine that affect the type of instrumentation required, and some information of prognostic value.

Two considerations have capital importance in the imaging of SCI: the clinical presentation and the assessment of the main functions and possible abnormalities of the spine. For asymptomatic patients that are conscious and can cooperate with the physical examination, less complex imaging is required than for those who are symptomatic or unconscious. Regarding the functions of the normal spine, which include support for the head and upper body, movement with flexion, extension, tilting and rotation, and protection for the spinal cord and the nerve roots, the radiological evaluation is not limited to the anatomic presence of fractures or dislocations, but also is of value in the assessment of movement and the integrity of the spinal cord and nerve roots.

However, useful CT and MRI imaging can be, liberal use of these expensive examinations should be avoided. This chapter will explore the advantages of each of the currently available techniques in general and their proper application to the most common spinal injuries, as well as their utility in surgical preparation.

Conventional radiology

After assessing and managing the airway of a trauma patient during an initial evaluation, immobilization devices most commonly implement protection of the patient's spinal cord until spine and SCI are ruled out. As part of the primary survey of the trauma patient, films of chest, pelvis, and lateral view of the cervical spine are immediately obtained without delaying the resuscitation process (Chapter 3). However, during a secondary survey, antero-posterior (AP) and open-mouth films of the cervical spine are performed in patients who are suspected to have a cervical spine injury.[1] When a lumbar or thoracic fracture is suspected, frontal, and cross table lateral radiographs are typically obtained in the immobilized patient. The integrity of the bone structures and alignment of the vertebral elements must be evaluated, and a preliminary diagnosis may be made in the resuscitation room. If the quality of the films is poor or inconclusive, a higher quality, thin section CT scan with sagittal and coronal reformations can be obtained to determine if a patient is an appropriate candidate for surgery. In patients that are severely injured, additional chest, abdominal, or pelvis CT scans that can be performed during this time. Patients severely injured can be better treated in a CT scanner than in an MRI suite. A CT scan is the ideal study for the evaluation of the spinal integrity.[2]

The stability of the spine is evaluated with conventional flexion and extension films. The thoracolumbar junction and lumbar region is evaluated with standing films in flexion and extension.

Spinal CT

CT studies of the spine can clearly identify subtle fractures and small osseous fragments not visible in plain films. They also show information regarding soft tissues, normally obscured in plain radiographs. Images obtained can be reconstructed in two- or three-dimensional reformations that can reveal dislocations and fractures (Figure 4.1). The development of spiral CT scanners permits faster evaluations of the cervical spine with acquisition times as short as 1 min.[3] The ideal thickness of the slices obtained in a post-trauma spine CT should be 1½mm to allow quality reformations in the sagittal and coronal plains without a significant stepping artifact. Although CT scan imaging possesses multiple advantages, it also has several drawbacks including harmful exposure to ionizing radiation and unintentional artifacts produced by movement during the acquisition of the images. CT scans also require the proper facilities to perform these studies, as well as trained personnel to obtain reformatted images that may not be immediately available.

Contrary to popular beliefs that CT evaluation is the first "one-step" in the diagnosis of the traumatic SCI, CT scans are valuable in several different scenarios: symptomatic or unconscious patients with incomplete cervical plain films are good candidates of having CT scans. Also, patients who have suspicious images in other radiographic studies can be better evaluated using this technique. Often CT will help to delineate fractures in such radiographically occult areas such as this case of traumatic spondylolisthesis that is hidden on plain lateral cervical radiograph but can be seen on CT and MRI. Those with surgically correctable injuries that would require a more detailed evaluation of the injury or information regarding the instrumentation needed for the repair should also be considered for CT scans.

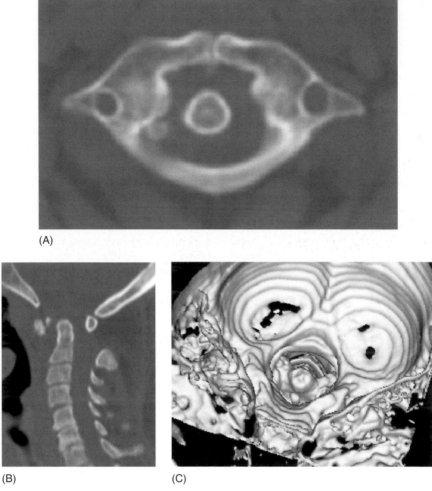

(A)

(B)   (C)

Figure 4.1 Thirty-five-year-old patient with history of down syndrome, who presents after a fall to the emergency department. The axial A, sagittal reconstruction B and 3D reconstruction illustrate the versatility of CT scans in evaluating spinal injuries. Notice the dramatic reduction in the size of the spinal canal as appreciated from the apical view of the 3D reconstruction.

Spinal MRI

Plain films are severely limited in their ability to detect soft tissue injuries of the surrounding ligaments and the spinal cord. A CT scan can show evidence of a herniated disk, hematoma or cord compression, especially if used with myelography. However, myelography is an invasive procedure that demands time and expert personnel to be performed. MRI on the other hand, has a unique role in evaluating of the soft tissues around the bony elements and the spinal cord.[4-6] MRI is capable of detecting abnormal intensities in the cord

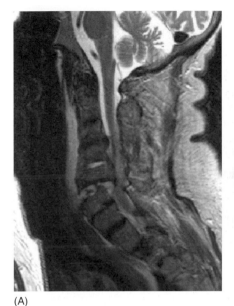

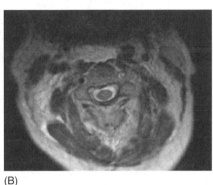

(A) (B)

Figure 4.2 Eighty-three-year-old male status post-fall with a blunt head injury. Patient developed immediately after his injury paraplegia of the lower extremities and severe weakness of the upper extremities. Sagittal T2-weighted MRI (A) demonstrates 10 mm retrolisthesis of C5 on C6 with disruption of the intervertebral disk and severe narrowing of the spinal canal. The cord has changes in intensity appearing hyperintense secondary to edema. The axial image (B) reveals a loss of flow-void in the left vertebral artery secondary to occlusion of the vertebral artery secondary to dissection.

secondary to edema, a feature that has important prognostic value. It also may show direct images of the anterior and posterior longitudinal ligaments. MRI scans are especially advantageous by showing changes in the intensity of the disk, bone edema, hematomas, and indirect evidence of ligamentous abnormalities which are visualized in prevertebral or dorsal interspinous edema (Figure 4.2). Disadvantages of MRI include the time needed to complete the study, the limited availability of technologists to perform the study at any time, and the elevated cost of such tests. For the critically ill patient, MRI may be difficult due to the need for special life support equipment and poor access to the patient by the medical personnel.[3]

In general, to perform a complete MRI study, T1- and T2-weighted spin-echo sequences should be obtained in sagittal and axial planes. These views allow a complete evaluation of possible hematoma, edema of the bony structures indicative of fractures, edema of the paravertebral soft tissues and evaluation of the intensity of the cord indicative of hemorrhages or cord edema, as well as the presence of narrow areas in the spinal canal and direct visualization of the longitudinal anterior and posterior ligaments.[7]

Cervical spine injuries

Emergency approach

As mentioned before, some of the most important aspects in the approach to trauma patients are the precautions to maintain and immobilize the cervical spine – measures that are usually initiated by paramedic personal. However, it is important to realize that the collars and immobilization board commonly employed by paramedics should not be used for prolonged periods of time because they are uncomfortable to the patient and have been associated with high intracranial pressures, pulmonary complications and the generation of pressure ulcers.[8,9] Therefore, it is important to establish a diagnosis of an injury, if any, as soon as possible and to start the medical or surgical treatments as soon as possible if indicated.

There have been long debates regarding the value of plain radiography in the initial evaluation of a patient with a possible cervical spine injury, and the type of views that are necessary to diagnose spine injuries in a sensitive and specific manner.

In the asymptomatic patient, for those who meet all of the following criteria: Glasgow Coma Scale score of 15, without any focal motor or sensory deficit, adequately oriented, without memory deficit and immediate response to external stimuli, not intoxicated (including alcohol levels higher than 0.08 mg/dl), without any neck pain or tenderness spontaneously or at palpation, without associated distracting injuries (e.g. long bone fractures, large lacerations, visceral injuries, burns), there is no recommendation for radiographic evaluation per the guidelines of the Joint Section on Disorders of the Spine and Peripheral Nerves of the American Association of Neurological Surgeons/Congress of Neurological Surgeons.[10,11]

In symptomatic patients, complete AP, lateral and odontoid plain films should be obtained.[12] Patients in this category include those who complain of neck pain or tenderness with palpation, and those who appear to have neurological deficits. Those that cannot be evaluated (unconscious, intoxicated, uncooperative patients, or those with large distracting injuries as mentioned above) can also be considered symptomatic patients. For these studies to be diagnostic, all the cervical vertebral bodies and the cervico-thoracic junction should be visualized.

A radiographic evaluation will define, when present, the majority of bony abnormalities, including fractures of the vertebra or the posterior elements and frequently can indicate ligamentous damage even though these structures are not directly seen. The three-view cervical studies in trauma patients alone have been reported to have a sensitivity between 62.5% and 84%, and a negative predictive value from 85% to 100%.[13–16] These values clearly indicate that, in symptomatic patients, plain films can miss a significant number of injuries. CT scans can increase the sensitivity and negative predictive value of the radiographic evaluation, depicting injuries in places not well visualized in plain films, especially the cranio-cervical and cervico-thoracic junctions. Also CT scans should be considered in patients with either suspicious findings in the plain films, persistently symptomatic patients with normal radiographs, or in those with discovered injuries that are surgical candidates.[17–20]

Conventional radiographic evaluation

Normally the cervical spine has a gentle lordosis; however, it is not unusual that, in trauma patients, this curvature is lost secondary to muscular spasm or the use of the collar. Therefore, the lack of lordosis is not always indicative of a cervical injury.[21] Kyphosis usually occurs as a result of reduction in the height of the vertebral bodies in compression and burst fractures.

Assessment of the lateral view of the cervical spine is done by observing and comparing the visible bone structures. One of the most important indications of cervical injury is misalignment of the vertebral bodies, facets, laminas, or spinous processes. Injury is evaluated based on the anterior aspect of the vertebral bodies, the posterior aspect of the vertebral bodies, the laminar-facet line, and the spino-laminar line (Figure 4.3). Another useful measurement is

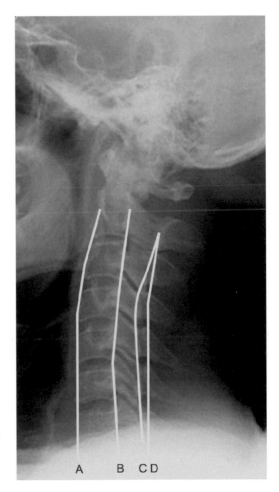

Figure 4.3 Lateral radiographic view of the cervical spine. The methodic observation of this radiographic view should start with the evaluation of the alignment of the anterior aspect of the vertebral bodies (A), the posterior aspect of the vertebral bodies (B), the laminar-facet line (C), and the spino-laminar line (D).

the prevertebral space that in general is less than 7 mm, and is highly suggestive of injury if wider than 10 mm.

The anterior–posterior view of the cervical spine is useful in the evaluation of subluxations of the facets that would manifest as misalignments of the spinous processes normally located in the midline.

The odontoid view is of special value in the detection of atlas and odontoid fractures, and atlanto-axial dislocations.

CT scans evaluation

As mentioned before, even with complete studies of the cervical spine, there is a significant chance of missing lesions. Several authors have reported high sensitivity in the evaluation of cervical spine injury in trauma patients using CT scans, with sensitivities between 90% and 98%, a negative predictive value of 95% and, if used in combination with the plain films, a sensitivity of almost 100%.[15,22,23]

In patients with abnormal mental status but with negative three-view films and CT scan, the chance of a relevant cervical spine injury is less than 1%.[12] Therefore, the decision to discontinue cervical immobilization can be made on the basis of the risk of having a cervical injury. Hanson *et al.* described a group of clinical factors that, when present, places the obtunded patient in the high-risk category for cervical spine injury.[24] This category indicates a 5% risk of cervical injury. These factors include high-speed motor vehicle accidents (more than 35 mph or 56 kmph), automobile accidents with a death at the scene, or fall from a height of more than 10 ft or 3 m. Other factors that classify as high risk can be significant closed head injuries, intracranial hemorrhages, neurological symptoms or signs referred to the cervical spine, pelvic or multiple extremity fractures.

Although these criteria were originally described as indicators for using CT scan, they can be used according to the clinical judgment to clear the neck of low risk obtunded patients with negative plain films and negative head CT, or to perform further evaluation with passive flexion/extension films or MRI.

In patients with persistent complaints of pain and negative plain films and CT scan, the possibility of ligamentous injury should be assessed with flexion/extension films or MRI.

Flexion/extension evaluation

Flexion/extension films are useful in evaluating the stability of the cervical spine and ruling out ligamentous injury. In conscious patients, such films can be taken safely without major inconvenience. Multiple series have been published without reported complications of the procedure.[13,25–27] Lewis *et al.* in a small retrospective study, found in a population of 141 patients that 8% ($n = 11$) had cervical instability in flexion/extension films. Of these 11 patients, four had normal plain films, which suggest the value of these studies.[26] The report had one false-negative flexion/extension study, however. Lewis reported that the negative predictive value of the combination of plain films and flexional extension views was more than 99%. Insko *et al.* found that, when adequate range of motion was obtained in the flexion–extension films, the number of false negatives was zero.[27] The main limitation however, was getting a full range of motion in acutely injured patients. They reported that 30% of studies were limited by inadequate motion, and in this group, 12.5% had injuries detected in cross-sectional imaging studies. Therefore, flexion/extension studies are valuable only if a complete range of movement is obtained.

In unconscious patients, several series have demonstrated the safety and value of flexion/extension studies.[13,28,29] These fluoroscopy guided studies are better obtained under the supervision of the radiology, orthopedic or neurosurgical staff to ensure that the manipulation of the neck is done in a safe but effective way. It has been also reported, however, that a higher number of inadequate studies were found in obtunded patients with rates as high as 59% of total cases.[30] This greatly limits the use of "passive" flexion/extension films. Griffiths *et al.* in a retrospective study on 479 patients with flexion/extension studies, suggested that flexion/extension films were of no benefit compared with CT scans and proposed a protocol to clear the cervical spine of trauma patients based on good quality plain films and CT scans with sagittal and coronal reformations.[30]

MRI evaluation

MRI of the cervical spine has an important role in the evaluation of soft tissue injuries of the cervical spine and can add valuable information about obtunded patients who are at high risk of having an SCI.[4,12,13,31,32]

MRIs have a sensitivity and negative predictive value close to 100% in the detection of injuries to the spinal cord.[4,32,33] MRIs are also very sensitive study to identifying other soft tissue injuries of the cervical spine for which it is considered the reference standard.[32–36] Holmes *et al.* reported that MRIs were helpful in finding the presence of ligamentous injury in all the patients of their series, a finding that has been consistently reported in the literature.[33,37]

However, MRIs are less effective in the identification of fractures, especially lesions of the posterior elements where CT scans are clearly superior. MRIs can miss between 45% and 50% of fractures, including many that can be clinically unstable.[33,38] This is probably due to the limited MRI spatial resolution associated with the lack of signal from cortical bone which not only limits the MRI's ability to detect fractures, but also to detect unilateral locked facets or vertebral subluxations. It is especially important to note that in the past, CT scans have also been reported to have low sensitivity in the detection of vertebral subluxations, missing up to 46% of this type of injuries in some series.[20] More recent series have shown that MRI and CT scans have similar effectiveness in detecting vertebral subluxations, identifying over 80% of diagnosed cases.

Specific cervical injuries
Atlanto-occipital dislocation
Atlanto-occipital dislocation has been traditionally considered an uncommon and almost always fatal injury.[39] However, improvements in the management

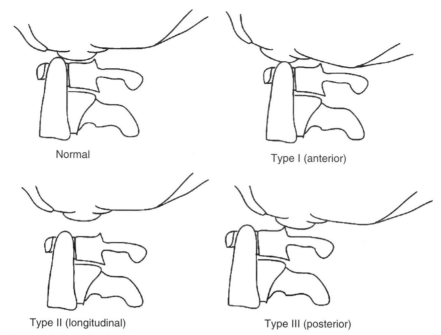

Normal   Type I (anterior)

Type II (longitudinal)   Type III (posterior)

Figure 4.4 Traynelis' classification of atlanto-occipital dislocations. The figure shows the normal relation between the occipital bone and the atlas (left upper corner), and the described three types of dislocation.

of emergency patients in the field and in rapid transport may increase the number of survivors that are seen with these lesions. Atlanto-occipital dislocations can be classified in three types: Type I (anterior), Type II (longitudinal), and Type III (posterior) (Figure 4.4).[40]

Although the diagnosis is at times obvious in plain films because the skull and the cervical spine do not properly align, frequently the initial diagnosis is missed in the original evaluation, and CT scans and MRIs may be required. This type of injury is frequently associated with significant retropharyngeal soft tissue edema (sensitivity of 90%), a finding that should prompt a high index of suspicion.[41,42] Several measurements have been proposed for the evaluation of atlanto-occipital dislocation,[41–43] but probably the most reliable method in patients in whom the landmarks can be identified is that proposed by Harris et al.[44–46] The basion-dental interval is considered abnormal when there is a displacement of more than 12 mm. Basion-to-posterior axial line distances are considered abnormal if the basion is greater than 12 mm anterior or greater than 4 mm posterior to the posterior axial line (Figure 4.5).

There is no information in the current literature regarding the specificity and predictive values of the available radiological studies in the diagnosis of atlanto-occipital dislocation. However, the sensitivity in the first set of plain films obtained in the emergency department has been reported as 57% (this is particularly applicable to nonlongitudinal dislocations), 84% for CT scan, and

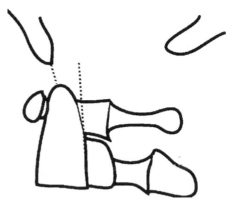

Figure 4.5 Basion–dental interval is the distance between the basion (short arrow) and the odontoid tip. The basion–dental interval is considered abnormal when there is a displacement of more than 12 mm. The posterior axial line is a line drawn tangential to the posterior aspect of the vertebral body of C2 (long arrow). The basion-to-posterior axial line distances are considered abnormal if the basion is greater than 12 mm anterior or greater than 4 mm posterior to the posterior axial line.

86% for MRI studies. The combined sensitivities after repeated films, CT scans, and MRIs are 83% for Type I, 72% for Type II, 75% for Type III, and 71% for other type of dislocation.[46]

In CT scans, the atlanto-occipital dislocation can be identified by a widening of the atlanto-occipital joints or lost of the relationship between the condyle and the atlas. These are images that are seen only in the reformatted coronal and sagittal views. A subtle aspect of importance in the evaluation of the atlanto-occipital dislocations is the alignment between the maxilla and the ring of C1. The demonstration on the axial images of rotation between C1 and the maxilla indicates anatomic abnormality.

In the MRI, it is also possible to visualize the widening between the basion and the dens in the sagittal images. The following have been described: disruptions of the anterior ligament and the tectorial membrane, hemorrhages or effusions in the atlanto-occipital facet joints, edema and contusion of the medulla, and spinal cord.[47–50]

Occipital condyle fractures

There are three types of occipital condyle fractures. Type I fractures are produced by axial load with comminution. Type II are basilar skull fractures that extends through the condyle, and type III fractures are avulsions of the medial portion of the condyle.[51–53]

Occipital condyle fractures are not usually identified in plain cervical films. The calculated sensitivity of plain radiography in the detection of these fractures is 3.2%.[54]

CT scans are very effective methods for detecting and evaluating occipital condyle fractures. CT scans clearly depict the morphology of the condyles and permit an easy evaluation of bone displacement, comminution, extension to the occipital bone and associated injuries.[55–57] Hanson *et al.* have reported an incidence of associated injuries to occipital condyle fractures of 29% for additional cervical spine fractures and 63% for diffuse head injury or intracranial hematomas.[57] CT scans are limited in the evaluation of the tectorial membrane and alar ligaments. In a similar study, MRIs were able to detect only 38% of the condyle fractures, but it was useful in the detection of prevertebral or nuchal ligament edema and hemorrhage, and cord edema and hemorrhage.[49,57]

Atlanto-axial dislocation

Atlanto-axial dislocations are not common in adults. There are only six cases reported in the literature of this injury.[58–62] All of them are individual case reports, which preclude the calculation of sensitivity, specificity, or predictive values in the use of the different diagnostic techniques.

There are two types of atlanto-axial dislocations: rotatory and anterior. A diagnosis is usually made on the lateral view of the cervical spine. In the case of rotatory subluxation, C1 is properly aligned with respect to the base of the skull, but C2 appears obliquely oriented. This diagnosis can be blurred in cases where torticollis adds some general rotation to the film.[2] In the case of anterior dislocation, the distance between the anterior arch of C1 and the dens is increased. CT scans also show the misalignment of C2 with respect to C1 and the widening of the distance between the anterior arch of C1 and the dens. Again, CT scans cannot evaluate the integrity of the ligaments, and MRI studies can add valuable information regarding this aspect, and the association with SCI.[63,64]

Atlas fractures

Atlas fractures represent 1–2% of all fractures of the spinal column and account for 2–13% of cervical spine injuries.[65,66]

The majority of atlas fractures are caused by transmission of forces by the occipital condyles onto the lateral masses of C1, shaped as wedges with the acute angle directed medially, which causes lateral displacement of the lateral masses and a burst of the C1 ring, usually in two places just anterior to and just posterior to one of the articular pillars. These are classic indications of a "Jefferson fracture."[67,68] The traditional evaluation of these fractures was done using the open-mouth odontoid view, where the lateral masses of C1 appear separated from the dens with lateral offset of the articular process. The "rule of Spence" has been used to help in the diagnosis of this injury.[69,70] The "rule of Spence" establishes that if the sum of the total overhang of both C1 lateral masses on C2 is equal or higher to 7 mm, the transverse ligament is probably disrupted. However, this rule, which was developed in cadavers, does not consider the magnification that normally occurs in plain films and that easily can increase the threshold to 8 mm and can be affected with several technical aspects in obtaining the plain films.[71,72]

Dickman *et al.* in a series of 39 patients comparing plain films and MRIs, reported that plain radiography alone is insufficient for detecting fractures associated with disruption of the transverse atlantal ligament.[73] The reported sensitivity of plain films alone was inferior to 30%. This has a very significant clinical importance because the injury of the transverse atlantal ligament is unstable and according to its type may require early surgery to be fixed. The

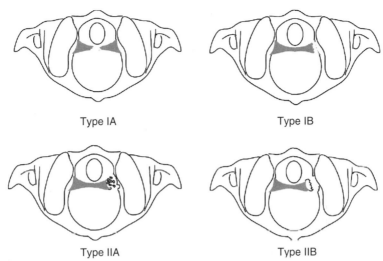

Type IA   Type IB

Type IIA   Type IIB

Figure 4.6 Classification of transverse ligament disruption based on MRI findings by Dickman *et al.*[73] Type I is a disruption of the substance of the ligament, IA midportion, and IB at the level of the periosteal insertion. Type II, associated with fractures of the lateral mass, IIA communited lateral mass fracture, and IIB avulsion of the tubercle from the lateral mass.

same authors, using MRI, classified the injuries of the transverse atlantal ligament in two types: type I, disruptions of the substance of the ligament (IA if the midportion is involved and IB if the disruptions is at the level of the periosteal insertion) and type II, associated with fractures of the lateral mass (IIA if there is a communited lateral mass fracture, and IIB if there is avulsion of the tubercle from the lateral mass) (Figure 4.6). Type I injuries require early surgical treatment with internal fixation while type II have a nonoperative successful rate of 74% and only require surgery after immobilization.

MRI has fundamental importance in the evaluation of patients in whom the plain films or the CT scans suggest the possibility of atlas fractures and transverse atlantal ligament fracture. The abnormal ligament appears discontinuous with high signal intensity and frequently hemorrhagic changes.[63,73]

Other unusually isolated fractures of C1 have been reported, including fractures of the transverse process that occasionally can extend to the transverse foramen and injure the vertebral arteries.[68,74–76]

Axis fractures

Axis fractures account for approximately 20% of cervical fractures.[77] They have been divided in three general categories: fractures of the odontoid process, hangman's fractures, and miscellaneous fractures.

Odontoid process
The odontoid fractures are the most common and represent 10–15% of cervical fractures.[78] Anderson *et al.* proposed a classification for the dens fractures

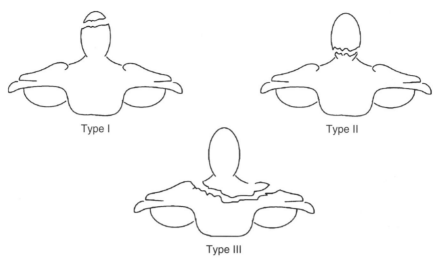

Type I

Type II

Type III

Figure 4.7 Odontoid fracture classification. Type I through the tip of the dens, type II through the base of the dens, and type III extending through the body of C2.

according to the location of the fracture that remains in use.[79] Type I fractures are situated through the tip of the dens, type II through the base of the dens, and type III extending through the body of C2. Later, Hadley *et al.* described an addition to the classical types (type IIA) in cases of comminution of the base of the dens with free fragments (Figure 4.7).[80]

Plain radiography has a reported sensitivity of 64–84% with a specificity of 46.2%.[81,82] Radiographically, the dens fractures are characterized by a transverse or oblique lucency through the tip of the dens, the lower portion of the dens or the vertebral body of C2, which is usually visualized in the lateral view and occasionally in the open-mouth view. CT scans can have some difficulty detecting horizontally oriented fractures, but after thin cut views are obtained, sagittal and coronal reformations can easily demonstrate the defect. Two common pitfalls in the detection of this injury that can be confused with fracture are the superimposition of the inferior margin of the posterior arch of C1, resulting in a radiolucent Mach effect in the AP views, and the presence of a subluxing congenital os odontoideum that results from nonfusion of the dens with the body of the axis. The view that the os odontoideum is a developmental variant is only accepted for an apex that is separated from the body of the dens. Other ossicles with sclerotic borders may represent old nonfused dens fractures.[83]

CT scans have a reported sensitivity of 71% and a sensitivity of 93.8% when the analysis of only axial images is considered. The diagnostic certainty increases when sagittal and coronal reformations are included.[83]

Hangman's fractures
Hangman's fracture or traumatic spondylolisthesis of the axis accounts for 4% of the cervical fractures.[78] Fractures of the axis are associated with other cervical

injuries in 4–18% of cases, specifically with atlas fractures in approximately 9% of cases according to some series.[84,85] In general, hangman's fractures are associated with low incidences of neurological symptoms; however, the presence of C1 fractures increases the risk of neurological damage.

Classically, hangman's fractures are classified in three groups.[86,87] Type I is characterized for a displacement of C2 on C3 of less than or equal to 3 mm. The fracture is usually stable and is rarely associated with neurological symptoms. It is thought that the mechanism is axial compression and extension. Type II is characterized for disruption of the posterior longitudinal ligament and C2–C3 disk with subluxation of 4 mm or more and angulation of 11 degrees or more of the C2–C3 endplates. The mechanisms are axial compression, extension, and rebound flexion. Neurological deficit is uncommon but may lead to early instability. Type IIA is characterized by less displacement but more angulation; it is usually caused by primary flexion and is clinically unstable. Type III is characterized by rupture of the C2–C3 facet joint capsules, isthmus fracture, extensive dislocation with rupture of both posterior and anterior longitudinal ligaments, or separation of the anterior longitudinal ligament from the body of C3. The mechanism is flexion and axial compression. This fracture may be fatal or can be associated with significant neurological deficit.

There is no available information in the literature regarding the sensitivity, specificity, and predictive values of plain films, CT scans, or MRIs in this particular kind of cervical fracture. The majority of cases are detected in plain radiography, in particular in the lateral view. As these fractures run in a predominantly vertical direction, they are eminently suited for display by CT. The reformatted images give valuable information regarding the displacement and angulation of C2 on C3. In patients with neurological deficits, MRIs are employed to evaluate the soft tissues, associated hematomas, or SCI. In plain lateral films, hangman's fractures can be associated with prevertebral swelling and, according with its type, will have specific findings. Type I fractures show fracture lines through the pars interarticularis or isthmus with normal intervertebral C2–C3 space and alignment of the dens. Type II will show the fracture of the C2 ring and abnormal displacement or angulation of the vertebral body of C2 on C3. Type III, in addition to the fracture and severe angulation and displacement, are associated with facet dislocation. Type I and Type II are not infrequently associated with tears fractures of the anterior aspect of C2 which gives further evidence of the hyperextension as mechanism of injury.[83,87,88]

This group of injuries is the most common type of traumatic lesions of the cervical spine representing, according to the different series, between 65.5% and 88.9% of cervical injuries.[22,24,33] There are a wide variety of subaxial cervical spine injuries, and there is no universally accepted method of classification. For these reason, the calculations of sensitivity of the different diagnostic techniques is not specific for the particular type of injuries but generalized to subaxial traumatic injuries. In the prospective cohort of 58 patients published by Berne *et al.*, if only subaxial injuries are considered, the initial plain films

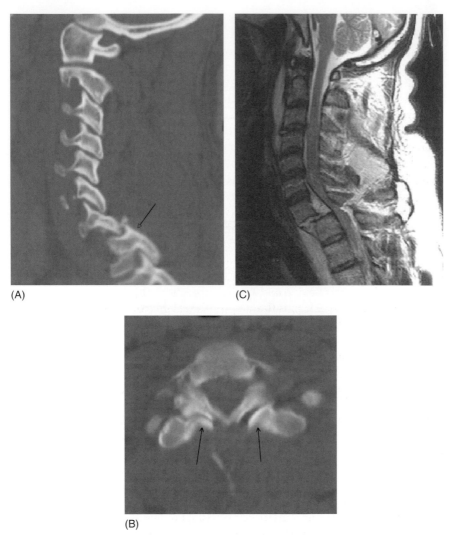

(A)

(C)

(B)

Figure 4.8 CT scan sagittal reformation (A), axial view (B), and sagittal T2-weighted MRI of the cervical spine (C) demonstrate a bilateral facet dislocation at the level C7–T1. The CT scan views demonstrate the naked facets (arrows), which are lying posterior to the lamina of C6. The MRI demonstrates disruption of the intervertebral disk with associated epidural hematoma, significant compression of the spinal canal and a large interspinous fluid collection. The anterior and posterior longitudinal ligaments appear intact.

identified only 50% of cases.[22] In the prospective cohort of 688 patient reported by Holmes *et al.*, if only subaxial injuries are considered, CT scan was able to identify 97.1% of fractures, and MRI had a sensitivity of 54.1% for fractures but 100% for soft tissue injuries.[33]

Although there is no consistent use and analysis per categories of different types of subaxial injuries, the most commonly used scheme is the Allen and

Ferguson classification.[89] According to this mechanistic classification, injuries of the subaxial spine can be grouped as follows considering the loading force and neck position at the moment of the injury:

C3–C7 injuries

When only flexion is the mechanism of trauma, unilateral (if associated with rotation) or bilateral (if pure flexion) facet dislocation is produced. In the plain films, the AP view will show asymmetry of the spinous process above the sub-luxation level, which would be rotated toward the side of the locked facet. The "bow-tie" sign has been described to depict the aspect of the right and left facets in the lateral view that, instead of being superimposed, are seen one besides the other.[90] CT scans are particularly useful showing the rotation of the vertebral body and the articular surface that, instead of being in contact with the one of the next level, appears alone or in the posterior aspect, a condition also known as "naked facet". MRI will show disruption of the facet joint liga-ments, ligamentum flavum, longitudinal and interspinous ligaments. In case of bilateral dislocation, it is common to find SCI and associated hematomas (Figure 4.8).[89]

If the mechanism of injury is flexion associated with compression, the injuries produced are anterior wedge vertebral body fractures with kyphosis, disrup-tion of the interspinous ligament, and teardrop fractures. Wedge fractures of the cervical spine usually occur in mid or lower cervical levels.[91] In the lateral radiograph, the main sign is decreased stature of the anterior aspect of the ver-tebral body usually not associated with prevertebral edema and with normal appearance in the AP view. The generation of a teardrop fracture requires a most severe flexion force and is clinically frequently associated with SCI, par-ticularly with anterior cord syndrome.[92,93] Radiographically, the teardrop frag-ment is a triangular piece of bone in the anteroinferior aspect of the vertebral body. The spinal canal narrows at the level of the injury, in part secondary to kyphosis, but also to posterior displacement of the fractured vertebral body. There is also widening of the interlaminar and interspinous spaces. Plain films tend to underestimate the degree of bony instability and degree of compression of the spinal canal; therefore, CT scans are very useful in demonstrating the fracture of the anterior aspect of the vertebral body, the frequently associated sagittal component of the fracture.[94] The reformatted images contribute to our understanding of the compression of the spinal canal. It is also useful to dis-tinguish this injury from burst fractures, which have a pure compression mechanism and have a prognosis that is completely different (Figure 4.9). While teardrop fractures are always unstable and have high association with quadriplegia, burst fractures can be seen in a wide spectrum from intact patients to patients with severe deficit, depending of the compression caused by the posteriorly displaced fragments.[83,95,96] MRIs are very useful to assess the integrity of the intervertebral disks (usually disrupted), the rupture of the anterior and posterior longitudinal ligaments, hemorrhagic changes and/or disruption of the facet joints, and injuries to the spinal cord.

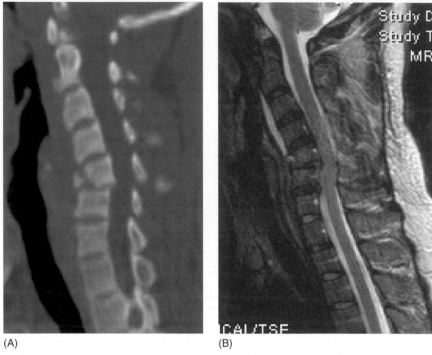

(A)   (B)

Figure 4.9 CT scan sagittal reformation (A) and sagittal T2-weighted MRI of the cervical spine (B) demonstrate a teardrop fracture in the anterior aspect of C5 with kiphotic deformity of the spine. Notice the narrowing of the spinal canal and hyperintensity of the spinal cord at the level of the injury, as well as the prevertebral hematoma evident in the MRI.

If the mechanism of lesion is flexion with distraction, injures produced include torn posterior longitudinal ligament and dislocated or locked facets, which imaging characteristics have been already discussed.

When extension acts alone without compression or distraction, it may produce fractures of the laminas or spinous processes. These lesions are stable and not associated with neurological deficits. However, extension of the cervical spine associated with pre-existing spinal canal stenosis may injure the spinal cord (central cord syndrome) without any evidence of bone lesion. Quencer *et al.* have demonstrated that the disruption of axons in the lateral white matter is the pathological hallmark of this injury.[97] These findings were supported in autopsy studies and MRI abnormalities that have been later confirmed by other authors.[98,99] In a majority of patients with central cord syndrome, MRIs demonstrate cervical spondylosis and bulging of the intervertebral disks causing stenosis of the canal. It has been reported that intramedullary abnormalities characterized by isointense signal on T1-weighted sequences and hyperintensity on T2-weighted sequences, predominantly from C3–C4 to C5–C6 but never below C6–C7 are consistently found in all patients with this clinical presentation. No evidence of hemorrhage in the echo gradient sequences has been found.[99]

Thoracolumbar spine injuries

Thoracolumbar spine injuries are relatively uncommon in the general population, with estimates ranging between 64 and 117 per 100,000/year.[100,101] However, they can be found in 2–6% of patients admitted to the hospital with blunt trauma and can be associated with significant morbidity and mortality in up to 30% of patients.[102–105]

The most common location of thoracolumbar spine injury is in the lumbar region, particularly at the L1 level (42%), followed by L2, L3, L4, and T12.[100,102,105–108]

As mentioned before, in the emergency approach to the trauma patient, it is important to provide the precautions to immobilize the spine and, in the case of the thoracolumbar spine, with a full-length backboard until injury has been ruled out or treatment is initiated. Once again however, prolonged immobilizations on the board should be avoided for the same reasons explained above

Although the indications for plain radiography of the thoracic and lumbar spine have not been extensively studied, it is reasonable to apply the same approach that we explained before for asymptomatic patients to defer the radiographic evaluation of the cervical spine. Specifically patients with Glasgow Coma Scale score of 15, without any focal motor or sensory deficit, adequately oriented, without memory deficit and immediate response to external stimuli, not intoxicated (including alcohol levels higher than 0.08 mg/dl), without any back pain or tenderness spontaneously or at palpation, without associated distracting injuries (long bone fractures, large lacerations, visceral injuries, burns) do not require radiographic evaluation. In patients with blunt trauma that cannot be considered asymptomatic according to these criteria, several authors recommend to obtain an AP and cross table lateral view of the thoracolumbar junction.[103,108–114] Recently, Gestring et al. have reported the use of AP and lateral digital scout views obtained in abdomino-pelvis CT scan in blunt trauma patients as screening tool for thoracolumbar injuries, with reported sensitivity and specificity of 100%, when compared with plain films.[115] This approach is interesting and practical, given the extensive use of CT scans in the evaluation of the abdomen and pelvis in obtunded patients. The interpretation of the digital radiographies was done blindly by the radiologists, which suggest that at least the sensitivity and specificity would be equivalent to plain films. The inconvenience of this study is the lack of current knowledge of the diagnostic efficiency of plain films.

There are no available studies assessing the sensitivity, specificity, and predictive values of the different diagnostic techniques. However, a recent epidemiology study by Holmes et al. reported that plain films were diagnostic in 93% of cases with thoracolumbar injuries when compared with CT scans and MRIs.[105] Interestingly, only one of the injuries detected in CT scans and not seen in the plain films was a chance fracture. The other injuries were transverse process fractures. CT scans were useful in the distinction between compression and burst fractures.

Several studies have addressed the role of MRIs in the evaluation of thoracolumbar injuries.[115–119] Many of the reported findings show a wide variation in part expected by the wide and diverse group of injuries grouped as thoracolumbar injuries. MRIs have demonstrated higher incidences of posterior and anterior ligament ruptures than expected on the basis of the CT scan images. The integrity of the posterior longitudinal ligament is very important in the planning of the reduction of posterior displaced fragments. As we will discuss in a following paragraph, the detection of soft tissue (ligaments, joint capsule, and disk) injuries in many cases have definitive prognostic value. Several MRI studies have shown difficulties in adapting the MRI findings with the traditional models of thoracolumbar injury based mainly in plan radiography and CT scan findings.[119]

The three-column model proposed by Denis is a helpful tool in the clinical and radiographic evaluation of fractures of the thoracic and lumbar region.[120] The anterior column consists of the anterior half of the vertebral body and intervertebral disk, and the anterior longitudinal ligament. The middle column consists of the posterior part of the vertebral body and intervertebral disk and the posterior longitudinal ligament. Finally, the third column consists of the complete vertebral arch along with the interspinous ligament, ligamentum flavum, and facet joint capsule (Figure 4.10). Minor injuries of the thoracolumbar spine compromise only part of a single column and include fractures of spinous or transverse process, articular process, or pars interarticularis.

Major injuries include compression fracture, burst fracture, flexion–distraction, and fracture dislocation.[121]

Compression fractures

Compression fractures are characterized by an intact middle column with compression of the anterior column. Plain films and sagittal reformations in CT scans show lost of stature in the anterior aspect of the vertebral body with intact posterior borders, no subluxations, and intact spinal canals (Figure 4.11).

Burst fractures

Burst fractures are generated by pure axial load and usually occur between T10 and L2. They are characterized by compression of both anterior and posterior columns. Denis proposed a classification of these fractures that has prognostic importance and help in the assessment of the surgical strategy.[121] Type A involve comminution of both endplates, usually associated with fractures of the posterior elements and more frequent in the lower lumbar levels where the axial load tends to be higher. Type B, usually produced by axial load and flexion, involve disruption of the superior endplate and retropulsion of the posterosuperior aspect of the vertebral body into the spinal canal. This is the most common type of burst fracture. Type C is a rare comminuted fracture of the inferior endplate produced by the same mechanism as type B. Type D are produced by axial load and rotation, and are more shear injuries, usually midlumbar. Type E is also uncommon and consists of lateral burst of the vertebral

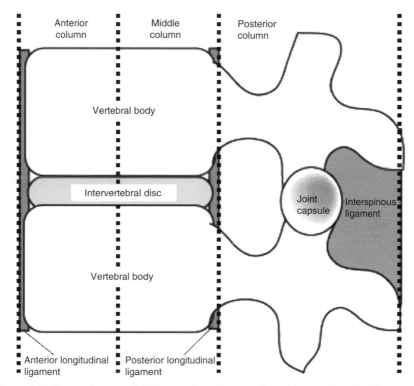

Figure 4.10 Three-column model. The anterior column consists of the anterior half of the vertebral body and intervertebral disk, and the anterior longitudinal ligament. The middle column consists of the posterior part of the vertebral body and intervertebral disk and the posterior longitudinal ligament. The third column consists of the complete vertebral arch along with the interspinous ligament, ligamentum flavum, and facet joint capsule.

body. Lateral films show the loss of height of the vertebral body compromising both anterior and posterior walls. Sometimes the retropulsed fragment can be identified, as well as associated pedicle fractures. The AP view shows increases in the interpeduncular distance that indicates failure of the middle column.[122] CT scans are useful in depicting the retropulsed fragments and, as mentioned before, can be very important for distinguishing compression from burst fractures in unclear cases.[123,124] MRI is especially valuable in the evaluation of burst fractures, given the high incidence of canal stenosis and SCIs. MRIs demonstrate associated ligamentous injury particularly of the posterior longitudinal ligament and interspinous ligament. MRIs can also clearly detect the degree of neural compression, intrinsic cord abnormality, extradural hematoma and the condition of the intervertebral disk (Figure 4.12).[125,126]

Flexion distractions

Flexion distraction mechanisms of injury generate horizontal fractures that can extend either through the bone only, through bone anteriorly and ligaments

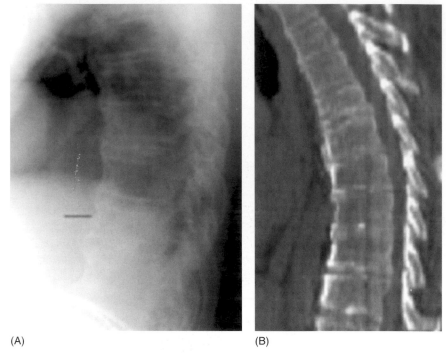

(A) (B)

Figure 4.11 Lateral radiographic view (A) and sagittal reconstruction of thoracic CT (B) scan show reduction in the height of the anterior aspect of the vertebral bodies of T6 and T7, due to compression fractures at these levels. There is no evidence of retropulsion of bone fragments into the spinal canal.

posteriorly, and through the disk, facet capsule, and the interspinous ligament. The first type that compromises bone exclusively, when limited to one level, are also known as chance fractures and, in general, have good prognosis for stability with primary healing. In the second type, mixed bone and ligament have intermediate prognosis, and in the third type are very severe injuries frequently associated with neurological deficits and are also known as bilateral facet dislocations.[127] Plain radiography shows increase in the interspinous process distance, pars fractures, and horizontal vertebral body fractures. CT scans can be of limited value if only axial views are obtained, given the horizontal direction of this injury. MRIs are important in the evaluation of the soft tissue injuries, being of particular relevance in the evaluation of the third type.

Fracture dislocations

Fracture–dislocation is caused by shear forces, which create very unstable and complex lesions. Plain films and CT scan show a wide spectrum of findings including subluxation or dislocation, increased interspinous space, jumped facets, reduction in the size of the spinal canal, and lesions that can resemble chance fractures but are always associated with dislocation or subluxation (Figure 4.13).

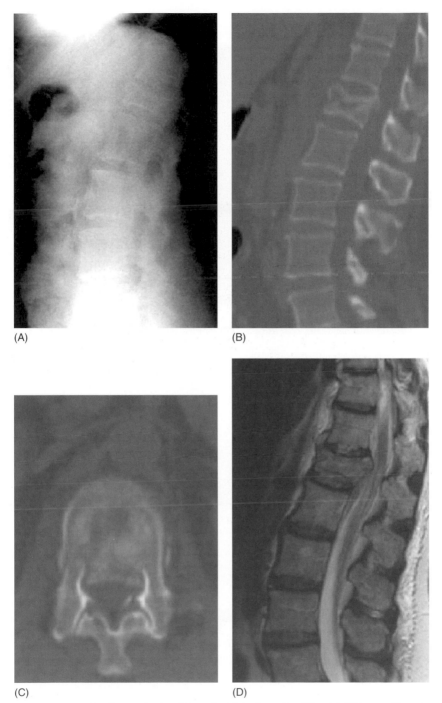

(A)   (B)

(C)   (D)

Figure 4.12 Lateral radiographic view (A), sagittal CT reformation (B), axial CT image (C), and
sagittal T2-weighted MRI of the lumbar spine (D) demonstrate significant (30%) loss of height of
the vertebral body of L1 (A), with a fracture that extends to the middle and posterior column
(B and C), causing significant compression of the spinal canal associated with changes in the
intensity of the conus medullaris (D).

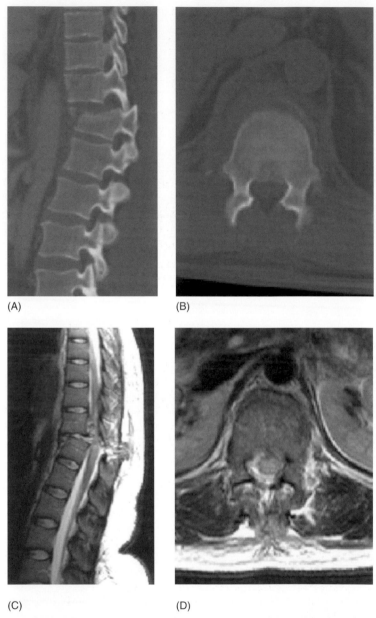

(A)

(B)

(C)

(D)

Figure 4.13 Sagittal CT scan reformation (A), axial CT scan view (B), sagittal (C), and axial (D) T2-weighted MRI of the lumbar spine demonstrate a fracture dislocation injury at the level T12–L1 with fracture of the anterior aspect of the vertebral body of L1, associated with bilateral facet dislocation. Notice the naked facets (B) as well as retropulsion of the L1 vertebral body with narrowing of the canal and changes in the intensity of the cord and disruption of the posterior longitudinal and interspinous ligaments (C,D).

Future of the radiological evaluation of SCI

Advancements in CT and MRI techniques are already affecting the diagnostic approach and even the pathophysiological interpretation of the SCI, as it has been explained in detailed in the prior sections. Of special importance toward the future are CT scan developments that allow faster acquisitions with less time and higher quality resolution of the axial images, as well as software advancements that allow faster and more efficient reformations that will play an important role in the evaluation of several of the injuries that have been mentioned.

Because of the small size of the cord, the susceptible difficulties generated by the surrounding bone and air, and pulsations of nearby vascular structures with longer acquisition times, MRIs still face several limitations in the evaluation of the cord. We should, however, expect that MRI techniques will evolve to the point of offering strategies, such as diffusion weighted imaging, perfusion studies, spectroscopy, etc., that are now commonly used in the brain. Such advances will constitute the future in the evaluation of patients with SCI with deep repercussions in the management and understanding of their pathology.

References

1 ACS. Initial assessment and management. In Surgeons ACo (ed.): *Advanced Trauma Life Support ATLS*. American College of Surgeons, Chicago, 1997, pp. 21–46.

2 Rothman S. Imaging of spinal trauma pearls and pitfalls. In Capen DA HW (ed.): *Comprehensive Management of Spine Trauma*. Mosby, St. Louis, 1998, pp. 39–95.

3 Young JW, Cure JK. Radiologic evaluation of the spine injured patient. In AM Levine FE, SR Garfin, *et al.* (eds): *Spine Trauma*. WB Saunders company, Philadelphia, 1998, pp. 28–60.

4 Kulkarni MV, McArdle CB, Kopanicky D, *et al.* Acute spinal cord injury: MR imaging at 1.5 T. *Radiology* 1987,164:837–843.

5 Mirvis SE, Geisler FH, Jelinek JJ, Joslyn JN, Gellad F. Acute cervical spine trauma: evaluation with 1.5-T MR imaging. *Radiology* 1988;166:807–816.

6 Tarr RW, Drolshagen LF, Kerner TC, Allen JH, Partain CL, James Jr AE. MR imaging of recent spinal trauma. *J Comput Assist Tomogr* 1987;11:412–417.

7 Kaiser MC, Ramos L. MRI of the Spine. *A Guide to Clinical Applications*. Thieme, New York, 1990.

8 Dodd FM, Simon E, McKeown D, Patrick MR. The effect of a cervical collar on the tidal volume of anaesthetised adult patients. *Anaesthesia* 1995;50:961–963.

9 Raphael JH, Chotai R. Effects of the cervical collar on cerebrospinal fluid pressure. *Anaesthesia* 1994;49:437–439.

10 Hoffman JR, Mower WR, Wolfson AB, Todd KH, Zucker MI. Validity of a set of clinical criteria to rule out injury to the cervical spine in patients with blunt trauma. National Emergency X-Radiography Utilization Study Group. *New Engl J Med* 2000; 343:94–99.

11 Joint Section on Disorders of the Spine and Peripheral Nerves of the American Association of Neurological Surgeons and the Congress of Neurological Surgeons. *Neurosurgery* 2002;50:S30–S35.

12 Joint Section on Disorders of the Spine and Peripheral Nerves of the American Association of Neurological Surgeons and the Congress of Neurological Surgeons. *Neurosurgery* 2002;50:S36–S43.

13 Ajani AE, Cooper DJ, Scheinkestel CD, Laidlaw J, Tuxen DV. Optimal assessment of cervical spine trauma in critically ill patients: a prospective evaluation. *Anaesth Intens Care* 1998;26:487–491.

14 MacDonald RL, Schwartz ML, Mirich D, Sharkey PW, Nelson WR. Diagnosis of cervical spine injury in motor vehicle crash victims: how many X-rays are enough? *J Trauma* 1990;30:392–397.

15 Borock EC, Gabram SG, Jacobs LM, Murphy MA. A prospective analysis of a two-year experience using computed tomography as an adjunct for cervical spine clearance. *J Trauma* 1991;31:1001–1005; discussion 1005–1006.

16 Freemyer B, Knopp R, Piche J, Wales L, Williams J. Comparison of five-view and three-view cervical spine series in the evaluation of patients with cervical trauma. *Ann Emerg Med* 1989;18:818–821.

17 Nunez Jr DB, Zuluaga A, Fuentes-Bernardo DA, Rivas LA, Becerra JL. Cervical spine trauma: how much more do we learn by routinely using helical CT? *Radiographics* 1996;16:1307–1318; discussion 1318–1321.

18 Acheson MB, Livingston RR, Richardson ML, Stimac GK. High-resolution CT scanning in the evaluation of cervical spine fractures: comparison with plain film examinations. *AJR Am J Roentgenol* 1987;148:1179–1185.

19 Kirshenbaum KJ, Nadimpalli SR, Fantus R, Cavallino RP. Unsuspected upper cervical spine fractures associated with significant head trauma: role of CT. *J Emerg Med* 1990;8:183–198.

20 Woodring JH, Lee C. The role and limitations of computed tomographic scanning in the evaluation of cervical trauma. *J Trauma* 1992;33:698–708.

21 Weir DC. Roentgenographic signs of cervical injury. *Clin Orthop* 1975;109:9–17.

22 Berne JD, Velmahos GC, El-Tawil Q, *et al.* Value of complete cervical helical computed tomographic scanning in identifying cervical spine injury in the unevaluable blunt trauma patient with multiple injuries: a prospective study. *J Trauma* 1999;47:896–902; discussion 902–903.

23 Mace SE. Emergency evaluation of cervical spine injuries: CT versus plain radiographs. *Ann Emerg Med* 1985;14:973–975.

24 Hanson JA, Blackmore CC, Mann FA, Wilson AJ. Cervical spine injury: a clinical decision rule to identify high-risk patients for helical CT screening. *AJR Am J Roentgenol* 2000;174:713–717.

25 Brady WJ, Moghtader J, Cutcher D, Exline C, Young J. ED use of flexion–extension cervical spine radiography in the evaluation of blunt trauma. *Am J Emerg Med* 1999; 17:504–508.

26 Lewis LM, Docherty M, Ruoff BE, Fortney JP, Keltner Jr RA, Britton P. Flexion–extension views in the evaluation of cervical-spine injuries. *Ann Emerg Med* 1991;20:117–121.

27 Insko EK, Gracias VH, Gupta R, Goettler CE, Gaieski DF, Dalinka MK. Utility of flexion and extension radiographs of the cervical spine in the acute evaluation of blunt trauma. *J Trauma* 2002;53:426–429.

28 Davis JW, Parks SN, Detlefs CL, Williams GG, Williams JL, Smith RW. Clearing the cervical spine in obtunded patients: the use of dynamic fluoroscopy. *J Trauma* 1995;39:435–438.

29 Sees DW, Rodriguez Cruz LR, Flaherty SF, Ciceri DP. The use of bedside fluoroscopy to evaluate the cervical spine in obtunded trauma patients. *J Trauma* 1998;45:768–771.

30 Griffiths HJ, Wagner J, Anglen J, Bunn P, Metzler M. The use of forced flexion/extension views in the obtunded trauma patient. *Skeletal Radiol* 2002;31:587–591.

31 D'Alise MD, Benzel EC Hart BL. Magnetic resonance imaging evaluation of the cervical spine in the comatose or obtunded trauma patient. *J Neurosurg* 1999;91:54–59.

32 McArdle CB, Crofford MJ, Mirfakhraee M, Amparo EG, Calhoun JS. Surface coil MR of spinal trauma: preliminary experience. *AJNR Am J Neuroradiol* 1986;7:885–893.

33 Holmes JF, Mirvis SE, Panacek EA, Hoffman JR, Mower WR, Velmahos GC. Variability in computed tomography and magnetic resonance imaging in patients with cervical spine injuries. *J Trauma* 2002;53:524–529; discussion 530.

34 Flanders AE, Schaefer DM, Doan HT, Mishkin MM, Gonzalez CF, Northrup BE. Acute cervical spine trauma: correlation of MR imaging findings with degree of neurologic deficit. *Radiology* 1990,177:25–33.

35 Keiper MD, Zimmerman RA, Bilaniuk LT. MRI in the assessment of the supportive soft tissues of the cervical spine in acute trauma in children. *Neuroradiology* 1998;40:359–363.

36 Katzberg RW, Benedetti PF, Drake CM, *et al*. Acute cervical spine injuries: prospective MR imaging assessment at a level 1 trauma center. *Radiology* 1999;213:203–212.

37 Geck MJ, Yoo S, Wang JC. Assessment of cervical ligamentous injury in trauma patients using MRI. *J Spinal Disord* 2001;14:371–377.

38 Levitt MA, Flanders AE. Diagnostic capabilities of magnetic resonance imaging and computed tomography in acute cervical spinal column injury. *Am J Emerg Med* 1991;9:131–135.

39 Gerlock Jr AJ, Mirfakhraee M, Benzel EC. Computed tomography of traumatic atlantooccipital dislocation. *Neurosurgery* 1983;13:316–319.

40 Traynelis VC, Marano GD, Dunker RO, Kaufman HH. Traumatic atlanto-occipital dislocation. Case report. *J Neurosurg* 1986;65:863–870.

41 Powers B, Miller MD, Kramer RS, Martinez S, Gehweiler Jr JA. Traumatic anterior atlanto-occipital dislocation. *Neurosurgery* 1979;4:12–17.

42 Lee C, Woodring JH, Goldstein SJ, Daniel TL, Young AB, Tibbs PA. Evaluation of traumatic atlantooccipital dislocations. *AJNR Am J Neuroradiol* 1987;8:19–26.

43 Wholey MH, Bruwer AJ, Baker HL. The lateral roentgenogram of the neck (with comments on the atlanto-odontoid-basion relationship). *Radiology* 1958;71:350–356.

44 Harris JH, Carson GC, Wagner LK. Radiologic diagnosis of traumatic occipitovertebral dissociation. 1. Normal occipitovertebral relationships on lateral radiographs of supine subjects. *AJR Am J Roentgenol* 1994;162:881–886.

45 Harris Jr JH, Carson GC, Wagner LK, Kerr N. Radiologic diagnosis of traumatic occipitovertebral dissociation. 2. Comparison of three methods of detecting occipitovertebral relationships on lateral radiographs of supine subjects. *AJR Am J Roentgenol* 1994;162:887–892.

46 Joint Section on Disorders of the Spine and Peripheral Nerves of the American Association of Neurological Surgeons and the Congress of Neurological Surgeons. *Neurosurgery* 2002;50:S105–S113.

47 Harmanli O, Koyfman Y. Traumatic atlanto-occipital dislocation with survival: a case report and review of the literature. *Surg Neurol* 1993;39:324–330.

48 Goldberg AL, Baron B, Daffner RH. Atlantooccipital dislocation: MR demonstration of cord damage. *J Comput Assist Tomogr* 1991;15:174–175.

49 Willauschus WG, Kladny B, Beyer WF, Gluckert K, Arnold H, Scheithauer R. Lesions of the alar ligaments. *In vivo* and *in vitro* studies with magnetic resonance imaging. *Spine* 1995;20:2493–2498.

50 Chaljub G, Singh H, Gunito Jr FC, Crow WN. Traumatic atlanto-occipital dislocation: MRI and CT. *Neuroradiology* 2001;43:41–44.

51 Anderson PA, Montesano PX. Morphology and treatment of occipital condyle fractures. *Spine* 1988;13:731–736.

52 Noble ER, Smoker WR. The forgotten condyle: the appearance, morphology, and classification of occipital condyle fractures. *AJNR Am J Neuroradiol* 1996;17:507–513.

53 Clayman DA, Sykes CH, Vines FS. Occipital condyle fractures: clinical presentation and radiologic detection. *AJNR Am J Neuroradiol* 1994;15:1309–1315.

54 Occipital condyle fractures. *Neurosurgery* 2002;50:S114– S119.

55 Raila FA, Aitken AT, Vickers GN. Computed tomography and three-dimensional reconstruction in the evaluation of occipital condyle fracture. *Skeletal Radiol* 1993;22: 269–271.

56 Bettini N, Malaguti MC, Sintini M, Monti C. Fractures of the occipital condyles: report of four cases and review of the literature. *Skeletal Radiol* 1993;22:187–190.

57 Hanson JA, Deliganis AV, Baxter AB, *et al.* Radiologic and clinical spectrum of occipital condyle fractures: retrospective review of 107 consecutive fractures in 95 patients. *AJR Am J Roentgenol* 2002;178:1261–1268.

58 Jones RN. Rotatory dislocation of both atlanto-axial joints. *J Bone Joint Surg Br* 1984;66:6–7.

59 Robertson PA, Swan HA. Traumatic bilateral rotatory facet dislocation of the atlas on the axis. *Spine* 1992;17:1252–1254.

60 Born CT, Mure AJ, Iannacone WM, DeLong Jr WG. Three-dimensional computerized tomographic demonstration of bilateral atlantoaxial rotatory dislocation in an adult: report of a case and review of the literature. *J Orthop Trauma* 1994;8:67–72.

61 Moore KR, Frank EH. Traumatic atlantoaxial rotatory subluxation and dislocation. *Spine* 1995;20:1928–1930.

62 Fuentes S, Bouillot P, Palombi O, Ducolombier A, Desgeorges M. Traumatic atlantoaxial rotatory dislocation with odontoid fracture: case report and review. *Spine* 2001;26: 830–834.

63 Dickman CA, Mamourian A, Sonntag VK, Drayer BP. Magnetic resonance imaging of the transverse atlantal ligament for the evaluation of atlantoaxial instability. *J Neurosurg* 1991;75:221–227.

64 Niibayashi H. Atlantoaxial rotatory dislocation. A case report. *Spine* 1998;23:1494–1496.

65 Hadley MN, Dickman CA, Browner CM, Sonntag VK. Acute traumatic atlas fractures: management and long term outcome. *Neurosurgery* 1988;23:31–35.

66 Levine AM, Edwards CC. Fractures of the atlas. *J Bone Joint Surg Am* 1991;73:680–691.

67 Jefferson G. Fractures of the atlas vertebra: repot of four cases and a review of those previously reported. *Br J Surg* 1920;7:407–422.

68 Hays MB, Alker Jr GJ. Fractures of the atlas vertebra. The two-part burst fracture of Jefferson. *Spine* 1988;13:601–603.

69 Spence Jr KF, Decker S, Sell KW. Bursting atlantal fracture associated with rupture of the transverse ligament. *J Bone Joint Surg Am* 1970;52:543–549.

70 Fielding JW, Cochran GB, Lawsing III JF, Hohl M. Tears of the transverse ligament of the atlas. A clinical and biomechanical study. *J Bone Joint Surg Am* 1974;56:1683–1691.

71 Heller JG, Viroslav S, Hudson T. Jefferson fractures: the role of magnification artifact in assessing transverse ligament integrity. *J Spinal Disord* 1993;6:392–396.

72 Isolated fractures of the atlas in adults. *Neurosurgery* 2002;50:S120–S124.

73 Dickman CA, Greene KA, Sonntag VK. Injuries involving the transverse atlantal ligament: classification and treatment guidelines based upon experience with 39 injuries. *Neurosurgery* 1996;38:44–50.

74 Barker Jr EG, Krumpelman J, Long JM. Isolated fracture of the medial portion of the lateral mass of the atlas: a previously undescribed entity. *Am J Roentgenol* 1976;126:1053–1058.

75 Jakim I, Sweet MB, Wisniewski T, Gantz ED. Isolated avulsion fracture of the anterior tubercle of the atlas. *Arch Orthop Trauma Surg* 1989;108:377–379.

76 Merianos P, Tsekouras G, Koskinas A. An unusual fracture of the atlas. *Injury* 1991; 22:489–490.

77 Hosten N, Liebig T. *CT of the Head and Spine*. Thieme, New York, 2002.

78 Greene KA, Dickman CA, Marciano FF, Drabier JB, Hadley MN, Sonntag VK. Acute axis fractures. Analysis of management and outcome in 340 consecutive cases. *Spine* 1997; 22:1843–1852.

79 Anderson LD, D'Alonzo RT. Fractures of the odontoid process of the axis. *J Bone Joint Surg Am* 1974;56:1663–1674.

80 Hadley MN, Browner CM, Liu SS, Sonntag VK. New subtype of acute odontoid fractures (type IIA). *Neurosurgery* 1988;22:67–71.

81 Ehara S, el-Khoury GY, Clark CR. Radiologic evaluation of dens fracture. Role of plain radiography and tomography. *Spine* 1992;17:475–479.

82 Weisskopf M, Reindl R, Schroder R, Hopfenmuller P, Mittlmeier T. CT scans versus conventional tomography in acute fractures of the odontoid process. *Eur Spine J* 2001;10:250–256.

83 Harris JH, Mirvis SE. *The Radiology of Acute Cervical Spine Trauma*. Williams and Wilkins, Baltimore, 1996.

84 Burke JT, Harris Jr JH. Acute injuries of the axis vertebra. *Skeletal Radiol* 1989;18:335–346.

85 Ryan MD, Henderson JJ. The epidemiology of fractures and fracture-dislocations of the cervical spine. *Injury* 1992;23:38–40.

86 Effendi B, Roy D, Cornish B, Dussault RG, Laurin CA. Fractures of the ring of the axis. A classification based on the analysis of 131 cases. *J Bone Joint Surg Br* 1981:319–327.

87 Levine AM, Edwards CC. The management of traumatic spondylolisthesis of the axis. *J Bone Joint Surg Am* 1985;67:217–226.

88 Garfin SR, Rothman RH. Traumatic spondylolisthesis of axis. *Cervical Spine Research Society. The Cervical Spine*. JB Lippincott, Philadelphia, 1983, pp. 223–232.

89 Allen Jr BL, Ferguson RL, Lehmann TR, O'Brien RP. A mechanistic classification of closed, indirect fractures and dislocations of the lower cervical spine. *Spine* 1982;7:1–27.

90 Andreshak JL, Dekutoski MB. Management of unilateral facet dislocations: a review of the literature. *Orthopedics* 1997;20:917–926.

91 White III AA, Johnson RM, Panjabi MM, Southwick WO. Biomechanical analysis of clinical stability in the cervical spine. *Clin Orthop* 1975;109:85–96.

92 Schneider RC, Kahn EA. Chronic neurological sequelae of acute trauma to the spine and the spinal cord. Part 1. The significance of the acute-flexion or "tear drop" fracture dislocation of the cervical spine. *J Bone Joint Surg* 1956;38A:985.

93 Schneider RC. The syndrome of anterior spinal cord injury. *J Neurosurg* 1955;12:95–98.

94 Lee C, Kim KS, Rogers LF. Sagittal fracture of the cervical vertebral body. *AJR Am J Roentgenol* 1982;139:55–60.

95 Apley AG. Fractures of e spine. *Ann R Coll Surg Engl* 1970;46:210–223.

96 Harris Jr JH, Edeiken-Monroe B, Kopaniky DR. A practical classification of acute cervical spine injuries. *Orthop Clin North Am* 1986;17:15–30.

97 Quencer RM, Bunge RP, Egnor M, *et al.* Acute traumatic central cord syndrome: MRI-pathological correlations. *Neuroradiology* 1992;34:85–94.

98 Martin D, Schoenen J, Lenelle J, Reznik M, Moonen G. MRI-pathological correlations in acute traumatic central cord syndrome: case report. *Neuroradiology* 1992;34:262–266.

99 Collignon F, Martin D, Lenelle J, Stevenaert A. Acute traumatic central cord syndrome: magnetic resonance imaging and clinical observations. *J Neurosurg* 2002;96:29–33.

100 Hu R, Mustard CA, Burns C. Epidemiology of incident spinal fracture in a complete population. *Spine* 1996;21:492–499.

101 Cooper C, Atkinson EJ, O'Fallon WM, Melton III LJ. Incidence of clinically diagnosed vertebral fractures: a population-based study in Rochester, Minnesota, 1985–1989. *J Bone Miner Res* 1992;7:221–227.

102 Samuels LE, Kerstein MD. "Routine" radiologic evaluation of the thoracolumbar spine in blunt trauma patients: a reappraisal. *J Trauma* 1993;34:85–89.

103 Cooper C, Dunham CM, Rodriguez A. Falls and major injuries are risk factors for thoracolumbar fractures: cognitive impairment and multiple injuries impede the detection of back pain and tenderness. *J Trauma* 1995;38:692–696.

104 Frankel HL, Rozycki GS, Ochsner MG, Harviel JD, Champion HR. Indications for obtaining surveillance thoracic and lumbar spine radiographs. *J Trauma* 1994;37:673–676.

105 Holmes JF, Miller PQ, Panacek EA, Lin S, Horne NS, Mower WR. Epidemiology of thoracolumbar spine injury in blunt trauma. *Acad Emerg Med* 2001;8:866–872.

106 Saboe LA, Reid DC, Davis LA, Warren SA, Grace MG. Spine trauma and associated injuries. *J Trauma* 1991;31:43–48.

107 Durham RM, Luchtefeld WB, Wibbenmeyer L, Maxwell P, Shapiro MJ, Mazuski JE. Evaluation of the thoracic and lumbar spine after blunt trauma. *Am J Surg* 1995;170:681–684; discussion 684–685.

108 Meldon SW, Moettus LN. Thoracolumbar spine fractures: clinical presentation and the effect of altered sensorium and major injury. *J Trauma* 1995;39:1110–1114.

109 Savitsky E, Votey S. Emergency department approach to acute thoracolumbar spine injury. *J Emerg Med* 1997;15:49–60.

110 Andreychik DA, Alander DH, Senica KM, Stauffer ES. Burst fractures of the second through fifth lumbar vertebrae. Clinical and radiographic results. *J Bone Joint Surg Am* 1996;78:1156–1166.

111 Buduhan G, McRitchie DI. Missed injuries in patients with multiple trauma. *J Trauma* 2000;49:600–605.

112 Enderson BL, Reath DB, Meadors J, Dallas W, DeBoo JM, Maull KI. The tertiary trauma survey: a prospective study of missed injury. *J Trauma* 1990;30:666–669; discussion 669–670.

113 Meek S. Lesson of the week: fractures of the thoracolumbar spine in major trauma patients. *BMJ* 1998;317:1442–1443.

114 Walters S. Fractures of the thoracolumbar spine in major trauma patients. It happened to me! *BMJ* 1999;318:1288.

115 Gestring ML, Gracias VH, Feliciano MA, *et al.* Evaluation of the lower spine after blunt trauma using abdominal computed tomographic scanning supplemented with lateral scanograms. *J Trauma* 2002;53:9–14.

116 Kliewer MA, Gray L, Paver J, *et al.* Acute spinal ligament disruption: MR imaging with anatomic correlation. *J Magn Reson Imaging* 1993;3:855–861.

117 Petersilge CA, Pathria MN, Emery SE, Masaryk TJ. Thoracolumbar burst fractures: evaluation with MR imaging. *Radiology* 1995;194:49–54.

118 Terk MR, Hume-Neal M, Fraipont M, Ahmadi J, Colletti PM. Injury of the posterior ligament complex in patients with acute spinal trauma: evaluation by MR imaging. *AJR Am J Roentgenol* 1997;168:1481–1486.

119 Oner FC, vd Rijt RH, Ramos LM, Groen GJ, Dhert WJ, Verbout AJ. Correlation of MR images of disc injuries with anatomic sections in experimental thoracolumbar spine fractures. *Eur Spine J* 1999;8:194–198.

120 Denis F. The three column spine and its significance in the classification of acute thoracolumbar spinal injuries. *Spine* 1983;8:817–831.

121 Denis F. Spinal instability as defined by the three-column spine concept in acute spinal trauma. *Clin Orthop* 1984:65–76.

122 Ballock RT, Mackersie R, Abitbol JJ, Cervilla V, Resnick D, Garfin SR. Can burst fractures be predicted from plain radiographs? *J Bone Joint Surg Br* 1992;74:147–150.

123 Atlas SW, Regenbogen V, Rogers LF, Kim KS. The radiographic characterization of burst fractures of the spine. *AJR Am J Roentgenol* 1986;147:575–582.

124 Fontijne WP, de Klerk LW, Braakman R, *et al.* CT scan prediction of neurological deficit in thoracolumbar burst fractures. *J Bone Joint Surg Br* 1992;74:683–685.

125 Blumenkopf B, Juneau III PA. Magnetic resonance imaging (MRI) of thoracolumbar fractures. *J Spinal Disord* 1988;1:144–150.

126 Saifuddin A, Noordeen H, Taylor BA, Bayley I. The role of imaging in the diagnosis and management of thoracolumbar burst fractures: current concepts and a review of the literature. *Skeletal Radiol* 1996;25:603–613.

127 Levine AM, Bosse M, Edwards CC. Bilateral facet dislocations in the thoracolumbar spine. *Spine* 1988;13:630–640.

CHAPTER 5

Controversies in surgical decompression: timing of decompressive surgery of the spinal cord

Mark S. Gerber and Volker K.H. Sonntag

Background

In the United States the annual incidence of traumatic spinal cord injury (SCI) is estimated at 40 per million population or 11,000 new cases each year.[1,2] Males between 16 and 30 years are at highest risk and represent almost 55% of the total injuries. Motor vehicle accidents are the leading cause of injury, followed by violence (gunshot wounds), falls, and recreational activities. The lifetime expense associated with care for an individual who is 25 years old when injured ranges from $500,000 to $2,000,000, depending on the level of injury.[1,3]

Improvements in the prehospital emergency medical system have helped decrease the morbidity and mortality rates associated with these injuries (Chapter 2). Despite ongoing research into pharmacological and spinal cord regeneration strategies (Chapter 1), surgery remains the only method of relieving the compressive effects of bone and disk fragments as well as epidural hematomas when closed reduction fails.

Surgery is and will continue to be a mainstay in the treatment paradigm of SCI, but the optimal timing of decompressive surgery remains controversial. The Joint Section of the American Association of Neurosurgeons and Congress of Neurological Surgeons recently published the *Guidelines for the Management of Acute Cervical Spine and Spinal Cord Injuries*.[4] This evidence-based review of the literature parallels the efforts of the Brain Trauma Foundation's Guidelines for the Management of Severe Head Injury.[5] The development of these guidelines required a meticulous review of the literature and classification of relevant papers as Class I, II, or III evidence based on the merits of the study. Based on the strength of the supporting evidence, standards, guidelines, and options were then developed. Additionally, the American Medical Association's list of attributes of clinical practice guidelines was also used to help determine the guidelines.[6] The issue of timing of spinal cord decompression was noted several times in the guidelines, but no single chapter specifically addressed this important and controversial issue.

Interestingly, in 1999 Fehlings and Tator[7] performed their own evidence-based review of the literature in an effort to address the issue of the timing of surgical decompression. Their analysis was conducted in the same fashion as the above evidence-based reviews. They identified numerous animal models of SCI and decompression that supported the theory that early decompression speeds return of neurological function.[8–18] Their analysis also included a thorough review of the literature evaluating neurological recovery in both operated and nonoperated spinal cord-injured individuals. They concluded that while Class II and III evidence supports that early decompression may improve neurological outcome, data are insufficient to support making it a standard or a guideline.

The case for and against early surgery

Injury to the spinal cord primarily results from the transfer of kinetic energy to the ligamentous and bony elements of the spine and to the spinal cord itself.[19] Continued secondary injury to the spinal cord is thought to be mediated by subsequent vascular and biochemical events, including vascular changes, electrolytic shifts, accumulation of excitotoxic neurotransmitters, free radical production, edema formation, and other inflammatory pathways.[20–29] Furthermore, the compressive effects of bone and disk fragments, hematomas, and malalignment of the spinal canal are thought to exacerbate this cascade.

As noted, data from models of SCI in cats, dogs, and primates support the hypothesis that early spinal cord decompression hastens recovery and improves neurological outcomes. Dolan et al.[8] used a small extradural clip to clamp the spinal cord of rats. Not only did the duration of clip compression directly affect functional recovery in the rats, but a clip with a greater closing force also led to a more severe deficit. Ducker et al.[30] also obtained similar findings in a primate SCI model. Using a canine model, Delamarter et al.[13] again demonstrated a statistically significant correlation between the duration of spinal cord compression and the degree of neurological recovery. Light and electron microscopic findings were also indicative of the duration of compression and led to the suggestion that persistent mass effect causes further cord injury.

In contrast, numerous clinical analyses have failed to find evidence supporting early decompressive surgery.[31–38] Many patients have either deteriorated or remained the same after surgical decompression. Wagner and Chehrazi[31] examined a cohort of 44 of 62 consecutive patients with cervical SCIs. During the 1-year follow-up, there were no differences in neurological outcomes in patients surgically decompressed within 8 h of injury and those treated between 9 and 48 h after injury. Furthermore, Marshall et al.[39] identified risks associated with early surgery in a prospective multicenter study of 283 spinal cord-injured patients. Fourteen (4.9%) patients experienced neurological deterioration after hospitalization. Of these 14 patients, four had undergone a surgical procedure within 5 days of injury. Two of these four patients were operated on the day of injury. Furthermore, none of the 64 patients operated on after the

10th day deteriorated neurologically. The authors suggested that surgery performed within the first 5 days of injury may increase patients' risk for neurological deterioration. They did note, however, that patients with worsening neurological function and evidence of compression may warrant aggressive intervention.

Others have noted neurological improvement in patients managed conservatively without surgery.[33,38,40–45] In 1969, Frankel et al.[41] reported their experience with 612 spinal cord-injured patients who were treated using the conservative techniques of Guttmann.[45] Using the force of gravity, realignment was achieved and fusion resulted from persistent bed rest. Of the patients with a complete SCI, 29% regained at least one Frankel grade during their hospitalization. Conservative nonoperative management is not without risk, however. Katoh et al.[42] reported a 10% incidence of progressive neurological deficit in their cohort of conservatively managed patients with incomplete SCIs.

Further data confounding the issue of timing are found in the work of Anderson and Bohlman.[46] They reported neurological improvement in motor functions of patients with both complete and incomplete SCIs who underwent surgery as long as 9 years after injury.[46,47]

None of these studies has been a controlled randomized trial. Furthermore, early surgery was defined loosely in these studies. Definitions have ranged from surgery within 8 h to as long as 5 days after injury. The surgical approach selected for decompression, that is anterior or posterior, also appears to affect the final neurological status of these patients.[48] Given the improvements in radiographic imaging, anesthesia, and anterior screw-plate fixation, earlier methods such as laminectomy may have increased the risk of continued injury to the spinal cord by further destabilizing patients. The neural elements also may have been decompressed inadequately. These issues likely confound attempts to draw firm conclusions based on the current literature.

Numerous authors have reported evidence supporting early decompressive surgery.[40,49–57] In particular, the rapid closed reduction of patients with bilateral locked facets has been reported to have had a remarkable effect on neurological recovery.[49,58–64] Hadley et al.[60] retrospectively reviewed 68 patients with facet fracture–dislocation injuries. With rapid closed reduction, 68% of the patients improved neurologically. Furthermore, of the 10 patients who showed "significant" neurological recovery, all underwent reduction within 8 h of injury; 6 of the 10 underwent reduction within 5 h of injury.

Other authors have attempted to clarify the issue of timing of decompression. Mirza et al.[65] retrospectively reviewed two groups of 15 patients who underwent early (within a mean of 1.8 days) or late (within a mean of 14.1 days) surgery. These patients were treated at separate hospitals because the treatment protocol differed based on the institution. All patients had neurological deficits. Compared to their preoperative motor scores, the early surgical group significantly improved after surgery whereas the late surgical group did not. Only one prospective randomized trial on the timing of surgery has been reported. Vaccaro et al.[35] found no differences in neurological outcomes in two randomized surgical cohorts. The early group was decompressed within 72 h of injury whereas the late group was decompressed after 5 days. Limitations of this study again included the definition of early surgery (mean, 1.8 days), the small number of patients enrolled, and the loss of patients to follow-up.

In addition to the potential neurological benefits of early decompression, several authors have noted these patients require shorter hospitalizations than conservatively treated patients. The most significant portion of the total expenditure for the care of spinal cord-injured patients occurs during their initial hospitalization.[3] Early surgery allows aggressive early mobilization, which appears to decrease a patient's stay in the intensive care unit (ICU). It also may decrease the complications associated with continued bedrest in the ICU: pneumonia, sepsis, deep venous thrombosis, decubitus ulceration, and urinary tract infections.[35] Furthermore, prolonged bedrest appears to exacerbate physical deconditioning. When deconditioning is minimized, patients have the opportunity to move to the rehabilitation phase of treatment with more energy and determination. The long-term neurological function of spinal cord-injured patients directly affects their lifetime cost of care.[66] Therefore, early surgery may offer both patients and society an economic benefit.

Logical arguments for early surgical decompression

The question regarding timing of decompressive surgery is as follows: Does early surgery, defined as within 8–12 h of injury, correlate with improved neurological outcomes? If the spinal cord and brain tissue are assumed to respond similarly to mass effect and ischemia, a direct analogy can be drawn between acute intracranial mass lesions and acute compressive lesions of the spinal cord. In the case of acute intracerebral, subdural, or epidural hematomas, most surgeons assess the degree of mass effect identified on imaging studies and the patient's neurological status before proceeding with surgery. One could argue that acute mass lesions of the spine associated with a neurological deficit should be addressed in a similar fashion.

For example, analogies can also be drawn between patients with a large dominant hemisphere subdural hematoma and a Glasgow Coma Scale (GCS) score of 4 and patients with a C6 burst fracture and a complete SCI. The likelihood of either group benefiting from a surgical procedure, although very low, is not zero. In an analogous situation, patients with a 40-ml acute right frontal hematoma and a GCS score of 10 could be compared to patients with a C5 anterior compression fracture who are able to wiggle their toes. In both groups, removal of the space-occupying mass affords patients a higher probability of attaining some neurological improvement.

A further comparison between intracranial and spinal pathology can be made. If it is assumed that the biochemical pathways that mediate secondary injury in the brain and spinal cord are similar, the renewed interest in decompressive hemicraniectomy in patients with an acute stroke can be likened to decompressing the spinal canal in trauma.[67]

Another analogy can be drawn from the results of the treatment of stroke. During the 1990s, large prospective randomized international trials with recombinant tissue plasminogen activator demonstrated the efficacy of *early* treatment of ischemic stroke.[68–71] The American Heart Association and the American Stroke Association in cooperation with stroke centers throughout the country have sought to educate the public regarding the symptoms of stroke and the need to seek emergent medical attention. Phrases such as "time is brain" continue to be part of the call to arms. If time is brain, why should we be so reticent to conclude that time is spinal cord?

Prospective trials

As a result of the data supporting improved neurological outcomes with early decompression, prospective trials have been entertained to answer this question definitively. In 1992, the Surgical Treatment for Acute Spinal Cord Injury Study (STASCIS) group was formed to conduct a randomized prospective controlled trial to evaluate formally the role and timing of decompressive surgery after acute SCI. Tator *et al.*[72] reported the results of the STASCIS multicenter retrospective study evaluating the role and timing of surgical intervention in patients with acute SCI. Such a trial, however, may be difficult to conduct because enrollment of a control group may prove challenging. Most individuals with a compressive lesion, regardless of their deficit, when presented the options for surgery or conservative management, would likely opt for surgery regardless of their chances for recovery. Surgeons might also find it ethically unconscionable not to operate on a patient randomized to the nonsurgical arm. These issues make the possibility of randomization difficult.

Tator *et al.*[72] identified another cause for concern in the design of a future randomized prospective study. In their multicenter study, magnetic resonance imaging (MRI) was performed in only 54% of the patients. Fehlings and colleagues recently reported that reliance on computed tomography (CT) alone in patients with SCIs can significantly underestimate the degree of spinal cord compression.[73,74] These issues need to be addressed before a prospective study can be organized so that an accurate and reliable standard imaging protocol could be performed at all participating centers.

Another controversial issue is how much time should be spent obtaining diagnostic studies. In many centers, several hours may elapse after admission before MRI can be obtained. Several groups have examined the utility of MRI for identifying compressive lesions before emergent surgical intervention. Papadopoulos *et al.* assessed the feasibility and outcome of patients undergoing immediate surgery for cervical spinal cord decompression.[75] Of 91 initial consecutive patients, 25 were excluded from the treatment protocol for several reasons: the need for other surgical procedures, presence of a contraindication on MRI, or the admitting surgeon's bias about the futility of surgical intervention. The mean time to MRI and operative decompression *after* arrival was 4.1 and 9.6 h, respectively. Compared to 24% of the reference patients, 50% of the protocol patients improved compared to their admitting Frankel grade. In fact, eight (12%) protocol patients improved from Frankel A or B (complete) to Frankel D or E (independent ambulation). The protocol patients also had shorter stays in the ICU and hospital. This study was part of a feasibility study for a National Institutes of Health Grant. A proposal for a national prospective randomized trial evaluating the timing of decompression and preoperative MRI findings has been rejected twice.

A retrospective analysis of the surgically treated patients enrolled in the National Acute Spinal Cord Injury Study (NASCIS) II trials led to the suggestion of a randomized study on the treatment and efficacy of surgical decompression.[40] As with pharmacological therapy, it seems likely that surgical decompression must be obtained within hours and not days to afford the greatest potential for significant neurological recovery.

Any future well-designed randomized trial must consider other variables that can confound data analysis and lead to inappropriate conclusions. In particular, age may significantly affect the ability of the patients to recover from acute SCI. Guest *et al.* retrospectively analyzed the surgical management of acute central cord syndrome.[76] Compared to older patients, motor scores improved significantly in patients younger than 60 years and in patients who underwent surgery for acute fracture dislocation within 24h of injury. The functional level of improvement also appears to be less in elderly patients despite longer periods of rehabilitation.[77]

Treatment strategies

At our institution, we favor aggressive management and treatment of patients with acute SCIs (Figure 5.1). In the trauma room, the patient is assessed neurologically and medically and then stabilized and treated according to the Advanced Trauma Life Support guidelines. Plain radiographs are then obtained. Gardner–Wells tongs and halo rings are kept nearby to allow the immediate application of traction when indicated. Despite the ongoing debate, solumedrol is administered to all spinal cord-injured patients according to the NASCIS protocol.[78–84] Patients with a complete neurological injury and bilateral locked facets have the highest probability of having traction applied in the trauma room. For many cases of bilateral locked facets, emergent manual reduction under fluoroscopic guidance is considered. Although concerns have been expressed about closed reduction of locked facets, none of our patients have deteriorated after reduction as a result of disk herniation.[85–87] In all cases of acute SCI, CT of the cervical spine with sagittal and coronal reformatted images is rapidly obtained. We often obtain a CT angiogram of the neck to evaluate injury to the vertebral arteries.[88]

The attending neurosurgeon and resident must coordinate and expedite the safe movement of the patient from the trauma room to the CT and/or MRI scanner. Unfortunately, the level of coordination required to obtain MRI can impede the care of patients. Based on the current speed and quality of imaging, plain

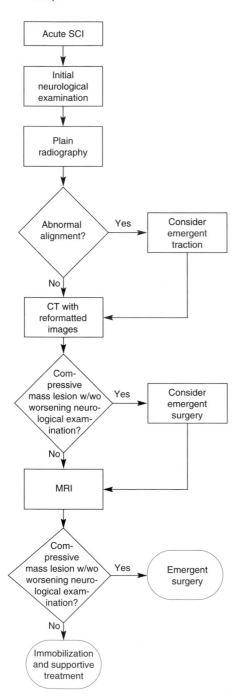

Figure 5.1 Treatment algorithm for patients presenting with traumatic acute SCI (Reproduced with permission from Barrow Neurological Institute).

radiography, and CT are the most worthwhile. Although MRI is preferred obtaining an MRI should not delay surgical decompression if plain radiography or CT already shows compression and the patient is deteriorating neurologically.

Depending on a patient's neurological examination, overall medical condition, and diagnostic images, closed reduction, further radiographic studies with MRI, emergent decompressive surgery, or all three may be considered. When patients are neurologically intact, their need for emergent treatment is moot. Typically, these patients are immobilized with traction or an external orthosis and undergo MRI to assess the extent of their injury and the need for surgical intervention. Barring any medical or surgical contraindication, patients with an incomplete SCI and evidence of persistent spinal cord compression are considered absolute emergencies and are scheduled for immediate surgery. In trauma patients, injuries to the chest, abdomen, and extremities as well as closed head injuries must be diagnosed and treated appropriately.

Once a decision has been made to perform surgery, an approach must be chosen. We tend to favor an anterior approach, especially in the cervical spine, for several reasons. An anterior approach allows removal of disk material and bone fragments originating from the vertebral body. Furthermore, two columns can be stabilized from an anterior approach because the anterior column can be reconstructed with a bone graft and screw plate. Offending soft tissue such as disk material or blood not clearly identified on CT can be addressed at surgery. When timely MRI is impossible or contraindicated, CT myelography may assist with surgical planning. We also prefer to monitor somatosensory evoked potentials in all patients.

In our experience, patients with unreduced unilateral or bilateral locked facets also can be reduced through an anterior approach. Under fluoroscopic guidance, the combined effects of muscular relaxation under anesthesia and distraction (either with traction and mild flexion or by directly spreading the vertebral bodies) make realignment significantly easier. An anterior graft must be the appropriate height to avoid distracting the facets until they no longer overlap. Depending on the surgical and radiographic findings, some patients wear a halo vest after anterior fusion. Postoperative supine and upright lateral radiographs of the cervical spine obtained while patients wear a halo or collar can help determine the need for posterior reinforcement after anterior reconstruction.

Spinal cord-injured patients seldom undergo a single reconstructive surgery through a posterior approach. If there is no evidence of anterior compression from a herniated disk, bone fragment, or hematoma and the anterior column appears to have retained its structural integrity, posterior fixation with interspinous wiring and lateral mass fixation is performed.

Patients with a complete SCI *tend* to be treated more conservatively than those with incomplete injuries. In general, as long as patients with a complete SCI are medically stable and have no other injuries that preclude surgery, they are offered urgent treatment, including surgical decompression. Imaging studies, age, medical history, premorbid function, and patient and family wishes are also considered when managing this challenging subset of patients.

Patients with an acute thoracic and lumbar SCI are assessed in a similar fashion. These patients often have other injuries related to their trauma, including pulmonary contusions, long bone fractures, and internal injuries. Thoracic fractures that cause complete SCIs tend to involve high-energy forces, leading to an increased likelihood of life-threatening internal injuries. These patients receive the necessary medical treatment until surgery, if indicated, can be performed.

Patients with evidence of both a SCI and traumatic brain injury are also evaluated as surgical candidates. Depending on the severity of the head injury, emergent decompressive surgery may still be indicated.

Conclusions

At present, there is a lack of Class I evidence supporting early decompression and stabilization in the setting of acute SCI in humans. Several compelling studies and anecdotal evidence suggest that early intervention does improve outcomes in patients with complete and incomplete SCIs. The current literature, surgeon preference, personal experience, and the wishes of patients and families help determine which patients are offered early surgical decompression. Until a well-designed prospective randomized trial is conducted, this issue will likely remain unresolved.

References

1 Spinal Cord Injury [Internet]. Facts and figures at a glance – May, 2001 Available from http://www.spinalcord.uab.edu/show.asp?durki=21446. Spinal Cord Injury Information Network, 2001.

2 Tator CH. Epidemiology and general characteristics of the spinal cord injury patient. In Benzel EC and Tator CH (eds): *Contemporary Management of Spinal Cord Injury: Neurosurgical Topics.* American Association of Neurological Surgeons, Park Ridge, IL, 1995, pp. 9–13.

3 Watts C, Esser GB. Economic overview of spinal disorders. In Menezes AH and Sonntag VKH (eds): *Principles of Spinal Surgery.* McGraw-Hill, New York, 1996, pp. 25–40.

4 Hadley MN, Walters BC, Grabb PA, *et al.* Guidelines for the management of acute cervical spine and spinal cord injuries (Suppl). *Neurosurgery* 2002;49:407–498.

5 Bullock R, Chestnut RM, Clifton GL, *et al.* Guidelines for the management of severe brain injury. *Brain Found* 1996;3:109–127.

6 Hadley M. Methodology of guideline development. *Neurosurgery* 2002;50:S2–S6.

7 Fehlings M, Tator CH. An evidence-based review of decompressive surgery in acute spinal cord injury: rationale, indications, and timing based on experimental and clinical studies. *J Neurosurg* 1999;91:1–11.

8 Dolan EJ, Tator CH, Endrenyi L. The value of decompression for acute experimental spinal cord compression injury. *J Neurosurg* 1980;53:749–755.

9 Tarlov IM (ed.). *Spinal Cord Compression: Mechanisms of Paralysis and Treatment.* Charles C Thomas, Springfield, IL, 1957.

10 Tarlov IM. Spinal cord injuries – early treatment. *Surg Clin North Am* 1955;35:591–607.

11 Tarlov IM, Klinger H. Spinal cord compression studies. II. Time limits for recovery after acute compression in dogs. *Arch Neurol Psych* 1954;71:271–290.

12 Brodkey JS, Richards DE, Blasingame JP, *et al*. Reversible spinal cord trauma in cats. Additive effects of direct pressure and ischemia. *J Neurosurg* 1972;37:591–593.

13 Delamarter RB, Sherman J, Carr JB. Pathophysiology of spinal cord injury. *J Bone Joint Surg Am* 1995;77:1042–1049.

14 Croft TJ, Brodkey JS, Nulsen FE. Reversible spinal cord trauma: a model for electrical monitoring of spinal cord function. *J Neurosurg* 1972;36:402–406.

15 Carlson GD, Minato Y, Okada A, *et al*. Early time-dependent decompression for spinal cord injury: vascular mechanisms of recovery. *J Neurotrauma* 1997;14:951–962.

16 Guha A, Tator CH, Endrenyi L, *et al*. Decompression of the spinal cord improves recovery after acute experimental spinal cord. *Paraplegia* 1987;25:324–339.

17 Nystrom B, Berglund JE. Spinal cord restitution following compression injuries in rats. *Acta Neurol Scand* 1988;78:467–472.

18 Zhang Y, Hillered L, Olsson Y, *et al*. Time course of energy perturbation after compression trauma to the spinal cord: an experimental study in the rat using microdialysis. *Surg Neurol* 1993;39:297–304.

19 Tator CH. Spine–spinal cord relationships in spinal cord trauma. *Clin Neurosurg* 1983;30:479–494.

20 Tator CH. Ischemia as a secondary neuronal injury. In Salzman SK and Faden AI (eds): *Neurobiology of Central Nervous System Trauma*. Oxford University Press, New York, 1994, pp. 209–215.

21 Demopoulos HB, Flamm ES, Pietronigro DD, *et al*. The free radical pathology and the microcirculation in the major central nervous system disorders. *Acta Physiol Scand Suppl* 1980;492:91–119.

22 Faden AI, Simon RP. A potential role for excitotoxins in the pathophysiology of spinal cord injury. *Ann Neurol* 1988;23:623–626.

23 Tator CH. Experimental and clinical studies of the pathophysiology and management of acute spinal cord injury. *J Spinal Cord Med* 1996;19:206–214.

24 Tator CH. Review of experimental spinal cord injury with emphasis on the local and systemic circulatory effects. *Neurochirurgie* 1991;37:291–302.

25 Tator CH, Fehlings M. Review of the secondary injury theory of acute spinal cord trauma with emphasis on vascular mechanisms. *J Neurosurg* 1991;75:15–26.

26 Wallace MC, Tator CH, Lewis AJ. Chronic regenerative changes in the spinal cord after cord compression injury in rats. *Surg Neurol* 1987;27:209–219.

27 Young W, Koreh I. Potassium and calcium changes in injured spinal cords. *Brain Res* 1986;365:42–53.

28 Anderson DK, Means ED, Waters TR. Spinal cord energy metabolism in normal and post-laminectomy cats. *J Neurosurg* 1980;52:387–391.

29 Wagner Jr FC, Stewart WB. Effect of trauma dose on spinal cord edema. *J Neurosurg* 1981;54:802–806.

30 Ducker TB, Salcman M, Daniell HB. Experimental spinal cord trauma. III. Therapeutic effect of immobilization and pharmacologic agents. *Surg Neurol* 1978;10:71–76.

31 Wagner Jr FC, Chehrazi B. Early decompression and neurological outcome in acute cervical spinal cord injuries. *J Neurosurg* 1982;56:699–705.

32 Larson SJ, Holst RA, Hemmy DC, *et al*. Lateral extracavitary approach to traumatic lesions of the thoracic and lumbar spine. *J Neurosurg* 1976;45:628–637.

33 Maynard FM, Reynolds GG, Fountain S, *et al*. Neurological prognosis after traumatic quadriplegia. Three-year experience of California Regional Spinal Cord Injury Care System. *J Neurosurg* 1979;50:611–616.

34 Tator CH, Duncan EG, Edmonds VE, *et al*. Comparison of surgical and conservative management in 208 patients with acute spinal cord injury. *Can J Neurol Sci* 1987;14:60–69.

35 Vaccaro AR, Daugherty RJ, Sheehan TP, *et al.* Neurologic outcome of early versus late surgery for cervical spinal cord injury. *Spine* 1997;22:2609–2613.

36 Vale FL, Burns J, Jackson AB, Hadley MN. Combined medical and surgical treatment after acute spinal cord injury: results of a prospective pilot study to assess the merits of aggressive medical resuscitation and blood pressure management. *J Neurosurg* 1997;87:239–246.

37 Waters RL, Adkins RH, Yakura JS, *et al.* Effect of surgery on motor recovery following traumatic spinal cord injury. *Spinal Cord* 1996;34:188–192.

38 Donovan WH, Kopaniky D, Stolzmann E, *et al.* The neurological and skeletal outcome in patients with closed cervical spinal cord injury. *J Neurosurg* 1987;66:690–694.

39 Marshall LF, Knowlton S, Garfin SR, *et al.* Deterioration following spinal cord injury. A multicenter study. *J Neurosurg* 1987;66:400–404.

40 Duh MS, Shepard MJ, Wilberger JE, *et al.* The effectiveness of surgery on the treatment of acute spinal cord injury and its relation to pharmacological treatment. *Neurosurgery* 1994; 35:240–249.

41 Frankel HL, Hancock DO, Hyslop G, *et al.* The value of postural reduction in the initial management of closed injuries of the spine with paraplegia and tetraplegia. I. *Paraplegia* 1969;7:179–192.

42 Katoh S, el Masry WS, Jaffray D, *et al.* Neurologic outcome in conservatively treated patients with incomplete closed traumatic cervical spinal cord injuries. *Spine* 1996;21:2345–2351.

43 Bedbrook GM. Spinal injuries with tetraplegia and paraplegia. *J Bone Joint Surg Br* 1979; 61B:267–284.

44 Harris P, Karmi MZ, McClemont E, *et al.* The prognosis of patients sustaining severe cervical spine injury (C2–C7 inclusive). *Paraplegia* 1980;18:324–330.

45 Guttmann L. Initial treatment of traumatic paraplegia and tetraplegia. In Harris P (ed.): *Spinal Injuries Symposium.* Morrison & Gibb, Edinburg, 1963, pp. 80–92.

46 Anderson PA, Bohlman HH. Anterior decompression and arthrodesis of the cervical spine: long-term motor improvement. Part II. Improvement in complete traumatic quadriplegia. *J Bone Joint Surg Am* 1992;74:683–692.

47 Bohlman HH, Anderson PA. Anterior decompression and arthrodesis of the cervical spine: long-term motor improvement. Part I. Improvement in incomplete traumatic quadriparesis. *J Bone Joint Surg Am* 1992;74:671–682.

48 Bohlman HH. Acute fractures and dislocations of the cervical spine. An analysis of three hundred hospitalized patients and review of the literature. *J Bone Joint Surg Am* 1979;61:1119–1142.

49 Aebi M, Mohler J, Zach GA, *et al.* Indication, surgical technique, and results of 100 surgically-treated fractures and fracture–dislocations of the cervical spine. *Clin Orthop* 1986; 203: 244–257.

50 Benzel EC, Larson SJ. Functional recovery after decompressive spine operation for cervical spine fractures. *Neurosurgery* 1987;20:742–746.

51 Krengel WF, Anderson PA, Henley MB. Early stabilization and decompression for incomplete paraplegia due to a thoracic-level spinal cord injury. *Spine* 1993;18:2080–2087.

52 Levi L, Wolf A, Rigamonti D, *et al.* Anterior decompression in cervical spine trauma: Does the timing of surgery affect the outcome? *Neurosurgery* 1991;29:216–222.

53 Murphy KP, Opitz JL, Cabanela ME, *et al.* Cervical fractures and spinal cord injury: outcome of surgical and nonsurgical management. *Mayo Clin Proc* 1990;65:949–959.

54 Weinshel SS, Maiman DJ, Baek P, *et al.* Neurologic recovery in quadriplegia following operative treatment. *J Spinal Disord* 1990;3:244–249.

55 Wiberg J, Hauge HN. Neurological outcome after surgery for thoracic and lumbar spine injuries. *Acta Neurochir (Wien)* 1988;91:106–112.

56 Wolf A, Levi L, Mirvis S, *et al*. Operative management of bilateral facet dislocation. *J Neurosurg* 1991;75:883–890.

57 Benzel EC, Larson SJ. Recovery of nerve root function after complete quadriplegia from cervical spine fractures. *Neurosurgery* 1986;19:809–812.

58 Lee AS, MacLean JC, Newton DA. Rapid traction for reduction of cervical spine dislocations. *J Bone Joint Surg Br* 1994;76:352–356.

59 Grant GA, Mirza SK, Chapman JR, *et al*. Risk of early closed reduction in cervical spine subluxation injuries. *J Neurosurg (Spine 1)* 1999;90:13–18.

60 Hadley MN, Fitzpatrick BC, Sonntag VKH, *et al*. Facet fracture–dislocation injuries of the cervical spine. *Neurosurgery* 1992;31:661–666.

61 Brunette DD, Rockswold GL. Neurologic recovery following rapid spinal realignment for complete cervical spinal cord injury. *J Trauma* 1987;27:445–447.

62 Sonntag VKH. Management of bilateral locked facets of the cervical spine. *Neurosurgery* 1981;8:150–152.

63 Evans DK. Reduction of cervical dislocations. *J Bone Joint Surg Br* 1961;43B:552–555.

64 Star AM, Jones AA, Cotler JM, *et al*. Immediate closed reduction of cervical spine dislocations using traction. *Spine* 1990;15:1068–1072.

65 Mirza SK, Krengel WF, Chapman JR, *et al*. Early versus delayed surgery for acute cervical spinal cord injury. *Clin Orthop* 1999;359:104–114.

66 Tator CH, Duncan EG, Edmonds VE, *et al*. Complications and costs of management of acute spinal cord injury. *Paraplegia* 1993;31:700–714.

67 Schwab S, Steiner T, Aschoff A, *et al*. Early hemicraniectomy in patients with complete middle cerebral artery infarction. *Stroke* 1998;29:1888–1893.

68 Hacke W, Kaste M, Fieschi C, *et al*. Intravenous thrombolysis with recombinant tissue plasminogen activator for acute hemispheric stroke. The European Cooperative Acute Stroke Study (ECASS). *JAMA* 1995;274:1017–1025.

69 Clark WM, Wissman S, Albers GW, *et al*. Recombinant tissue-type plasminogen activator (Alteplase) for ischemic stroke 3 to 5 hours after symptom onset. The ATLANTIS Study: A randomized controlled trial. Alteplase Thrombolysis for Acute Noninterventional Therapy in Ischemic Stroke. *JAMA* 1999;282:2019–2026.

70 The National Institute of Neurological Disorders and Stroke rt-PA Stroke Study Group. Tissue plasminogen activator for acute ischemic stroke. *New Engl J Med* 1995;333: 1581–1587.

71 Hacke W, Kaste M, Fieschi C, *et al*. Randomized double-blind placebo-controlled trial of thrombolytic therapy with intravenous alteplase in acute ischaemic stroke (ECASS II). Second European–Australasian Acute Stroke Study. *Lancet* 1998;352:1245–1251.

72 Tator CH, Fehlings M, Thorpe K, *et al*. Current use and timing of spinal surgery for management of acute spinal cord injury in North America: results of a retrospective multicenter study. *J Neurosurg* 1999;91:12–18.

73 Rao SC, Fehlings MG. The optimal radiologic method for assessing spinal canal compromise and cord compression in patients with cervical spinal cordy injury. Part I. An evidence-based analysis of the published literature. *Spine* 1999;24:598–604.

74 Fehlings MG, Rao SC, Tator CH, *et al*. The optimal radiologic method for assessing spinal canal compromise and cord compression in patients with cervical spinal cord injury. Part II. Results of a multicenter study. *Spine* 1999;24:605–613.

75 Papadopoulos SM, Selden NR, Quint DJ, *et al*. Immediate spinal cord decompression for cervical spinal cord injury: feasibility and outcome. *J Trauma* 2002;52:323–332.

76 Guest J, Eleraky MA, Apostolides PJ, *et al*. Traumatic central cord syndrome: results of surgical management. *J Neurosurg* 2002;97(1 Suppl):25–32.

77 Seel RT, Huang ME, Cifu DX, *et al.* Age-related differences in length of stays, hospitalization costs, and outcomes for an injury-matched sample of adults with paraplegia. *J Spinal Cord Med* 2001;24:241–250.

78 Bracken MB, Shepard MJ, Collins WF, *et al.* A randomized, controlled trial of methylprednisolone or naloxone in the treatment of acute spinal-cord injury. Results of the Second National Acute Spinal Cord Injury Study. *New Engl J Med* 1990;322:1405–1411.

79 Bracken MB, Shepard MJ, Collins WF, *et al.* Methylprednisolone or naloxone treatment after acute spinal cord injury: 1-year follow-up data. Results of the Second National Acute Spinal Cord Injury Study. *J Neurosurg* 1992;76:23–31.

80 Bracken MB, Holford TR. Effects of timing of methylprednisolone or naloxone administration on recovery of segmental and long-tract neurological function in NASCIS 2. *J Neurosurg* 1993;79:500–507.

81 Bracken MB, Shepard MJ, Holford TR, *et al.* Administration of methylprednisolone for 24 or 48 hours or tirilazad mesylate for 48 hours in the treatment of acute spinal cord injury. Results of the Third National Acute Spinal Cord Injury Randomized Controlled Trial. National Acute Spinal Cord Injury Study. *JAMA* 1997;277:1597–1604.

82 Bracken MB, Shepard MJ, Holford TR, *et al.* Methylprednisolone or tirilazad mesylate administration after acute spinal cord injury: 1-year follow up. Results of the Third National Acute Spinal Cord Injury Randomized Controlled Trial. *J Neurosurg* 1998;89: 699–706.

83 Bracken MB, Aldrich EF, Herr DL, *et al.* Clinical measurement, statistical analysis, and risk-benefit: controversies from trials of spinal injury. *J Trauma* 2000;48:558–561.

84 Bracken MB, Holford TR. Neurological and functional status 1 year after acute spinal cord injury: estimates of functional recovery in National Acute Spinal Cord Injury Study II from results modeled in National Acute Spinal Cord Injury Study III. *J Neurosurg* 2002;96: 259–266.

85 Harrington JF, Likavec MJ, Smith AS. Disc herniation in cervical fracture subluxation. *Neurosurgery* 1991;29:374–379.

86 Olerud C, Jónsson Jr H. Compression of the cervical spine cord after reduction of fracture dislocations. Report of 2 cases. *Acta Orthop Scand* 1991;62:599–601.

87 Doran SE, Papadopoulos SM, Ducker TB, *et al.* Magnetic resonance imaging documentation of coexistent traumatic locked facets of the cervical spine and disc herniation. *J Neurosurg* 1993;79:341–345.

88 Willis BK, Greiner F, Orrison WW, *et al.* The incidence of vertebral artery injury after mid-cervical spine fracture or subluxation. *Neurosurgery* 1994;34:435–442.

CHAPTER 6

Biomechanics of spinal column failure

Eric P. Roger, G. Alexander Jones and Edward C. Benzel

All figures in this chapter taken from Benzel, EC. *Biomechanics of Spine Stabilization*, New York: Thieme; 2001. Reprinted by permission.

Spinal stability

The classic definition of clinical stability is: "the ability of the spine under physiological loads to limit patterns of displacement so as not to damage or irritate the spinal cord or nerve roots and, in addition, to prevent incapacitating deformity or pain caused by structural changes".[1] Normal physiological loads vary significantly. Therefore, stability should be interpreted as circumstance dependent, rather than an all-or-none phenomenon. For example, spinal stability should be provided when landing from a jump; conversely, a certain degree of spinal laxity is required to stoop for tying the laces of one's shoes.

The inherent structure of the spine provides a physiological and functional degree of freedom of motion, referred to as the neutral zone (see later discussion). Normal range of motion (ROM) includes translation and rotation about the three cardinal anatomical axes (Figure 6.1), providing six potential movements referred to as degrees of motion. Segmental motions at the various spinal levels (Figure 6.2) are generally determined by facet orientation, bony anatomy, associated ligaments, and supporting structures (e.g. the rib cage).

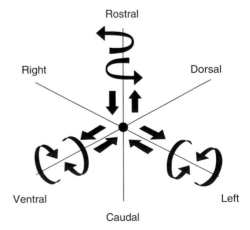

Figure 6.1 The Cartesian coordinate system with the instantaneous axis of rotation (IAR) as the center. Translation and rotation can occur in both of their respective directions about each axis. (Reprinted by permission. See full reference above.)

Rostral

Right

Dorsal

Ventral

Left

Caudal

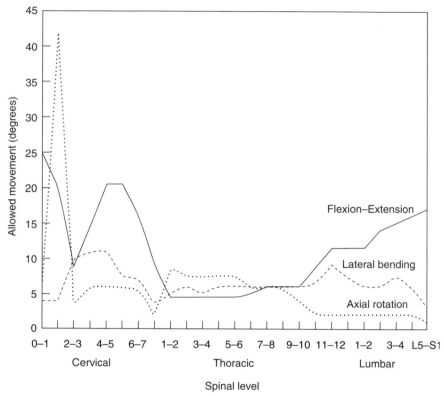

Figure 6.2 Segmental motions allowed at the various spinal levels (combined flexion and extension, *solid line*; unilateral lateral bending, *dashed line*; and unilateral axial rotation, *dotted line*). (Reprinted by permission. See full reference on p. 95.)

Flexion and extension are most prominent in the cervical and lumbar spine, while rotation is greatest in the cervical spine.

Spinal stability is maintained by a variety of anatomical structures that have evolved to provide resistance against deforming forces. These structures include both hard and soft tissues.

Vertebral body

The vertebral body is the main axial load-bearing structure of the spine. Its cylindrical shape, bounded peripherally by cortical bone and rostro-caudally by end-plates, confers it with superior biomechanical properties. The width and depth of vertebral bodies increase as one descends in the spine to accommodate increased axial load (Figures 6.3 and 6.4). The relative weakness of the L5 vertebrae can be explained by the height asymmetry between the ventral and dorsal cortical walls.

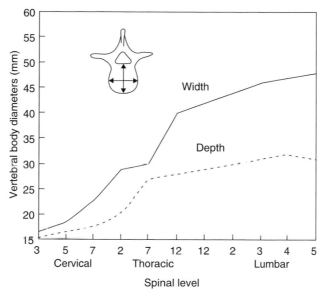

Figure 6.3 Vertebral body diameter versus spinal level. The width (*solid line*) and depth (*dashed line*) of the vertebral bodies are depicted separately. (Reprinted by permission. See full reference on p. 95.)

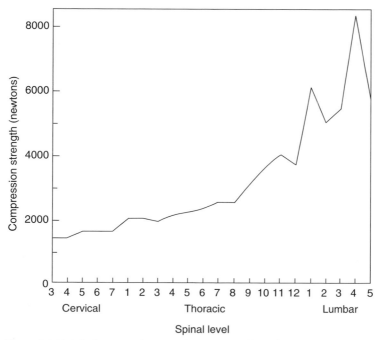

Figure 6.4 Vertebral compression strength versus spinal level. (Reprinted by permission. See full reference on p. 95.)

Intervertebral disks

The intervertebral disk is composed of the nucleus pulposus (a hydrated core that serves as a shock absorber), and the annulus fibrosus (a fibrocartilaginous ring designed to provide structural support). Concentric axial loads cause equally distributed forces within the disk, while eccentrically placed loads cause bulging of the annulus on the side of the applied force, with associated displacement of the nucleus to the opposite side (Figure 6.5). Shearing and rotational forces are resisted by the annular fibers that are placed in a 30-degree angle in respect to each other (Figure 6.6).

Facet joints

In conjunction with the intervertebral disk, the facet joints provide additional articulation between segmental levels. Their orientation (Figure 6.7) serve to facilitate or limit degrees of motion (Figure 6.2), and therefore play an important role in spinal stability. Cervical facets are coronally oriented. Therefore, they

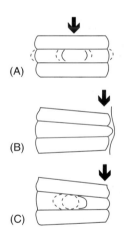

Figure 6.5 (A) An axial load causes an equally distributed force application to the disk. (B) An eccentric force application results in annulus fibrosus bulging on the side of the greatest force application (i.e. the concave side of the bend). (C) The nucleus pulposus moves in the opposite direction. Dashed lines indicate the positions of structures during force application. (Reprinted by permission. See full reference on p. 95.)

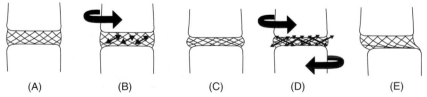

Figure 6.6 (A) Annular fibers are oriented in a 30-degree orientation with the endplate. (B) This permits a significant torsion prevention potential (*arrows*). In fact, they are more optimally oriented for torsion prevention than for distraction (or compression) prevention. If the annular fibers are lax (C), torsion resistance diminishes (*arrows*) (D). Chronic instability and mechanical pain may result. (E) Lax annular ligaments also predispose to the more commonly observed imaging correlate of chronic instability, subluxation. (Reprinted by permission. See full reference on p. 95.)

resist translation, while facilitating flexion, extension, and rotation. Conversely, lumbar facets are sagittally oriented (with the exception of L5-S1), resisting rotation, while allowing significant flexion and extension. Thoracic facets are intermediately oriented, thus providing an "intermediate" restriction in translation and rotation.

Ligaments

Spinal ligaments provide passive stabilization of the vertebral column. Their bone-to-bone interface and elastic properties provide both tension-band and translational support. The tension-band contribution to spinal stability is related to both the ligament's tensile strength (Figure 6.8), as well as the moment arm through which it acts. As is discussed later, the moment arm is the perpendicular distance from the instantaneous axis of rotation (IAR) to the applied force vector. The amount of resistance (counter bending moment) a ligament provides is proportional to its distance from the IAR (Figure 6.9).

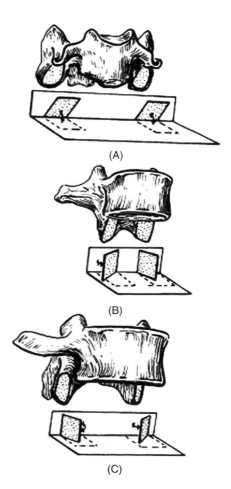

(A)

(B)

Figure 6.7 Facet joint orientation. (A) The relative coronal plane orientation in the cervical region, (B) the intermediate orientation in the thoracic region, and (C) the relative sagittal orientation in the lumbar region. (Reprinted by permission. See full reference on p. 95.)

(C)

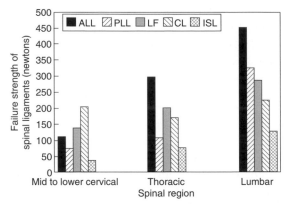

Figure 6.8 Failure strength of spinal ligaments versus spinal region (ALL: anterior longitudinal ligament; PLL: posterior longitudinal ligament; LF: ligamentum flavum; CL: capsular ligament; ISL: interspinous ligament.) (Reprinted by permission. See full reference on p. 95.)

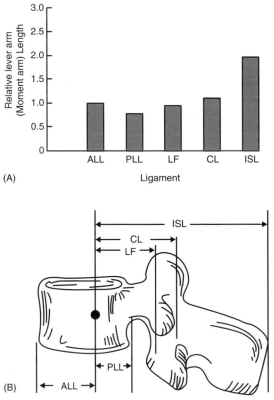

Figure 6.9 (A) The relative lever arm (moment arm) length of ligaments causing flexion (or resisting extension). (B) The ligaments and their effective moment arms. Note that this length depends on the location of the IAR. An "average" location is used in this illustration. (Dot: IAR; ALL: anterior longitudinal ligament; PLL: posterior longitudinal ligament; LF: ligamentum flavum; CL: capsular ligament; ISL: interspinous ligament.) (Reprinted by permission. See full reference on p. 95.)

Muscles

As opposed to skeletal muscles effecting long bone motion (which span one or two articulations), the paraspinous musculature (and associated abdominal musculature) span multiple segments (Figure 6.10). The primary function of the paraspinous musculature is to stabilize the spinal column, rather than to effect motion. An exception to this is the action of the erector spinae muscles when arising from a forward flexed position. In general, any imbalance of muscular forces causes movement about an axis. Conversely, a balancing of muscle and other intrinsic forces about an axis results in no net movement. The ventral abdominal musculature is critical in counterbalancing the erector spinae muscles to provide stability.[2] It has been suggested that neuromuscular control of abdominal muscle tone may provide stability, thus reducing the need for reflex muscle contraction.

Rib cage

The rib cage, acting as a barrel attached to the spine, adds significant stability to the upper and middle thoracic segments. Both the costovertebral and costosternal joints are essential to this contribution (Figure 6.11).

Spinal alignment

A perfectly straight spine would theoretically be an ideal axial loading spinal configuration. It, however, would tolerate eccentric loads poorly and would provide limited flexibility. The spine has, therefore, evolved to adopt a curvilinear sagittal conformation – with a primary kyphotic thoracic curve, compensated by secondary cervical and lumbar lordotic curves of equal summative magnitude. This results in a balanced configuration that is necessary for a bipedal upright posture (Figure 6.12). Any increase in thoracic kyphosis (or loss of lumbar lordosis) leads to an increased moment arm (i.e. perpendicular distance from the IAR to the gravitational force vector), generating a greater bending moment at each vertebral segment (Figure 6.13). The moment arm (M) is equal to the force (F) multiplied by its perpendicular distance (D) from the IAR ($M = F \times D$). The greater the deformity, the greater the moment arm length. Hence, "Deformity begets deformity." The same mechanism applies to deformities in the coronal plane (scoliosis).

Spinal instability

Definition

Instability is the inability to limit excessive or abnormal spinal displacement in any plane. The term "excessive" underlies the difficulty in quantifying abnormal displacement. The extensive literature on acute spinal instability clearly illustrates the difficulties associated with such a definition process.[1,3–7]

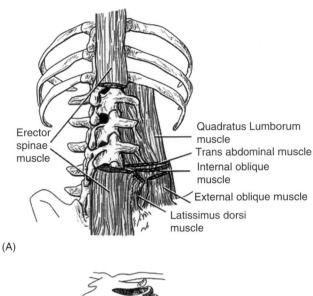

(A)

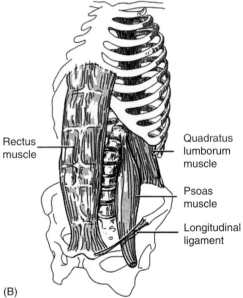

(B)

Figure 6.10 The effects of muscles on stability. (A) Muscles provide stability by virtue of the orientation of their attachments to the spine. (B) In some situations, as with the rectus abdominis muscle, the muscle may influence spinal movement indirectly (i.e. without direct attachment to the spine). Similarly, this muscle (as well as others) may stabilize the spine by balancing opposing muscle function, thus resulting in no movement. A significant degree of stability is thus provided. Lateral bending is achieved via the contraction of muscles attached to the lateral aspect of the spine; for example, the quadratus lumborum, attached to the right and the left muscle actions likewise results in no movement. (Reprinted by permission. See full reference on p. 95.)

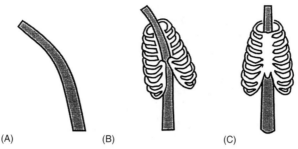

Figure 6.11 An illustration of the stability provided to the spine by the rib cage. (A) The spine without a rib cage can bend excessively. (B) The addition of the rib cage moderately increases stability. (C) Sternal attachments are required for achievement of the full stabilization potential of the rib cage. Removal of the effects of either the sternum or the ribs causes a significant diminution of stability. (Reprinted by permission. See full reference on p. 95.)

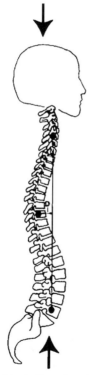

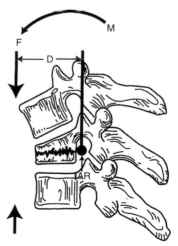

Figure 6.12 A kyphotic posture (as is present in the thoracic spine) increases the length of the natural moment arm (D) and thus, the magnitude of the bending moment resulting from an eccentrically placed (with respect to the IAR) axial load (*arrows*). (Reprinted by permission. See full reference on p. 95.)

Figure 6.13 A depiction of the injury force vector causing a ventral wedge compression fracture. F: applied force vector; D: length of moment arm (from IAR to plane of F); M: bending moment. (Reprinted by permission. See full reference on p. 95.)

Table 6.1 Instability categorization scheme.

Acute instability
- Overt instability
- Limited instability

Chronic instability
- Glacial instability
- Dysfunctional segment motion

Classification

Many classification schemes of instability have been introduced over the last few decades. In general, instability is referred to as either acute or chronic (Table 6.1). As previously discussed, instability is not an all-or-none phenomenon, but rather an array of increments, ranging from stable to grossly unstable. Moreover, acute instability can be described as overt or limited. Both of these (more commonly overt) may progress to a more chronic state if left unattended. Acute instability is most frequently encountered in traumatic, infectious, and/or neoplastic conditions. Chronic instability may, as previously suggested, be a sequela of an acute process, but may also result from degenerative changes. Chronic instability may be subdivided into glacial instability (in which the deformity progresses slowly, like the motion of a glacier), and/or dysfunctional segment motion. In the latter, there is no progression of deformity, but rather a pain syndrome generated by "dysfunctional motion." This is synonymous with mechanical instability. The focus of this chapter is on the subdivisions of acute instability, particularly in the context of trauma.

Overt instability

Overt instability is defined as the inability of the spine to support the torso during normal activity. For such instability to occur, a loss of vertebral body or disk integrity must be combined with a loss of integrity of the dorsal elements. This results in a circumferential loss of spinal integrity. Loss of ventral column integrity, as is observed with wedge compression or burst fractures, can be readily illustrated with lateral plain radiographs and sagittal computerized tomography (CT) or magnetic resonance imaging (MRI). The loss of dorsal integrity may be more challenging to assess. Plain films or sagittal tomograms may show splaying of the spinous processes or frank dorsal element fractures. Dorsal pathology may also be noted on clinical examination by pain on palpation or loss of midline soft tissue definition (Figure 6.14). MRI, especially sagittal T2 images, may be most useful in assessing dorsal ligamentous integrity.[8] The addition of fat suppression or short inversion time inversion recovery (STIR) sequences may offer even superior quality images.[9] Overt instability is synonymous with gross instability and should be treated surgically in nearly all cases.

Limited instability

Limited instability is defined as the loss of either ventral or dorsal spinal integrity, with the preservation of the other. Such is sufficient to support

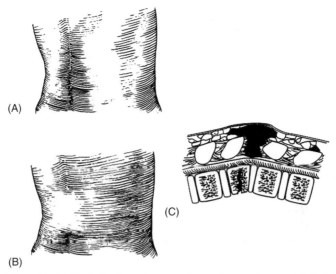

(A)

(B)

(C)

Figure 6.14 Dorsal instability in the thoracic and lumbar region can be suggested, particularly in thin patients, by physical examination. (A) The presence of tenderness over the spinous processes or the absence of the normal midline crease, (B) on account of swelling or hematoma formation below the skin, (C) suggests underlying soft tissue injury. This, in turn, suggests but does not prove the presence of dorsal spinal instability. (Reprinted by permission. See full reference on p. 95.)

most normal activities. Isolated laminar fractures or ligamentous disruption (as illustrated on fat suppression T2) with intact ventral elements are such an example. Conversely, isolated wedge or burst vertebral fractures, with preserved integrity of dorsal elements, are considered as constituting "limited" instability. Occasionally, underestimation of dorsal ligamentous injury may lead to overt instability being mistaken for limited instability. This is less likely if MRI is used liberally. Dynamic flexion/extension radiographs may also be useful in the context of limited instability (see criteria in further discussion). Dynamic radiographs may be misleading when guarding is present, and may even be dangerous when underlying overt instability is present. Clinical judgment must guide the use of such imaging. Limited instability is usually managed non-operatively with bracing. Surgery may be indicated if there is a significant risk of chronic instability.

Spine fractures (classification, mechanism, and associated instability)

Fracture classification

Spinal fracture classification is a formidable topic that can comprise an entire book. Fractures may be classified by spinal column involvement, or by mechanism of injury. Cervical fractures and dislocations are addressed in a later chapter and, therefore, are not addressed here.

Spinal column classification

Spinal column classifications are usually devised in an attempt to "visualize" complex fractures in a simple, yet meaningful anatomical fashion. The "column" concept is clinically useful since it facilitates the conceptualization and categorization of case-specific phenomena. Louis[10] suggested that the spine bears loads through three columns – the vertebral body and both facet joint complexes. Although this is true, his theory addresses only axial load transmission, and is limited in its ability to assess distraction, flexion, and extension components of injury. In addition, it does not address the integrity of ligamentous structures. Holdsworth[11] and Kelly[12] had initially suggested a two-column concept (ventral and dorsal). This theory provided specific information regarding angular deformation. In his seminal article, Kelly describes the two columns as: "one of solid bone and one composed of neural arches … Working together, these two columns support the body's weight."[12] He also points to the importance of the dorsal ligamentous complex in the assessment of overall stability.

In his three-column theory, Denis[13] introduces the concept of a middle column, containing the dorsal vertebral body, posterior longitudinal ligament, and dorsal annulus fibrosus (Figure 6.15). Depending on the constellation of column injuries, he identified four fracture types: compression, burst, seat-belt type, and fracture dislocation (Table 6.2).

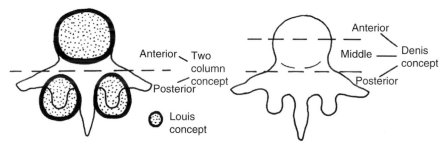

Figure 6.15 The "column" concepts of spinal stability. The concept described by Louis (*left*) assigns significance to the vertebral body and the facet joint complexes (lateral masses) on either side of the dorsal spine. Denis's three-column concept (*right*) assigns significance to the region of the neutral axis and the integrity of the posterior vertebral body wall (the middle column). The two-column construct (*left*) relies on anatomically defined structures, the vertebral body (anterior column) and the posterior elements (posterior column). Denis's three-column concept (*right*) similarly relies on anatomically defined structures. (Reprinted by permission. See full reference on p. 95.)

Table 6.2 Basic modes of failure of the three columns in the four types of spinal injuries.[13]

	Columns		
Types of fracture	Anterior	Middle	Posterior
Compression	Compression	None	None or severe distraction
Burst	Compression	Compression	None
"Seatbelt"	None or compression	Distraction	Distraction
Fracture-dislocation	Compression rotation shear		Distraction rotation shear

The middle column allows for the specific assessment of the neutral axis. The neutral axis (not to be confused with the neutral zone), is that longitudinal region of the spinal column that bears a significant portion of the axial load, and about which spinal element distraction or compression does not excessively occur with flexion or extension (Figure 6.16). The IAR is generally located within the neutral axis. It has been suggested that compromise of any two of the three columns constitutes an unstable fracture.

Mechanism of injury classification

The most widely discussed mechanistic scheme is the AO classification.[14] The AO classification breaks fractures down by types, which are further subdivided by groups, subgroups, and specifications. This classification scheme is extensive and provides categories for the majority of spine fractures. Mechanism of injury is deduced by plain radiographs and CT, with attention paid to both bony and ligamentous integrity. The dorsal ligamentous complex is indirectly assessed and interpreted as being intact or deficient. This classification scheme breaks down injuries into three fundamental categories (using the two-column theory). Type A are ventral column injuries resulting from axial loading with or without flexion (Table 6.3). Type B are ventral and dorsal column injury from flexion or extension, with distraction (Table 6.4). Type C are ventral and dorsal column injury from rotational forces (Table 6.5).

Type A injuries are subdivided into impaction fractures (wedge), split fracture (including pincer), and burst fractures. Type B injuries are subdivided into ligamentous flexion distraction (ligamentous Chance fracture), bony-flexion distraction (bony Chance fracture), and hyperextension shear injury. Type C injuries are subdivided into rotation plus Type A, rotation plus Type B and rotational shear.

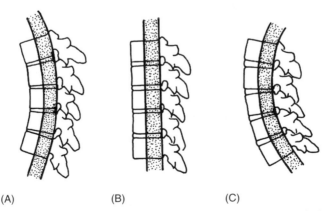

(A) (B) (C)

Figure 6.16 The depiction of the neutral axis (*shaded areas*). The neutral axis is the longitudinal region of the spinal column that bears much of the axial load and about which spinal element distraction or compression does not significantly occur with the assumption of (A) flexed, (B) neutral, or (C) extension postures. This is a dynamic and theoretical concept. (Reprinted by permission. See full reference on p. 95.)

Type A fractures are considered to have intact dorsal bony and ligamentous integrity, while Type B and C do not. It has been suggested that MRI may improve the reproducibility of the AO classification scheme.[15,16] Attempts to classify fractures based purely on MRI findings correlates poorly with the AO scheme.[15]

Table 6.3 AO classification. Type A injuries: groups and subgroups.[14]

Type A: Vertebral body compression
A1 Impaction fractures
    A1.1 Endplate impaction
    A1.2 Wedge impaction features
    A1.3 Vertebral body collapse
A2 Split fractures
    A2.1 Sagittal split fracture
    A2.2 Coronal split fracture
    A2.3 Pincer fracture
A3 Burst fractures
    A3.1 Incomplete burst fracture
    A3.2 Burst split fracture
    A3.3 Complete burst fracture

Table 6.4 AO classification. Type B injuries: groups and subgroups.[14]

Type B: Anterior and posterior element injury with distraction
B1 Posterior disruption predominantly ligamentous (flexion-distraction injury)
    B1.1 With transverse disruption of the disk
    B1.2 With Type A fracture of the vertebral body
B2 Posterior disruption predominantly osseous (flexion–distraction injury)
    B2.1 Transverse bicolumn fracture
    B2.2 With disruption of the disk
    B2.3 With Type A fracture of the vertebral body
B3 Anterior disruption through the disk (hyperextension-shear injury)
    B3.1 Hyperextension-subluxations
    B3.2 Hyperextension-spondylolysis
    B3.3 Posterior dislocation

Table 6.5 AO classification. Type C injuries: groups and subgroups.[14]

Type C: Anterior and posterior element injury with rotation
C1 Type A injuries with rotation (compression injuries with rotation)
    C1.1 Rotational wedge fracture
    C1.2 Rotational split fracture
    C1.3 Rotational burst fracture
C2 Type B injuries with rotation (distraction injuries with rotation)
    C2.1 B1 injuries with rotation (flexion–distraction injuries with rotation)
    C2.2 B2 injuries with rotation (flexion–distraction injuries with rotation)
    C2.3 B3 injuries with rotation (hyperextension–shear injuries with rotation)
C3 Rotational-shear injuries
    C3.1 Slice fracture
    C3.2 Oblique fracture

It has been suggested that describing fractures in such an onerous fashion (e.g. Type B2.3.2), although highly appropriate for research, may not be most suitable for clinical decision-making and discussion. It may perhaps be more appropriate to simply describe the injury mechanism (compression, distraction, translation/rotation, with or without burst), integrity of dorsal ligamentous complex, and neurological status.[17] An associated point system can easily be built in to assess stability and guide treatment approach (see later discussion).

Fracture mechanism

The configuration and mechanism of a spine fracture can be determined by understanding the magnitude and direction of the force vector in relationship to the IAR. Compressive forces applied ventral to the IAR often result in wedge compression fractures. Pure axial loading (i.e. in line with the IAR) results in a pure burst fracture. Distraction forces placed dorsal to the IAR result in a ligamentous or bony Chance fracture, while a compressive force in that same area (behind the IAR) results in a hyperextension-shear injury. The extent of the fracture depends on the magnitude of the bending moment, which is proportional to both the magnitude and the perpendicular distance of force application in relation to the IAR (moment arm). Likewise, an alteration of the IAR, as observed for example in a kyphotic deformity, can significantly affect the bending moment.

The amount of bony disruption may be predicted by the stress/strain curve (Figure 6.17). When assessing a spinal segment as a complex composed of bone, disk and ligaments, most of the initial strain is dissipated

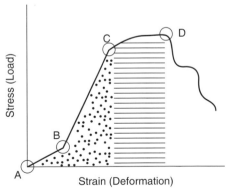

Figure 6.17 A typical stress/strain curve for a biological tissue, such as a ligament. AB, the neutral zone. BC, the elastic zone. When the elastic limit (yield point) (C) is reached, permanent deformation can occur (permanent set). CD, the plastic zone where a permanent set occurs. Past D, failure occurs and the load diminishes. Hashed plus dotted area represents strength, whereas the dotted area represents resilience. (Reprinted by permission. See full reference on p. 95.)

through the ligaments and disk. This is referred to as the neutral zone. Once the maximal strain capacity of the neutral zone is reached, the tissues are then deformed according to Hooke's law, which states that for small displacements, the size of deformation is proportional to the deforming force. The magnitude of this "elastic zone" is dependent on the elastic modulus of each specific tissue, and is obviously greater for ligaments than bone. Once the elastic limit is reached, any further stress application results in permanent deformation (i.e. plastic zone), until failure occurs. After damage has occurred, the segment is left in a state of relative laxity, with an expanded neutral zone. This increase in the neutral zone is synonymous with segmental instability.

In an attempt to surgically stabilize fractures, the surgeon must first assess the weight-bearing capacity of the ventral column. Elements such as the extent of comminution, dispersion of comminuted fragments, and angular deformation may be indicative of this axial weight-bearing capacity.[18]

Ventral wedge compression fractures

Wedge compression fractures are a product of forced flexion with axial loading, resulting in a compressive force vector placed ventral to the IAR located in the neutral axis (within the middle column of Denis) (Figure 6.13). The resultant bending moment generates compression of the vertebral elements ventral to the IAR with preservation, or even distraction, of dorsal elements. The dorsal distraction is not significant, and is well resisted by the dorsal ligamentory complex. Segments of the spine that are in a naturally kyphotic posture, such as thoracic and thoracolumbar regions, are predisposed to wedge compression fractures. They are biomechanically disadvantaged by a ventral gravitational bending moment. The thoracolumbar junction is at especially high risk, since it interfaces between two relatively solid segments – the thoracic segment and rib cage rostrally, and the relatively unyielding lumbar segment caudally.

Burst fractures

True burst fractures are the product of pure axial loading and no eccentric load application outside of the IAR (i.e. no or minimal bending moment) (Figure 6.18). Any eccentric load placement results in an angular deformity (ventral or lateral compression wedge). Burst fractures result in a pancaking of the vertebral body, with the cortical cylinder "bursting" outwards and often into the spinal canal. Burst fractures occur most commonly in segments where the IAR is located along the anatomic "plumb-line," as the gravitational force vector passes through their respective IARs. This is most commonly observed in the upper and middle cervical and lumbar spine, although cervical flexibility often results in eccentric load placement.

Burst fractures compromise both the anterior and middle columns of Denis,[13] suggesting instability. However, most burst fractures are not overtly unstable,

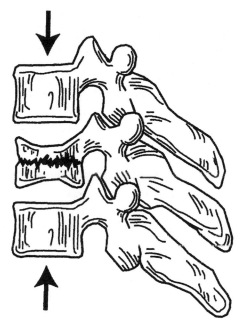

Figure 6.18 The mechanism of injury of a burst fracture: true axial loading without a bending moment ($D = 0$). (Reprinted by permission. See full reference on p. 95.)

since the dorsal elements are preserved. Non-operative management may suffice if no neurological compromise exists.

Flexion–distraction (Chance) fractures

Flexion–distraction load applications are much less common than axial (concentric or eccentric) loads. This requires a force vector directed both ventrally and rostrally. The most common mode of this type of force vector application is in deceleration injuries, where there patient is restrained by a single lap belt (Figure 6.19). The injury most commonly affects the cervical and upper thoracic spine. This fracture was first described by Chance in 1948.[19] A Chance fracture may occur through a bony cleavage plane, or through the vertebral end-plate. Conversely, the force vector may be directed dorsally in distraction, as observed in hyperextension-shear injuries (see AO Type B3). Overall, flexion–distraction-type fractures are considered overtly unstable, as they involve both the ventral and dorsal columns.

Dorsal element fracture

Dorsal element fractures are akin to wedge compression fracture, but with the load application dorsal to the IAR – as seen with hyperextension injury with axial loading. This is most commonly observed in the cervical spine and results in laminar, spinous process, and/or facet fractures.

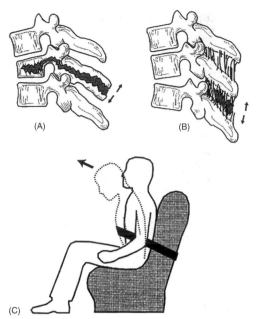

(A)

(B)

(C)

Figure 6.19 There are two fundamental types of Chance (flexion–distraction) fracture. (A) Diastasis fracture through the pedicles and vertebral body. (B) Fracture through the vertebral endplate or disk. (C) The mechanism of injury is depicted. (Reprinted by permission. See full reference on p. 95.)

Criteria for fracture instability

Classifying spine fractures as stable or unstable is like determining whether an object is black or white, when in fact it may be a shade of gray. In an attempt to employ this dichotomous scheme, one must often agree to disagree. In reality, the key issue is in determining which fractures are overtly unstable and require surgical stabilization, and which fractures have limited instability but have a high likelihood of chronic progression and should also be treated surgically – versus which fractures are grossly stable and may simply be treated with an external orthosis.

As a prelude, it is noteworthy that all fractures, independent of column involvement or mechanism of injury that impinge upon neural elements should be considered as candidates for a decompressive procedure. An exception to this may be the case of a complete cord lesion, where neurological recovery is highly unlikely.

Fractures involving both ventral and dorsal columns should be considered overtly unstable and often require surgical stabilization. With the AO classification scheme,[14] this applies to all non-Type A fractures. This approach to surgical stabilization is discussed in the next chapter. The Denis 3-column classification[13] may lead to confusion in this specific instance, since it considers the involvement of both the anterior and middle columns as a sign of instability. Suffice it to say that these fractures are not overtly unstable. Optimal management is, at this time, still controversial.

AO Type A fractures involve only anterior column compromise and are considered to be associated with "limited instability." Conversely, isolated posterior longitudinal complex disruptions, as documented on MRI, are minimally unstable.

The main difficulty arises in determining which fractures with limited instability have a significant risk of chronic deformity progression and/or neurological compromise. It may be useful in these cases to compile all predisposing risk factors for instability in the form of a point system, or checklist criteria. Most "point systems" attempt to objectify stability (or lack of thereof) by assigning relative scores to the involved column, the amount of resting (static) and dynamic displacement (both angular and transitional), the amount of neural element injury, as well as the circumstances surrounding the patient at hand. In White and Panjabi's point system[1] (Table 6.6), a score of 5 or more is suggestive of overt instability, while a score of 2 to 4 is suggestive of limited instability. The corresponding translation and angulation cut-offs for resting and dynamic films have been compiled in Table 6.7 for cervical, thoracic, and lumbar levels. These

Table 6.6 Quantitation of acute instability for subaxial cervical, thoracic, and lumbar injuries.[1]

Condition	Points assigned
Loss of integrity of anterior (and middle) column	2
Loss of integrity of posterior column(s)	2
Acute resting translational deformity	2
Acute resting angulational deformity	2
Acute dynamic translational deformity exaggeration	2
Acute dynamic angulational deformity exaggeration	2
Neural element injury	3
Acute disk narrowing at level of suspected pathology	1
Dangerous loading anticipated	1

Table 6.7 Resting and dynamic radiological guidelines.[1]

	Resting	Dynamic
Subaxial cervical spine	>3.5 mm displacement >11 degree angulation	>3.5 mm translation >20 degree angulation
Thoracic spine	>2.5 mm displacement >5 degree angulation	
Lumbar spine	>4.5 mm displacement >22 degree angulation	>4.5 mm translation >15 degree L1-L4 >20 degree L4-L5 >25 degree L5-S1

values arise from cadaveric biomechanical studies, as well as meta-analyses of normal physiological values.[1]

A more recent point system attempts to guide surgical versus non-surgical management.[17] In this scheme, points are assigned to injury mechanism, neurological involvement, and compromise of the posterior ligamentous complex.

As useful as these point systems may be, the spine surgeon must still rely on common sense, combined with clinical astuteness.

References

1 White AA, Panjabi MM (eds). *Clinical Biomechanics of the Spine*, 2nd edn. Lippincott, Philadelphia, 1990, pp. 30–643.

2 Garner-Morse MG, Stokes AF. The effects of abdominal muscle coactivation on lumbar spine stability. *Spine* 1998;23:86–92.

3 Cope R, Kilcoyne RF, Gaines RW. The thoracolumbar burst fracture with intact posterior elements. Implications for neurologic deficit and stability. *Neuro-Orthopedics* 1989; 7:83–87.

4 Holdsworth FW. Fractures, dislocations, and fracture-dislocations of the spine. *J Bone Joint Surg* 1970;52A:1534–1551.

5 White III AA, Panjabi MM. Update on the evaluation of instability of the lower cervical spine. *Instr Course Lect* 1987;36:513–520.

6 Aulisa L, Di Segni F, Tamburrelli F, *et al*. Surgical management of instability of the lumbar spine. *Rays* 2000;25(1):105–114.

7 Benzel EC (ed.). *Biomechanics of Spine Stabilization*. AANS Publication, Rolling Meadows, IL, 2001, pp. 29–82.

8 Benzel EC, Hart BL, Ball PA, *et al*. Magnetic resonance imaging for the evaluation of patients with occult cervical spine injury. *J Neurosurg* 1996;85:824–829.

9 Saifuddin A. MRI of acute spine trauma. *Skeletal Radiol* 2001; 30:237–246.

10 Louis R. Spinal stability as defined by the three-column spine concept. *Anat Clin* 1985; 7:33–42.

11 Holdsworth FW. Fractures, dislocations, and fracture-dislocations of the spine. *J Bone Joint Surg* 1963;45B:6–20.

12 Kelly RP, Whitesides TE. Treatment of lumbodorsal fracture-dislocations. *Ann Surg* 1968;167:705–717.

13 Denis F. The three column spine and its significance in the classification of acute thoracolumbar spinal injuries. *Spine* 1983;8:817–831.

14 Magerl E, Aebi M, Gertzbein SD, *et al*. A comprehensive classification of thoracic and lumbar injuries. *Eu Spine J* 1994;3:184–201.

15 Oner FC, van Gils APG, Dhert WJA, *et al*. MRI findings of thoracolumbar spine fractures: a categorisation based on MRI examinations of 100 fractures. *Skeletal Radiol* 1999;28:433–443.

16 Saifuddin A, Noordeen H, Taylor BA, *et al*. The role of imaging in the diagnosis and management of thoracolumbar burst fractures: current concepts and a review of the literature. *Skeletal Radiol* 1996;25:603–613.

17 Vaccaro AR, Zeiller SC, Hulbert RJ, *et al*. The thoracolumbar injury severity score: a proposed treatment algorithm. *J Spinal Disord Tech* 2005;18:209–215.

18 McCormack T, Karaikovic E, Gaines RW. The load sharing classification of spine fractures. *Spine* 1994;19:1741–1744.

19 Chance CQ. Note on a type of flexion fracture of the spine. *Br J Radiol* 1948;21:452–453.

CHAPTER 7

Principles of spine stabilization

G. Alexander Jones, Eric P. Roger and Edward C. Benzel

All figures in this chapter taken from Benzel, EC. *Biomechanics of Spine Stabilization*. New York: Thieme; 2001. Reprinted by permission.

Introduction

The surgical management of a patient with a spine injury includes neural decompression as well as stabilization of the vertebral column. The latter includes either the treatment of acute, overt instability (as discussed in the previous chapter), or the treatment of limited instability for the management or prevention of deformity, and/or the treatment of persistent pain. This chapter addresses the biomechanical concerns associated with achieving spinal stability. In clinical practice, the concerns for protection of neurological function may necessarily cause the surgeon to modify or supplant an intervention that was designed solely to attain or preserve stability.

Principles of stabilization by spinal level

The occipitocervical junction

The occipitocervical junction differs from all other regions of the spine, both regarding the significant motion it allows, and its unique anatomic features. This combination creates the setting for a variety of injuries. The goal in treating spinal instability at any level is to restore stability with a minimum loss of motion. This is especially important at the occipitocervical junction, since these segments permit significant mobility. Because of both of these factors, namely the mobility and unique anatomy, solid bony arthrodesis can be difficult to achieve.

Ventral stabilization

Ventral stabilization of the occipitocervical junction, with the exception of odontoid screw fixation, is generally not indicated in the trauma setting. Anatomic barriers are significant. Sites for screw insertion and arthrodesis are usually inadequate. The infection risk with transoral approaches is high, as are the neurological exposure and visceral complications associated with the high extrapharyngeal approach (Figure 7.1).

Odontoid screw fixation for the treatment of type II odontoid fractures is by far the most common and popular ventral craniocervical and upper cervical spine stabilization technique.[1] It facilitates compression of the dens against

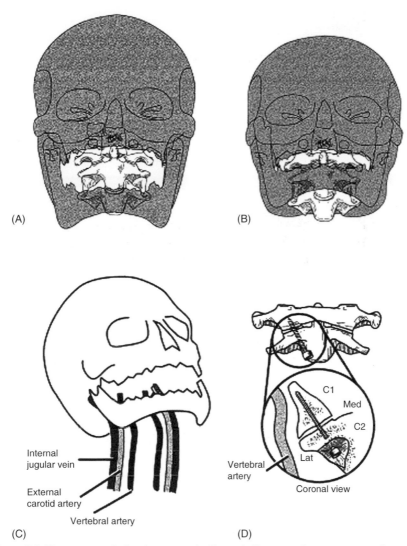

(A)

(B)

(C)

Internal
jugular vein

External
carotid artery

Vertebral artery

(D)

C1

Med

C2

Vertebral
artery

Lat

Coronal view

Figure 7.1 The upper cervical region poses significant challenges to the surgeon regarding ventral fixation. The factors involved include (A) risk of infection with transoral approaches, (A and B) the suboptimal trajectory with transoral and extrapharyngeal approaches, (C) juxtaposed vascular and neural structures, and (D) the adequacy of bone in which to place screws. (Reprinted by permission. See full reference on p. 116.)

the body of the axis via use of the lag screw effect (Figure 7.2). Increased compression across a fusion bed (as opposed to onlay fusion), according to Wolff's law, leads to greater chance of arthrodesis. The following anatomical factors are relative contraindications for this technique: (1) old fractures in which a fibrous nonunion has developed are associated with suboptimal

(A)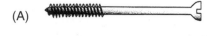

(B)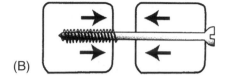

(C)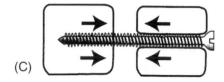

Figure 7.2 The partially threaded screw (lag screw) can be used to achieve a lag effect (A and B), which can also be achieved by overdrilling the proximal bone and using a fully threaded screw (C). (Reprinted by permission. See full reference on p. 116.)

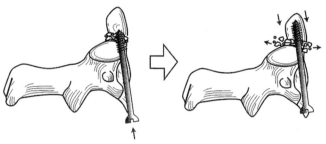

Figure 7.3 Comminuted fractures of the dens or rostral C2 body do not allow the application of significant compression forces to the bone fragments. This is so because they are displaced rather than compressed, as depicted. (Reprinted by permission. See full reference on p. 116.)

arthrodesis rates; (2) diagonal fractures predispose to angulation and translation of the bone fragments during compression; and (3) significantly comminuted fractures (type IIA) do not allow for a proper compression effect, with further dispersion of the fragments with compression (Figure 7.3).

Dorsal stabilization

Dorsal craniocervical stabilization includes techniques for occipitocervical fixation, atlantoaxial fixation, and the caudal extension of each. These techniques include wires, clamps, hooks, screws, and plates. The latter three are available in many universal spine instrumentation systems.

Wires and cables have been employed for occipitocervical region fixation for some time. In general, cables are stronger and more resistant to fatigue failure than wires. The Gallie technique is relatively poor at preventing flexion, extension, lateral bending, and rotation compared to the Brooks technique, clamps, and transarticular screw fixation.[2] Wires have a tendency to "cheese-cut"

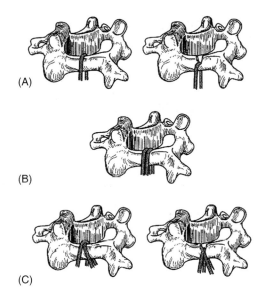

Figure 7.4 Wires and cables can "cheese-cut" through bone (A). This is related in part to its relatively small surface area of contact with bone. This can be effectively doubled if parallel wires or cables are used (B). If the wires are crossed at their contact point with bone, this effect is diminished (C). (Reprinted by permission. See full reference on p. 116.)

(A)

(B)

(C)

through bone, especially osteoporotic bone. Using double wires minimizes, but does not eliminate, this risk (Figure 7.4). Spinous process wiring acts as an effective tension band, but provides little stability in any other plane (e.g. axial loading) (Figure 7.5).

Dorsal atlantoaxial fixation may be accomplished via several methods. Transarticular screw fixation may be used in the setting of laminectomy, and provides significant resistance against translation and rotation. Segmental C1–C2 fixation may also be used.[3] A variant of this technique employs translaminar screws at the C2 level; this has proven to be biomechanically equivalent.[4]

Occipitocervical fixation may be accomplished with the use of a Luque box and wiring, or with an occipital plate and caudal fixation with a universal spine system. Of note is that the best occipital implant–bone interface is located in the midline. However, if this is the only point of fixation, control over rotation is diminished (Figure 7.6). A securely fitting occipital plate (i.e. the plate is bent so that "rocking" is eliminated), minimizes such rotation.

Sub-axial cervical spine

The sub-axial cervical spine is anatomically less complicated than the occipitocervical junction. It does not possess the complex ligamentous and bony structures of the upper cervical region, and the structure of the vertebral bodies is relatively monotonous, as it is in the thoracic and lumbar regions. It is also readily accessible from both ventral and dorsal approaches, thus opening a wider range of surgical options.

The majority of traumatic spinal cord injuries (SCIs) in the United States are associated with cervical fracture–dislocations. Spine stabilization in this setting involves reduction of the deformity, followed by stabilization. Of patients who undergo an attempt at closed reduction, 26% fail to achieve reduction.[5] When

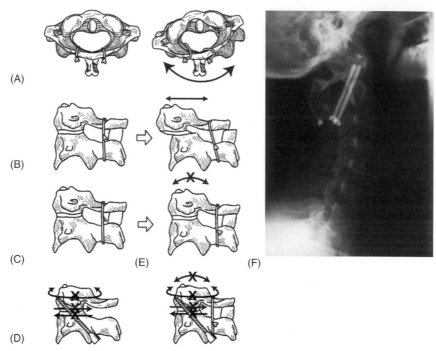

Figure 7.5 Dorsal C1–C2 wire fixation strategies resist rotation and translation poorly (A and B). They, however, resist flexion well. In addition, extension is resisted if a dorsal bone graft (spacer) is included in the construct (C). Pars interarticularis screws act as a cantilever and resist rotation (D) relatively well. Pars interarticularis screws may be augmented by C1–C2 wire fixation. This adds to the flexion and extension resistance (E). Such a construct is depicted in (F). (Reprinted by permission. See full reference on p. 116.)

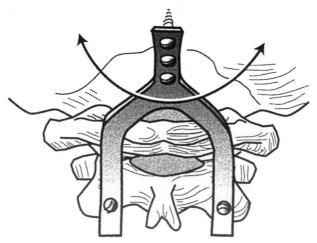

Figure 7.6 Midline occipital screw fixation provides solid fixation, but less than optimal rotation prevention ability. Because a single implant is used, a precise fit to lateral cervical spine fixation points may be suboptimal. (Reprinted by permission. See full reference on p. 116.)

reduction is accomplished, it is subsequently lost in 28% of those patients. Open reduction may be required in such cases, and can be performed either dorsally or ventrally.[6] Following this, arthrodesis and fixation are performed.

Ventral stabilization

Ventral cervical stabilization consists of corpectomy or discectomy, to provide spinal cord decompression or restore anatomic alignment, followed arthrodesis and plate application (Figure 7.7). This may be required for fracture–dislocation injuries (with disruption of anterior and posterior columns), or compression fracture (with disruption of the anterior and middle columns). Ventral stabilization without use of a plate, especially in the setting of flexion–distraction-type injuries, is associated with a high incidence of postoperative kyphosis.[5] If there is significant disruption of the dorsal structures (facet joints, ligaments), some form of dorsal tension-band fixation should be considered as well.

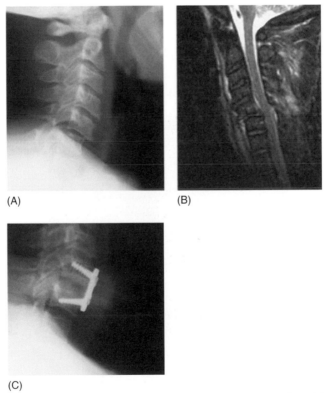

(A) (B)

(C)

Figure 7.7 The lateral radiograph (A) of a patient who had incurred a circumferential disruption of the spinal column 2 weeks before. Both subluxation and neural compression are demonstrated (A and B). This necessitated decompression (discectomy) reduction, fusion, and instrumentation (C). (Reprinted by permission. See full reference on p. 116.)

Dorsal stabilization

In flexion–distraction injuries without ventral spinal cord compression and without significant disruption of ventral bony and ligamentous stability, a dorsal stabilization procedure alone may be sufficient. This uses either polyaxial lateral mass screws with connecting rods, a lateral mass screw/plate system, or interspinous wiring. If a long-segment dorsal cervical construct is used, care should be taken to avoid placing the terminus at the cervicothoracic junction (Figure 7.8). Extending the construct caudally to the T2 or T3 level will significantly reduce the stress placed on the junction, and thereby

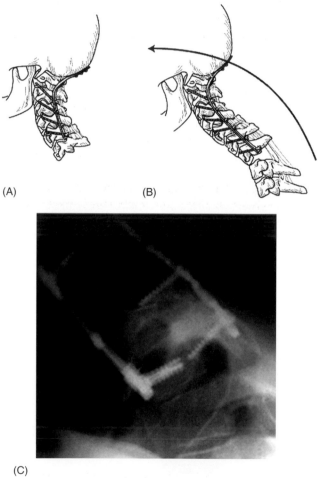

(A)   (B)

(C)

Figure 7.8 Occipitocervical constructs can be extended caudally to C5 or C6 without significant concern (A). However, extension to C7 places a significant stress on the cervical thoracic junction, potentially resulting in a junctional instability (B). This concept is illustrated by a case of a 20-year-old male who was "instrumented" to C7. A progressive kyphosis ensued (C). (Reprinted by permission. See full reference on p. 116.)

the chance of postoperative deformity. This occurs at the expense of some mobility.

Thoracic spine

The thoracic spine is the most stable portion because of its firm attachment to the rib cage. Operative management for the restoration of stability in the acute setting is seldom required, though neural decompression may be. Open treatment is generally reserved for progressive kyphosis or intractable pain. Dorsal stabilization of the thoracic spine generally involves a longer segment, since mobility is not an issue. Care must be taken to avoid placing the terminus of a construct at the apex of the natural thoracic kyphosis, which is generally around T6, lest an iatrogenic deformity may result (Figure 7.9). A variety of techniques for ventral stabilization exist as well, although the approaches are usually more involved.

Thoracolumbar junction

The thoracolumbar junction is especially prone to trauma (Figure 7.10). It is a junctional region bounded rostrally by the thoracic spine (which can apply a significant bending moment on account of its rigid nature across a great length) and caudally by the lumbar spine (which is composed of vertebrae of greater size and strength).

McCormack and Gaines documented the factors that may predispose a fracture of the thoracolumbar junction to develop progressive kyphosis postoperatively.[7]

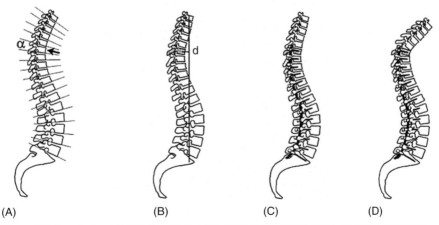

(A)   (B)   (C)   (D)

Figure 7.9 An apical vertebra is the vertebra in a curve (in any plane) that is associated with the greatest angle (α) between adjacent vertebrae of all vertebra in the curve (A). This vertebra and adjacent disk interspaces are exposed to significant stresses because of the application of a bending moment (length *d*) (B). Extending a long construct up to, but not beyond, an apical vertebra exaggerates this effect (C) and causes a tendency toward further deformation (D). (Reprinted by permission. See full reference on p. 116.)

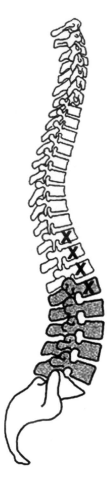

Figure 7.10 The vulnerability of the thoracolumbar region (*Xs*) to trauma is related to the relatively small size of the vertebral bodies (compared to the lumbar region (*shaded areas*)), the absence of protection from the rib cage, and its kyphotic posture. This causes a significant bending moment to be applied to relatively weak and unprotected vertebra. (Reprinted by permission. See full reference on p. 116.)

Injuries that are associated with a substantial disruption of spinal stability require extensive (longer) spinal instrumentation constructs (i.e. three levels above and two below the injured level). Often, the fracture pattern, as well as the location and degree of neural element compromise, dictates the surgical approach in this region. With ventral dural sac compression at the level of the spinal cord or the conus medullaris, such as with a burst fracture, a ventral approach for decompression is advised. This may be followed by the placement of an interbody strut. One of a variety of ventral and ventrolateral plates may be used to span the operated levels. Alternatively, patients with an extension–distraction injury and fractured dorsal elements may benefit from a dorsal approach, since the dura mater and/or neural elements may be "caught" between laminar fragments. This is especially true at the level of the cauda equina. In patients without neurological deficit, thoracolumbar fractures that are generally stable are amenable to nonoperative management.

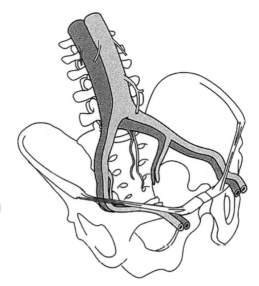

Figure 7.11 Ventral exposure of the low lumbar and lumbosacral regions are limited by visceral (predominantly vascular) structures. The pelvic brim poses an obstacle to low lateral retroperitoneal exposures, as depicted. (Reprinted by permission. See full reference on p. 116.)

Lumbar and lumbosacral spine

The lower lumbar (L3 and below) region and the lumbosacral junction are less frequently involved with traumatic spine injuries. However, they are susceptible to degenerative changes, as well as pathological fractures resulting from malignancy. Ventrolateral access to this region may be hampered by the iliac wing, and ventral access carries the risk of damage to the aorta, vena cava, and proximal iliac vessels (Figure 7.11). Additionally, ventral access to the lumbosacral junction in men carries at least some risk of retrograde ejaculation. Nevertheless, ventral stabilization can often employ a shorter-segment construct than would be required for equivalent stability with a dorsal construct.

Timing of stabilization

The two main goals of surgery in spinal trauma are decompression of neurological elements, and stabilization of a destabilized segment. Timing of stabilization is most often dictated by the need for decompression, but may be limited by the patient's condition, especially in the context of multi-system trauma.

In the context of limited instability, where only one of the columns is compromised, decompression may further destabilize the affected segment by creating a circumferential instability. In such cases, stabilization procedures are indicated. Failure to do so may lead to further neurological compromise, pain, or progressive deformity.

In complete spinal cord lesions, it is highly unlikely that decompression would lead to return of function, even though bony fragments may be severely distorting the neural elements.[8] Therefore, urgent decompression and stabilization is rarely indicated. Early surgery, however, may facilitate earlier mobilization and aggressive spinal rehabilitation. Earlier mobilization may reduce bed rest-induced complications including, but not limited to, pulmonary complications, venous thrombosis, and decubitus ulcers. Furthermore, stabilization of complete SCIs may reduce pain and offer improved sagittal alignment,[9] thus facilitating activities of daily living and wheelchair use.

Finally, limited instability, or unrecognized overt instability, may lead to chronic or glacial instability with subsequent progressive deformity, pain, and/or neurological dysfunction. In such cases, delayed stabilization may be required.

Role of orthotic devices

As stated previously, the goals of management in the setting of spinal cord and vertebral column injury are twofold: adequate decompression of neural elements and stabilization of the vertebral column. External splinting may serve as a primary means of achieving the latter, or as a useful adjunct to operative treatment. This section considers the use of orthotics strictly from the standpoint of instability. If operative neural decompression is indicated, such clearly must be considered a higher priority.

Fundamental properties of spinal bracing

Prior to an in depth consideration of the various types of orthotics, one must first consider some of the fundamental properties and limitations of spinal bracing.

First, the efficacy of external immobilization is inversely proportional to the distance between the spinal column and the inner surface of the brace (Figure 7.12). Thus, more effective immobilization may be achieved in regions where

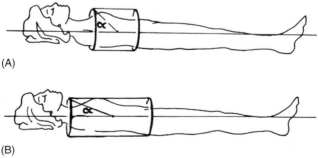

(A)

(B)

Figure 7.12 The effectiveness of spinal bracing is inversely related to the axial distance between the spine and the inner surface of the brace. This is theoretically defined by the following relationship: efficacy of bracing is related to the cosine of α in which α is the angle defined by the edge of the brace, the instantaneous axis of rotation at the unstable segment, and the long axis of the spine. This angle is dictated by both the length of the brace and the thickness of tissue between the spine and the inner surface of the brace. A short brace ($\alpha = 45$ degrees; cosine $\alpha = 0.707$) (A). A long brace ($\alpha = 15$ degrees; cosine $\alpha = 0.966$) (B). Obviously, a significant reduction of efficacy comes with the use of a shorter, wider brace; that is, the length-to-width ratio of the brace is too small. (Reprinted by permission. See full reference on p. 116.)

this distance is relatively small, as in the cervical spine. Conversely, the lumbosacral region is considerably more difficult to stabilize with splinting because of the significant amount of soft tissue between the spinal column and the brace.

Second, splinting of a long bone fracture involves immobilization of one joint proximal and one joint distal to the site of injury. While this does not apply directly to the vertebral column, an analogy can be made as follows: the "long bones" are the cranium, the cervical spine, the thoracic spine, the lumbar spine, and the sacro-pelvic complex, and the "joints" may be considered the boundaries or junctions between each of these regions (Figure 7.13). This leads to the observation that, in many circumstances, longer braces (which traverse more than one junction) offer greater stability than shorter braces. This is so because, in addition to immobilizing several junctional areas, the longer brace has the effect of decreasing the angle α over a shorter brace of the same length (Figure 7.12).

Cervical, cervicothoracic, and craniothoracic bracing

The cervical spine is, perhaps, the region of the spine that is most amenable to effective bracing. This is due to the relative paucity of soft tissue surrounding the vertebral column, as well as the availability of substantial points of fixation above and below (i.e. the cranium and the thoracic cage).

One unique attribute of the cervical spine is the significant difference in form and function between the occipitoaxial complex and the sub-axial portion. Because of this anatomic arrangement, complex movements of the neck are possible. From the standpoint of bracing, this implies that movement in the sagittal plane can occur in the sub-axial spine (true flexion–extension) or at the atlanto-occipital joint (capital flexion–extension, Figure 7.14). When a cervical spine brace is placed without sufficient points of fixation in the low cervical or

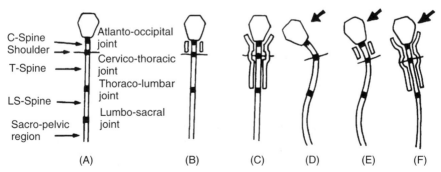

Figure 7.13 The consideration of the axial skeleton as consisting of five segments. The segments are depicted and defined (A). A cervical collar (B) and a brace embracing the mandible and the thoracic regions (C) are depicted. Responses to externally applied forces are depicted for the unbraced (D) and the collar (E) and extensively braced (F) spines. Note the relative augmentation of protection provided by longer braces. (Reprinted by permission. See full reference on p. 116.)

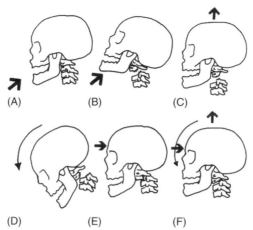

Figure 7.14 A very unstable hangman's fracture can be managed by application of a complex set of forces to the unstable segment. The fracture itself is a result of a hyperextension loading to failure (A). This usually results in a subluxation of C2 on C3 and disruption of the pars interarticularis of C2 (B). Neither simple distraction (C), capital flexion (D), nor true neck extension (E) alone provides adequate reduction. However, a combination of slight simple distraction, moderate capital flexion, and moderate true neck extension provides an optimal force complex application for reduction (F). Arrows depict forces and moments applied. (Reprinted by permission. See full reference on p. 116.)

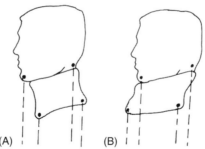

Figure 7.15 The parallelogram-like bracing effect is a unique aspect of cervical spine bracing that is associated with the combination of capital and true neck movements and the unique points of fixation available. When inadequate low cervical or thoracic fixation is attained, true neck flexion–extension is relatively unimpeded. Thus the compensatory relationship between the capital and the true neck movements is not significantly thwarted. In this case, low cervical flexion is accompanied by compensatory capital extension. This, in fact, may be encouraged somewhat by the brace itself (A). The converse is also true (B). The vertical dashed lines highlight these parallelogram movements. (Reprinted by permission. See full reference on p. 116.)

high thoracic region, a parallelogram-like effect may occur (Figure 7.15). This is a result of true flexion–extension being relatively unimpeded by the brace, with a compensatory movement (capital extension or flexion, respectively) at the atlanto-occipital joint. Fixation of the cervical spine with a more substantial

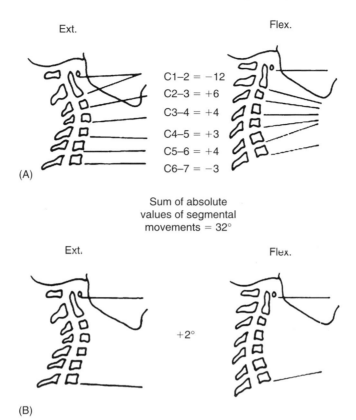

$$\begin{array}{ll}
\text{C1--2} = -12 \\
\text{C2--3} = +6 \\
\text{C3--4} = +4 \\
\text{C4--5} = +3 \\
\text{C5--6} = +4 \\
\text{C6--7} = -3
\end{array}$$

Ext. Flex.

(A)

Sum of absolute
values of segmental
movements = 32°

Ext. Flex.

+2°

(B)

Figure 7.16 The assessment of segmental movement at each individual level (in degrees) can be measured and calculated from flexion and extension radiographs. The total movement is the sum of angles. The overall movement between the cranium and the low cervical region (lowest segment assessed) is the measured movement. The difference is an objective assessment of snaking. The differences at segmental levels are depicted in this hypothetical example (A). "Ext." identifies the extension intersegmental angles, and "Flex." identifies the flexion intersegmental angles. The sum of angles is 32 degrees. The overall movement between the cranium and the lowest segment assessed is 2 degrees (B). Therefore, in this case, the objective measure of snaking is 30 degrees. (Reprinted by permission. See full reference on p. 116.)

thoracic component, or with rigid operative fixation, is the most effective way to eliminate this phenomenon.

Rigid fixation, however, introduces an additional problem; that is that of *snaking*. This term applies to a serpentine movement of the cervical spine, resulting from simple flexion or extension, when both the cranium and the thoracic cage are rigidly immobilized (Figure 7.16). This may be observed on lateral radiographs as small flexion or extension movements at each segmental level during an attempt at flexion or extension. The measurements of each of these movements, when added up, may be significantly greater than the overall flexion or extension observed between the occiput and the thorax.[10]

The greater the difference between these values, the greater the degree of snaking. Snaking can thus be quantified as the difference between the sum of the absolute values of all the segmental movements, and the amount of overall movement between the head and the thorax.

Soft cervical collars

Soft cervical collars provide the least stability of any device available. They generally offer, at least to some extent, a mandibular point of fixation. But they do not provide any low cervical or thoracic points of fixation. Because of this, they do very little to limit range of motion in flexion and extension, and there is no indication for their use in posttraumatic stabilization.

Hard cervical collars

Combining a more rigid collar with a secure mandibular extension rostrally and shoulder/thoracic extension caudally, hard cervical collars (Philadelphia or Aspen) provide greater limitation of motion in all planes than soft collars. They are less effective at stabilizing the occipitocervical junction,[10,11] but do provide some stability in this region. Hard collars have been shown to provide effective stabilization in various atlantoaxial or sub-axial injuries, including isolated atlas fractures with intact transverse atlantal ligament, various atlantoaxial fractures, and sub-axial fractures without displacement or overt instability. More stable injuries of the occipitocervical junction, such as occipital condyle fractures, may be treated with hard collar immobilization as well. Of note, the Philadelphia and Aspen collars have been shown to provide equivalent stability.[12]

Cervicothoracic bracing

Extending the caudal extent of a collar to include a rigid vest, cervicothoracic braces include sternal occipital mandibular immobilization (SOMI), four-poster, and cervicothoracic orthosis (CTO) braces. These provide greater stability than hard collars, especially in the low cervical and upper thoracic regions. This increased control over true flexion–extension provides for less parallelogram-like movement than hard cervical collars. These devices are useful for the treatment of sub-axial cervical and high thoracic injuries.

Craniothoracic fixation

This category includes the halo device (rigid) and the Minerva brace (semi-rigid) for stabilization of the cervical spine. These braces have in common the stabilization of the cervical spine by fixing the cranium and the thoracic cage. This reduces overall cervical spine motion, as well as motion at the segmental level. Additionally, because of the limitation of both capital and true flexion and extension, the propensity of the cervical spine to move in a parallelogram manner is reduced considerably.

Various studies have evaluated the halo and the Minerva braces, both individually and together.[13–19] Both tend to function very well in controlling overall spine motion in all planes and at all levels of the cervical spine. Motion at the segmental level, however, is probably greater with the halo than with the Minerva brace. This, when combined with the generally small amount of total motion allowed by the halo, implies that a considerable amount of snaking is permitted with this device. Conflicting reports exist regarding the efficacy of stabilization at the occiput-C1 joint. It is not clear which device is superior.

Peculiar to the halo are several serious complications, which have not been reported with other types of spinal orthoses. These include pin site infections, cerebrospinal fluid leaks, skull penetration, brain abscess, and cranial nerve palsy. These risks, while uncommon, must nevertheless be considered when deciding on which type of orthosis to use.

The senior author has reported on a series of 10 patients who were treated serially with immobilization with a halo vest, then Minerva brace, then, thus served as their own controls.[15] Eight of the ten patients preferred the Minerva brace to the halo.

The published data on halos generally comes from spine surgeons experienced in their application. Application of the Minerva brace, unlike the halo, is generally performed by an orthotist. It is possible that the skill level and experience of the orthotist with Minerva braces represents another variable in the data presented on the technique to date.

In the setting of posttraumatic stabilization, the use of craniothoracic immobilization of the cervical spine is indicated for injuries at the occipitocervical junction where a hard collar is deemed insufficient, or postoperatively for injuries at this level. The use of this type of immobilization for sub-axial injuries, which are deemed too unstable for treatment with a hard collar, however, should be approached with extreme caution. This is because of the amount of segmental motion allowed by these devices.

Thoracic bracing

Bracing of the upper thoracic spine overlaps with the sub-axial cervical spine. In fact, bracing through this region can be considered either as the caudal extension of cervical immobilization techniques (hard collar or halo) with a longer vest, or as the inclusion of rostral points (by rigid or semi-rigid means) in a thoracic fixation orthosis. In fact, to this end, Koch and Nickel demonstrated the progressively greater stability afforded by a halo vest as the cervical spine is descended through the sub-axial region and into the rostral thoracic spine (Figure 7.17).[18]

The remainder of the thoracic spine is unique, in that it is associated with long spinal segments both rostral and caudal to the pathology, thus affording the opportunity to apply conventional splinting techniques. The distance from the inner surface of the brace to the spine is less relevant here, because of the significant stability provided by the rib cage. Bracing is a viable treatment alternative for patients with thoracolumbar compression or burst fractures who are neurologically intact.[20–22] Patients managed in this manner have a reasonably low probability of requiring surgery.

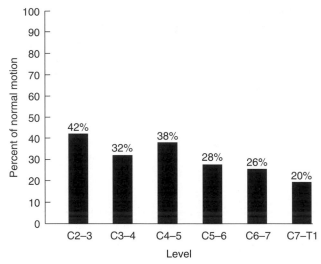

Figure 7.17 Koch and Nickel determined the percentage of normal cervical spine motion allowed in a halo. The average was 31%; the range was from 42% in the upper cervical spine to 20% in the low cervical spine. The restriction of segmental motion increased as the spine was descended, as depicted. (Reprinted by permission. See full reference on p. 116.)

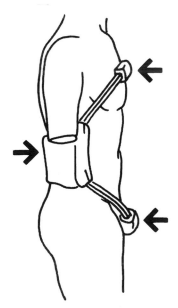

Figure 7.18 The three-point bending forces applied by the Jewett brace (*arrows*). These forces are similar to those applied by spinal implants (e.g. Harrington distraction rod). (Reprinted by permission. See full reference on p. 116.)

A thoracolumbosacral orthosis (TLSO) is generally preferred. The Jewett brace has been used for this injury as well. The Jewett brace has the advantage of helping to maintain posture by the application of a three-point bending moment (Figure 7.18). However, this brace has several shortcomings. First, while providing effective stabilization in the sagittal plane, it does little to retard motion in rotation or lateral bending. Second, and possibly more importantly from the patient's point of view, it can be quite uncomfortable. The dorsally directed force vectors are applied by pads on (or near) the manubrium and pubic symphysis, and the ventrally directed force is centered on the thoracolumbar junction. This is generally the site of injury for which this type of brace is most useful.

Lumbar and lumbosacral bracing

The lumbar and lumbosacral regions are difficult to brace effectively. This is the result of the significant amount of soft tissue between the brace and the vertebral column, even in lean people, as well as the lack of availability of adequate points of fixation. For a brace to be effective, there must be at least four or five vertebral levels both rostrally and caudally to provide fixation. The pelvis has proven to be a difficult region to secure, and hip flexion, even with the application of a hip spica, allows an unacceptable amount of motion in the lumbosacral region. Therefore, the efficacy of lumbar bracing is suspect.[23] The value of low lumbar and lumbosacral bracing in the trauma patient has not been established. However, it seems clear that the expectation of immobilizing an unstable spine with these techniques is perhaps overly optimistic. The use of these bracing techniques in the postoperative period must rely on the experience and judgment of the surgeon.

References

1 Apfelbaum RI, Lonser RR, Verres R, et al. Direct anterior screw fixation for recent and remote odontoid fractures. *J Neurosurg (Spine 2)* 2000;93:227–236.
2 Grob D, Crisco JJ, Panjabi MM, et al. Biomechanical evaluation of four different posterior atlantoaxial fixation techniques. *Spine* 1992;17(5):481–490.
3 Harms J, Melcher RP. Posterior C1–C2 fusion with polyaxial screw and rod fixation. *Spine* 2001;26(22):2467–2471.
4 Gorek J, Acaroglu E, Berven S, et al. Constructs incorporating intralaminar C2 screws provide rigid stability for atlantoaxial fixation. *Spine* 2005;30(13):1513–1518.
5 Hadley MN, Walters BC, Grabb PA, et al. Guidelines for the management of acute cervical spine and spinal cord injuries. *Clin Neurosurg* 2002;(49):407–498.
6 Ordonez BJ, Benzel EC, Naderi S, et al. Cervical facet dislocation: techniques for ventral reduction and stabilization. *J Neurosurg (Spine 1)* 2000;92:18–23.
7 McCormack T, Karaikovic E, Gaines RW. The load sharing classification of spine fractures. *Spine* 1994;19(15):1741–1744.
8 Boerger TO, Limb D, Dickson RA. Does "canal clearance" affect neurological outcome after thoracolumbar burst fractures? *J Bone Joint Surg* 2000;82:629–635.
9 Gertzbein SD. Scoliosis Research Society. Multicenter spine fracture study. *Spine* 1992;17(5):528–540.
10 Johnson RM, Hart DL, Simmons EF, et al. Cervical orthoses: a study comparing their effectiveness in restricting cervical motion in normal subjects. *J Bone Joint Surg [Am]* 1977;59A:332–339.

11 Kauppi M, Neva M, Kautiainen H. Headmaster collar restricts rheumatoid atlantoaxial subluxation. *Spine* 1999;24(6):526–528.

12 Hughes SJ. How effective is the Newport/Aspen collar? A prospective radiographic evaluation in healthy adult volunteers. *J Trauma* 1998;45(2):374–378.

13 Mirza SK, Moquin RR, Anderson PA, *et al.* Stabilizing properties of the halo apparatus. *Spine* 1997;22(7):727–733.

14 Sharpe KP, Rao S, Argyrios Z. Evaluation of the effectiveness of the Minerva cervicothoracic orthosis. *Spine* 1995;20(13):1475–1479.

15 Benzel EC, Hadden TA, Saulsbery CM. A comparison of the Minerva and halo jackets for stabilization of the cervical spine. *J Neurosurg* 1989;70:411–414.

16 Maiman D, Millington P, Novak S, *et al.* The effect of the thermoplastic Minerva body jacket on cervical spine motion. *Neurosurgery* 1989;25:363–368.

17 Tomonaga T, Krag MH, Novotny JE. Clinical, radiographic, and kinematic results from an adjustable four-pad halovest. *Spine* 1997;22(11):1199–1208.

18 Koch RA, Nickel VL. The halo vest. An evaluation of motion and forces across the neck. *Spine* 1978;3:103–107.

19 Lind B, Sihlbom H, Nordwall A. Forces and motions across the neck in patients treated with the halo-vest. *Spine* 1988;13:162–167.

20 Cantor JB, Lebwohl NH, Garvey T, *et al.* Nonoperative management of stable thoracolumbar burst fractures with early ambulation and bracing. *Spine* 1993;18(8):971–976.

21 Chow GH, Nelson BJ, Gebhard JS, *et al.* Functional outcome of thoracolumbar burst fractures managed with hyperextension casting or bracing and early mobilization. *Spine* 1996;21(18):2170–2175.

22 Mumford J, Weinstein JN, Spratt KF, *et al.* Thoracolumbar burst fractures: the clinical efficacy and outcome of nonoperative management. *Spine* 1993;18(8):955–970.

23 Axelsson P, Johnsson R, Stromqvist B. Effect of lumbar orthosis on intervertebral mobility. *Spine* 1992;17:678–681.

CHAPTER 8

Controversies in the management of cervical spinal cord injury

Paul G. Matz and Mark N. Hadley

Introduction

Cervical spinal cord injury (SCI) is an entity commonly encountered by most practicing neurosurgeons. Management of patients with cervical SCI has four main goals:

1 Timely recognition of the extent of injury to the spinal cord and spinal column.
2 Optimization of the potential for neurological recovery.
3 Cervical spinal stabilization.
4 Mobilization and physical rehabilitation.

To achieve these goals, neurosurgeons have traditionally relied on rapid recognition of spinal injuries employing plain radiographs with or without computed tomography (CT), followed by realignment. Stabilization of the spinal column injury has been achieved by either external fixation or internal fixation and fusion. Supplemental bone as a fusion substrate is employed with the latter.[1] Prior to the widespread use of methylprednisolone within 8h of acute SCI, little other than hopeful observation has routinely been offered to patients as a medical management strategy to optimize their potential for neurological recovery.

With the availability of magnetic resonance imaging (MRI) along with improvements in the medical and surgical care of SCI patients, new management paradigms have been offered in contrast to historical, traditional management. This chapter discusses these issues and the controversies that surround them.

Fracture patterns associated with cervical SCI

Cervical SCI in adults is nearly always associated with injury to the cervical vertebrae and/or their supporting ligaments. In contrast, traumatic injury to the cervical spine does not always produce SCI. In the overall population of blunt trauma victims, cervical spinal injury has an incidence of 2.4%.[2] Twenty-four percent of cervical fracture injuries involve the axis. Thirty-nine percent of cervical fracture injuries include C5, C6, and C7.[2] In this same traumatic injury population, almost 30% of cervical injuries have been clinically insignificant. The specific mechanisms producing cervical spinal injury are multiple. A broad generalization is that fractures of the cervical vertebrae are a consequence of compression superimposed upon flexion or extension bending moments.[3] In contrast, ligamentous disruption is often associated with distraction forces, with superimposed bending moments playing a role. In all likelihood, combinations of these forces play a role in most injuries of the cervical spinal column.

Although few controversies have been associated with the categorization of cervical spine fractures, a brief overview bears mentioning. The upper cervical spinal vertebrae serve flexion and extension along with rotation. The C1 vertebrae functions much like a washer superimposed between the skull as transmitted through the occipital condyles, and the support structure of the spine beginning at the axis. The C1–2 joint serves as a pivot which allows for approximately 50% of head rotation. The subaxial spine, C3 through C7, primarily functions in positions of flexion and extension and shares in load bearing.

Fracture patterns of the cervical spine have been characterized based on their location. Fractures of the atlas represent approximately 7% of all acute cervical fractures and involve either disruption of the ring in two places or displacement of the ring from the lateral masses (Jefferson fracture).[4] The combination of movement, location, and anatomy of the axis predisposes it to multiple and varied fracture/dislocation injuries, distinct form other vertebrae. Axis fractures represent 17–24% of all cervical spine fractures.[2,5] They have been subdivided into fractures involving the odontoid (Types I, II, IIA, and III), those involving the pars (Hangman's fracture), and miscellaneous fractures.[5,6] Although not always separately classified, clinical management of Type II odontoid fractures and Hangman's fractures may be modified depending on the degree of subluxation, initial dens displacement (odontoid fracture), or angulation (Hangman's fractures). It is not unusual to find simultaneous injuries to the atlas and axis.[4,7] Combination injuries of the atlas and axis are more likely to be associated with neurological morbidity.[7]

Subaxial cervical spine fractures may involve the lamina, lateral masses, facets, or vertebral bodies of vertebrae C3 through C7. These injuries are often a consequence of compressive forces with superimposed flexion or extension.[3] Distraction forces have been associated with ligamentous disruption and posterior element fractures. Subluxation of the facet joints is typically associated with flexion, rotation, and distraction forces.[8] Because of its larger spinal canal diameter, the upper cervical spine (C1–2 levels) often tolerate a greater degree of subluxation before neurological injury occurs compared to the narrower canal diameter of the subaxial cervical spine. However, SCI involving the upper cervical cord has been associated with higher morbidity than that involving lower cervical levels.[9] The greater the degree of compression of the subaxial vertebrae and/or the greater the degree of subluxation of the subaxial cervical vertebrae, the greater is the likelihood of acute cervical SCI.

Evaluation and "clearance" of the cervical spine

In the overall population of trauma victims, acute cervical spinal injury has an incidence of 2.4%.[2,10] Appropriately, emergency medical technicians (EMT) and emergency department (ED) personnel are trained to practice strict spinal immobilization until the structural integrity (vertebrae and ligaments) of the cervical spine can be ensured. Although the necessity of spinal immobilization in every trauma patient may be argued, immobilization of the cervical spine remains the standard practice for the pre-hospital treatment of the acute trauma victims by EMT personnel.[11] The initial evaluation of the cervical spine begins in the ED and traditionally involves both the clinical examination followed by plain radiographs of the cervical spine from the occiput through T1. Neurological assessment of traumatic injury patients involves determination of cognitive impairment and sensorimotor deficits, if any. In the neurologically intact and alert, fully oriented patient without substance impairment or an associated distracting injury, an assessment is done for cervicalgia, tenderness, and impairment in range-of-motion (ROM). If these abnormalities are *not* present in the neurologically normal, alert, coherent patient as described above, the cervical spine may be cleared without radiographic assessment.[12] If any of the above abnormalities or physical findings are present, the acute trauma victim should be assessed with a three-view cervical spine radiograph series including anteroposterior, lateral, and odontoid views.[13] Radiographs should be of sufficient quality to view the occiput through the T1 vertebra adequately. In a large series of trauma patients, Davis *et al.* identified a 2.3% incidence of cervical spinal injuries. Within this group, 4.6% of patients had delayed or missed diagnoses. These authors noted that the single most common reason for a missed initial diagnosis was the failure to obtain adequate cervical spine radiographs. Davis *et al.* concluded that the delayed diagnosis of cervical injury could have been avoided in 31 of 34 patients had they been assessed with an adequate three-view cervical spine X-ray series.[10]

To determine if oblique views of the cervical spine played a role in the evaluation of cervical spinal trauma, Freemyer *et al.* prospectively compared five-view plain radiographs with three-view radiographs in a series of 58 patients.[14] Fractures were identified in 33 patients and were confirmed using conventional tomography. These authors found no difference between three-view and five-view plain radiographic series in terms of sensitivity. They concluded that there was no advantage in obtaining oblique cervical spine radiographs in the initial assessment of acute trauma patients.[14]

To identify the optimal role of CT following trauma, Ross *et al.* studied 204 patients at high risk for cervical spine injury after trauma. Thirteen patients sustained upper cervical spinal injuries. The initial sensitivity of three-view plain radiographs in this series was 85%. With the use of supplemental CT, the sensitivity and specificity were markedly increased.[15] In a similar series, cervical CT was used to examine 123 patients who were unable to have their cervical spines "cleared" using plain radiographs. In these patients, supplemental CT through poorly visualized cervical levels or levels suspicious for injury, allowed "clearance" of the cervical spines of 93% of patients within 24 h of admission. CT studies detected 98% of the injuries in this series and when combined with three-view plain radiographs, 100% of all injuries were identified.[16]

Cervical CT studies have also been used to better define the nature and extent of post-traumatic cervical spine fractures in a series of 88 patients.[17] In 36% of these patients, plain radiographs either missed or did not properly define the fracture site. Cervical CT studies revealed all of the fractures in these patients, most of which occurred at the C1–2 or C6–7 levels and involved the posterolateral elements.[17] Berne and colleagues prospectively evaluated 58 patients using plain radiographs and cervical CT after blunt trauma. The use of CT in addition to plain C-spine radiographs increased the sensitivity of diagnosing a cervical fracture in this series from 60% to greater than 90%.[18] Each of these series demonstrated that CT was feasible in the acute trauma setting, and that it had utility in supplementing the plain radiographic assessment of the cervical spines of symptomatic acute trauma victims.

One controversy on this issue is whether or not CT alone (without three-view X-rays) is adequate in the assessment of the cervical spine in symptomatic trauma victims. While the use of supplemental CT studies has increased sensitivity and specificity in the diagnosis of traumatic fracture injury compared to three-view radiographs alone, CT scanning of the cervical spine alone is not as specific or sensitive as three-view X-rays supplemented with CT as needed.[19] In an exhaustive literature review of and medical-evidence based guidelines production on this subject, Hadley et al. concluded that the medical literature supports the three-view X-ray series with supplemental CT as the diagnostic gold standard for the assessment of the cervical spine in symptomatic trauma patients.[20]

The likelihood of occult ligamentous instability of the cervical spine after blunt trauma is extremely low, estimated to be less than 0.1% in one large series.[21] In this same group of study patients, plain radiographs were able to identify 93% of these injuries. However, in the rare patient with cervical SCI and normal plain radiographs supplemented with CT as necessary, dynamic X-rays (flexion and extension views) or MRI may be considered to assess for cervical spinal ligamentous injury and instability. Ajani et al. and Lewis et al. each prospectively examined patients using dynamic cervical spine films after major trauma. Ajani et al. identified one patient of 100 they studied who had an unstable cervical spine detected using dynamic films.[22] Lewis et al. identified 3% of 141 patients who had normal plain radiographs, but abnormal, unstable dynamic films. All of these patients were symptomatic with cervicalgia.[23] Geck et al. examined a series of 89 patients with suspected occult ligamentous injury of the cervical spine with MRI. In their series, 7.9% of patients had ligamentous injuries as diagnosed by MR, two of which required operative stabilization.[24] Benzel and colleagues used cervical MRI to evaluate 174 acute trauma patients in whom physical findings indicated the potential for cervical spinal injury or in whom radiographic findings suggested ligamentous injury.

Thirty-five patients (20%) were found to have isolated ligamentous injuries by MRI, only one of whom required surgery.[25] In contrast, Patton et al. did not find one instance of occult ligamentous injury by MRI in 26 cognitively abnormal patients who suffered blunt injury to the head and spine.[26] If MRI is utilized to assess for ligamentous injury of the cervical spine of acute trauma victims, it is suggested that the imaging be obtained within 48 h of injury for greatest potential accuracy.[24,25] MRI is extremely useful in the assessment of the cervical spinal cord for compression and/or intrinsic cord injury or edema, with or without hemorrhage.[19,27,28]

At our institution, we follow the recommendations on imaging of the cervical spine following acute trauma as offered in the Guidelines for the Management of Acute Cervical Spine and Spinal Cord Injuries by Hadley et al.[20]

Awake, alert, unintoxicated, neurologically intact patients without symptoms, or other distracting injury (as described by rigid criteria and documented on repeated assessment) are not imaged with any X-rays of the spinal column, irrespective of the mechanism of the traumatic event. All other acute trauma patients with the potential of a cervical spine or SCI are radiographically assessed with a three-view cervical X-ray series supplemented with thin-section bone window CT through areas poorly or incompletely visualized on the standard X-rays or through areas suspicious for injury on the standard X-rays. If this combination of diagnostic imaging studies is negative for cervical spinal injury we "clear" the patient's cervical spine and remove immobilization devices. In patients with persistent cervicalgia or in patients with any suggestion of ligamentous injury on the standard X-rays (soft tissue swelling, minor changes in alignment, splaying of spinous processes, odd angulation at an interspace) or on the CT images (widened facet joints), we obtain dynamic flexion and extension lateral X-rays in the radiology department. If these studies reveal normal motion and maintenance of alignment in flexion and extension, we "clear" the patient's cervical spine.

Patients with neurological symptoms or signs referable to their cervical spinal cord or cervical nerve roots are imaged with cervical MRI. We have not been impressed with acute MRI (within 48 h of injury) and its ability to identify clinically significant ligamentous injury of the cervical spine not otherwise identified by standard C-spine X-rays, supplemental CT images, and the selected addition of lateral dynamic flexion and extension X-rays, and therefore do not use MRI for this purpose.

The role of early MRI after cervical SCI

Continued improvements in image quality and resolution along with ever-increasing availability, has allowed MRI to assume an increasing role in the evaluation of patients with acute cervical SCI. Early after its inception, Kulkarni et al. examined the utility of MRI to determine the type of cord injury following cervical SCI (hemorrhagic or non-hemorrhagic). In their series, MRI was not performed acutely – the earliest MRI was attained was 1 day after

injury. MRI was able to discern contusion/edema from intraspinal hemorrhage. Furthermore, patients who suffered intraspinal hemorrhage had a poorer
prognosis.[27] These findings were corroborated in a more recent series of 104
patients in whom acute cervical MRI was performed after trauma. The presence of hemorrhage within the spinal cord substance was a negative predictive
factor for improvement in neurological function after cervical SCI.[28] The early
use of cervical MRI after SCI to predict prognosis is valuable but is not the most
crucial issue. Instead, it is the ability of MRI to determine the presence or absence
of cord compression by bone, disk, or hematoma that is at the heart of surgical
decision-making early in the management of patients following acute SCI.[19]

The ability of MRI to depict locked facets, disruption of ligaments, acute disk
herniation, cord compression, and cord edema was studied in several series of
patients with cervical facet subluxation injuries.[29–31] In the acute setting, MRI
was effective at diagnosing facet subluxation and was superior to all other
imaging modalities at revealing acute disk herniation, cord compression, cord
edema, and posterior longitudinal ligament disruption.[29–31] The early use of
MRI in these series permitted rapid identification of spinal canal compromise
related to bone, disk, or epidural hematoma while simultaneously identifying
the potential for cervical spinal instability.[19,30,31] MRI has become the imaging
modality of choice if and when the cervical spinal cord (in particular) or the
ligamentous structures or disk spaces of the cervical spinal column need rapid
and accurate assessment following acute traumatic injury.

One of the controversies in the management of patients with acute SCI is
whether every patient with a cervical SCI and vertebral subluxation warrants
an acute cervical MRI prior to attempted closed or open reduction of their
fracture–dislocation injury. To the practitioner, the obvious advantage of an
early MRI is a clear determination of both the degree of spinal canal and cord
compromise and the presence of a ventral mass compressing the spinal cord.[19]
The disadvantage of an MRI prior to reduction is the delay in returning the
subluxed vertebral column to normal alignment, an event thought to be associated with improved neurological recovery.[32] Vaccaro *et al.* prospectively
examined a series of alert patients with acute cervical SCI and subluxation.
Eleven patients met enrollment criteria and underwent MRI examination
prior to reduction. Nine of eleven patients experienced successful subsequent
closed reduction. In this group, two patients had ventral disk herniation prior
to reduction and five patients had ventral disk herniation subsequent to reduction. None of these patients with disk herniations experienced neurological
compromise due to the disk herniation.[33] In this series of alert patients, early
MRI did not produce a diagnostic benefit but did result in delays in accomplishing reduction of the cervical subluxation injury.

In a literature review of and medical evidence-based guideline production
on the topic of closed reduction of acute cervical fracture–dislocation injuries,
Hadley *et al.* concluded that no awake, alert patient with a cervical disk herniation in conjunction with a cervical facet-dislocation injury has been reported
to deteriorate (worsen neurologically) as a result of the disk herniation during

closed reduction.[34] The role of pre-reduction MRI in this patient group remains unclear and may result in a substantial delay in realignment of the spinal column and decompression of the spinal cord in these patients.[32, 34–36]

Since early reduction of cervical fracture–dislocation injuries appears to hold some promise for improved neurological recovery, we attempt reduction as early as possible at our institution. In the alert patient, closed reduction is attempted while monitoring the patient's neurological status, without the assistance of a pre-reduction MRI. Once closed reduction has been accomplished or if neurological deterioration ensues, or if closed reduction cannot be accomplished, cervical MRI is obtained. Early operative decompression is offered to any patient with cord compression (even if the bony injury has been effectively reduced) who has MR evidence of persistent cord compromise.

In the patient who is not alert or cognitively normal, the patient's neurological status and examination cannot be monitored. In these instances, we obtain a cervical MRI as soon as the patient is medically stable (early in their hospital course). If no ventral disk herniation is evident, we proceed promptly with closed reduction. If a ventral mass is present on MRI, operative decompression and open reduction are performed followed by stabilization and fusion, all during the same operative setting. This protocol, also utilized by others, allows for rapid reduction of the dislocated cervical spine in a safe, effective manner in the maximum number of patients while minimizing the delay in treatment patients might experience waiting for and accomplishing MRI in circumstances when MRI is likely to be of little diagnostic benefit.[37]

Timing and method of reduction after cervical SCI

Empirically, the concept of reduction of cervical spinal fracture–dislocation injuries is simple. Having sustained a primary SCI due to the fracture deformity, the dysfunctional spinal cord may contain viable but malfunctioning neurons and compressed, but not severed, long tracts. If subluxation of cervical vertebrae is superimposed upon SCI, these vulnerable neurons and axons may become non-viable due to continued compression, distortion, and ischemia. If the vertebral subluxation deformity is reduced and the spinal canal space (area and diameter) returned to normal, the secondary insults of compression, pressure, and distortion will be eliminated and ischemia may be ameliorated. These considerations should be at the forefront of the practitioner's mind when neurological function in the SCI patient is diminished but remains evident, as in the neurologically "incomplete" patient. Even in absence of spinal cord neurological function after acute SCI (i.e. the neurologically "complete" patient) these matters are of paramount importance.

With regard to reduction of acute cervical spinal fracture–dislocation injuries, there are two main controversies. The first is the need for and value of pre-reduction cervical MRI as addressed above. The second controversy is the means by which reduction and realignment is accomplished, open versus closed. It is possible that attempted closed reduction may be futile in certain instances and with certain injuries, and would therefore only delay the opportunity for early reduction of the fracture–dislocation injury by open means. The issue raised therefore, is whether certain acute SCI patients with fracture–dislocation injuries should go immediately to the operating room for open reduction, decompression, and realignment, or should all patients be offered a trial of closed reduction prior to consideration of operative treatment?

In 1975, Yashon and colleagues described a series of patients with cervical fracture–dislocations who underwent successful rapid closed reduction.[35] Their protocol included the aggressive use of sequential weights to more rapidly accomplish deformity reduction. They did not report any complications associated with this practice in awake, alert patients as long as continuous neurological monitoring was accomplished during the process of closed reduction.[35] Others have described similar experiences and have suggested that neurological recovery has been optimized in patients managed with rapid closed reduction.[36] Hadley et al. examined a series of 68 patients with fracture–dislocations of the cervical spine. Closed reduction was attempted in almost all of these patients with a 58% success rate. Open reduction was performed in those who failed closed reduction and was successful in 83% of procedures. Significant neurological improvement rates were observed in patients after both successful closed (78%) and open (60%) reduction. However, the greatest neurological benefit identified among patients in their series was among the 10 patients who had their facet-dislocation injuries reduced most rapidly after injury.[32] Similarly, Wolf and colleagues reviewed a series of 52 patients with bilateral locked facets and neurological injury. Closed reduction was successful in 77% of these patients. The remainder underwent open reduction and realignment. At 1 year, significant improvement was evident in 15 patients.[38] The authors concluded that early reduction offered the best chance for neurological improvement after cervical spinal fracture–dislocation injury. These clinical series suggest a benefit to early reduction of cervical fracture–dislocation injuries by open or closed means with the duration of time between injury and reduction being of the essence. In a series of 131 patients examined retrospectively and then followed prospectively, Rizzolo and colleagues used a protocol of early rapid closed reduction in alert, cognitively normal patients with acute SCI due to cervical fracture–dislocation. Patients who were not cognitively normal underwent cervical MRI. Open reduction was accomplished in non-alert patients with a ventral mass, closed reduction in those patients without a ventral mass. The authors compared their results against historical controls of series of other investigators. They concluded that early closed reduction remained the treatment of choice for alert cooperative patients with acute cervical spine-dislocation injuries. They advocated cervical MRI for those patients not cognitively normal, and in this group, the presence of a ventral mass by pre-reduction MRI mandated surgical decompression of the mass prior to open reduction.[37] The findings of Rizzolo et al. as well as the series cited above support the principle of rapid spinal realignment following cervical fracture–dislocation injury.[32,37,38]

Despite these reports, the most effective and practical means to accomplish early reduction of cervical fracture–dislocation injuries remains an issue. In a prospective multi-institutional study, Marshall and colleagues examined 283 patients with traumatic SCI, 14 of whom deteriorated neurologically during hospitalization. Deterioration in 12 of 14 patients was related to a specific management event. Several of the patients who deteriorated underwent early surgery for open reduction, while others deteriorated during attempted closed reduction with traction or were treated in a halo vest.[39] Although the authors described a trend against early surgery and better outcome, it was evident that neurological deterioration could be associated with both open and closed reduction of acute fracture–dislocation injuries. Wilberger and colleagues examined a subgroup of patients from the NASCIS II trial who underwent surgery (295 patients) for incomplete SCI. They noted that good outcomes were observed with very early surgery (less than 25 h after injury) and with late surgery (greater than 200 h after injury). The complication rate associated with open reduction in this subgroup was 8.4%. In contrast, the complication rate associated with non-surgical treatment was 10.3%, not a significant difference.[40] These two large multi-center reviews document that reduction of cervical fracture–dislocation injuries by open or closed means are associated with high-success rates and low-failure complication rates.

As noted previously, Hadley *et al.* and Wolf *et al.* retrospectively examined similar protocols of initial early closed reduction followed by open reduction if necessary. Hadley *et al.* described a 4% mortality rate among patients who required open reduction. There were no deaths related to closed reduction.[32] Wolf *et al.* described an overall mortality rate of 6.1% (open and closed reduction methods). Most deaths were due to respiratory failure.[38] Mirza and colleagues retrospectively compared patients at one institution who underwent early open reduction of cervical fracture–dislocation injuries to similar patients at another institution who underwent successful early closed reduction with elective stabilization. In their report, early open reduction was not associated with a higher morbidity, nor were there any major differences in neurological outcome among patients treated by open or closed means. These authors concluded that early open reduction diminished the overall length of hospitalization.[41] Several studies have demonstrated the efficacy of both early open and closed reduction of acute cervical fracture–dislocation injuries. Both methods have been associated with morbidity and mortality, yet both have been reported with improved neurological outcome if accomplished in a timely fashion.

Because of the potential profound benefits of early spinal reduction and spinal cord decompression, we attempt closed reduction in the monitored intensive care unit (ICU) setting as soon as possible after injury in the alert, cognitively normal patient with a cervical fracture–dislocation.[42] In this scenario, cervical MRI may pose a significant delay to spinal realignment and offer little or no additional diagnostic benefit. We proceed with rapid succession weight administration with the use of halo ring, cranial cervical traction, and closely monitor the patient's neurological examination. Patients who are cognitively abnormal undergo urgent pre-reduction cervical MRI evaluation. If a ventral mass is present on MRI, open decompression is performed followed by reduction, stabilization, and fusion. If no ventral mass is present, closed reduction is undertaken promptly as described above. For those patients who fail attempted closed reduction, cervical MRI is performed (if not done previously) once the patient is immobilized in a formal halo ring-vest device. If the cervical MRI indicates a ventral mass in this setting, prompt open decompression precedes open reduction. While others have reported the safe use of closed reduction under general anesthesia, the true efficacy of these techniques have not been well established if passive closed reduction fails.[43] Our protocol as defined above permits the safe and timely reduction of cervical fracture–dislocation injuries in the maximum number of acutely injured SCI patients.

Medical management of acute SCI patients

The controversies about this topic are not whether acute SCI patients should be managed by trained medical specialists in a hospital setting. They are whether or not acute SCI patients should receive early aggressive blood pressure support (and potential augmentation) to potentially improve spinal cord perfusion, and whether acute SCI patients should be managed in a monitored setting (ICU or step-down unit) to best identify (and subsequently treat) potentially deleterious cardiac and hemodynamic disturbances and pulmonary insufficiency. While great emphasis has been placed on the pharmacological treatment of acute SCI patients and on the timing of reduction of cervical spinal-dislocation injuries or on the timing of surgical treatment following acute SCI (each of these topics are reviewed elsewhere in this book), there is no consensus among clinicians as to a "standard medical treatment paradigm," nor is there consistency in the medical management of acute SCI patients within institutions, within major cities or within regions of the country.

Both issues appear very important to patients following acute SCI. Hypotension is common following acute traumatic SCI even among isolated acute SCI patients. The likelihood of hypotension increases with the severity of the associated neurological injury even without complete spinal cord disruption and loss of sympathetic autonomic input. Hypotension is deleterious in the setting of acute SCI and augmentation of systemic blood pressure to a mean of 85–90 mmHg appears to improve spinal cord perfusion and increase the potential for neurological improvement and recovery.[44–47]

Likewise, cardiac disturbances, typically profound bradycardia, and pulmonary insufficiency are common after acute SCI. Cardiac instability and arrhythmias contribute to hypotension and poor perfusion and pulmonary insufficiency contributes to poor oxygen exchange and hypoxia, both deleterious following acute SCI. Aggressive medical care in a monitored setting (ICU or step-down unit) will allow rapid detection of cardiac, hemodynamic, or pulmonary instability and should trigger prompt intervention to maximize perfusion and oxygen delivery to the injured spinal cord.

After extensive literature review and medical evidence-based guideline production on these two topics, Hadley *et al.* concluded that the existing medical evidence did not support either a standard or a guideline level recommendation on the medical management of acute SCI patients.[42,44] Class III medical evidence in the literature does support option level recommendations on these issues:

• Management of patients with acute SCI, particularly with severe cervical level injuries, in an ICU or similar monitored setting is recommended.

• Use of cardiac, hemodynamic, and respiratory monitoring devices to detect cardiac dysfunction and respiratory insufficiency in patients after acute SCI is recommended.

• Hypotension (systolic blood pressure <90 mmHg) should be avoided if possible or corrected as soon as possible after acute SCI.

• Maintenance of mean arterial blood pressure at 85–90 mmHg for the first 7 days after acute SCI to improve spinal cord perfusion is recommended.

At our institution, the management of patients with acute cervical SCI is multi-faced, often simultaneous. Immediately upon arrival spinal immobilization is maintained or reinforced. The patient is rapidly and thoroughly assessed and resuscitated. Mean arterial blood pressure is maintained at 85 mmHg from the outset and supplemental oxygen is applied often via an endo- or nasotracheal tube and mechanical ventilation (as necessary), to ensure adequate systemic oxygenation. These immediate medical assessment and treatment measures are initiated in the ED and occur simultaneously with the initial radiographic and (potential) acute MR assessment of the acute SCI patient.

Once stabilized from a cardiopulmonary–hemodynamic standpoint and the initial radiographic assessment completed, the immobilized patient is rapidly transferred to our neurosurgical ICU where invasive monitoring devices are inserted (if not already placed in the ED) and rapid halo ring cranio-cervical traction is utilized in an attempt at early closed reduction (as appropriate), or a halo ring-vest orthosis is applied, either as definitive treatment if spinal reduction is unnecessary, or as a prequel to prompt open decompression and open reduction with stabilization and fusion.

We monitor acute SCI patients and maintain mean arterial blood pressure at 85 mmHg for 7 days following acute injury. Invasive monitoring devices include arterial pressure lines, central venous catheters, indwelling bladder catheters, and often endo- or nasotracheal tubes with mechanical ventilation. Depending on the patient's age, cardiac history, cardiac performance, and other associated injuries, a Swan–Ganz catheter may be employed. Maintenance of (and potential augmentation of) mean arterial blood pressure is accomplished first with crystalloid and colloid as indicated, then with pressors as required depending on the patient's specific cardiovascular–hemodynamic status. With this aggressive, combined medical/surgical approach to acute SCI patients, we feel we maximize each patient's potential for neurological recovery.

Conclusions

The acute management of cervical SCI appears to involve both contemporary medical and surgical strategies yet continues to be updated and refined through further clinical experience and study. Most of the options offered in this chapter are based on large collective case series of patients, with few controlled trials from which to draw definitive, meaningful conclusions. Consequently, most of the recommendations we describe are educated opinions and are offered as *options* for management, not *guidelines* or *standards* for care. The options we have described in this chapter are based on our clinical experience, which has been influenced by on the collective experience of others as reported in the literature. Our goal when treating acute SCI patients is to stabilize the patient medically and maintain/improve their spinal cord perfusion, identify the nature of their spinal and SCIs as rapidly as possible, reduce spinal column deformity, and eliminate spinal cord compression as promptly as practical, and ultimately to stabilize an unstable spine as soon as it is appropriate. The rationale behind this combined medical/surgical management protocol is to optimize the acute injury patient's potential for maximal, favorable neurological outcome.

References

1 Committee on Trauma of the American College of Surgeons. Hospital and pre-hospital resources for optimal care of the injured patient. *Bulletin Am Coll Surg*, 1986;71:4–23.
2 Goldberg W, Mueller C, Panacek E, *et al*. Distribution and patterns of blunt traumatic cervical spine injury. *Ann Emerg Med* 2001;38:17–21.
3 Southern EP, Oxland TR, Panjabi MM, *et al*. Cervical spine injury patterns in three modes of high-speed trauma: a biomechanical porcine model. *J Spinal Disord* 1990;3:316–328.
4 Hadley MN, Dickman CA, Browner CM, *et al*. Acute traumatic atlas fractures: management and long-term outcome. *Neurosurgery* 1988;23:31–35.
5 Hadley MN, Browner C, Sonntag VKH. Axis fractures: a comprehensive review of management and treatment in 107 cases. *Neurosurgery* 1985;17:281–290.
6 Hadley MN, Browner CM, Liu SS, *et al*. New subtype of acute odontoid fractures (type IIA). *Neurosurgery* 1988;22:67–71.
7 Dickman CA, Hadley MN, Browner C, *et al*. Neurosurgical management of acute atlas-axis combination fractures: a review of 25 cases. *J Neurosurg* 1989;70:45–49.
8 Cybulski GR, Douglas RA, Meyer PR, *et al*. Complications in three-column cervical spine injuries requiring anterior–posterior stabilization. *Spine* 1992;17:253–256.
9 Myllynen P, Kivioja A, Rokkanen P, *et al*. Cervical spinal cord injury: the correlations of initial clinical features and blood gas analyses with early prognosis. *Paraplegia* 1989;27:19–26.
10 Davis JW, Phreaner DL, Hoyt DB, *et al*. The etiology of missed cervical spine injuries. *J Trauma* 1993;34:342–346.
11 Hadley MN, Walters BC, Grabb PA, *et al*. Joint section on disorders of the spine and peripheral nerves of the American Association of Neurological Surgeons and the Congress of Neurological Surgeons. Guidelines for the management of acute cervical spine and spinal cord injuries. *Neurosurgery* 2002;50(Suppl)S7–S17.
12 Hoffman JR, Mower WR, Wolfson AB, *et al*. Validity of a set of clinical criteria to rule out injury to the cervical spine in patients with blunt trauma. National Emergency X-Radiography Utilization Study Group. *New Engl J Med* 2000;343:94–99.

13 MacDonald RL, Schwartz ML, Mirich D, *et al*. Diagnosis of cervical spine injury in motor vehicle crash victims: How many X-rays are enough? *J Trauma* 1990;30:392–397.

14 Freemyer B, Knopp R, Piche J, *et al*. Comparison of five-view and three-view cervical spine series in the evaluation of patients with cervical trauma. *Ann Emerg Med* 1989;18:818–821.

15 Ross SE, Schwab CW, David ET, *et al*. Clearing the cervical spine: initial radiologic evaluation. *J Trauma* 1987;27:1055–1060.

16 Borock EC, Gabram SG, Jacobs LM, *et al*. A prospective analysis of a two-year experience using computed tomography as an adjunct for cervical spine clearance. *J Trauma* 1991;31: 1001–1005.

17 Nunez DB, Zuluaga A, Fuentes-Bernardo DA, *et al*. Cervical spine trauma: How much more do we learn by routinely using helical CT? *Radiographics* 1996;16:1307–1318.

18 Berne JD, Velmahos GC, El-Tawil Q, *et al*. Value of complete cervical helical computed tomographic scanning in identifying cervical spine injury in the unevaluable blunt trauma patient with multiple injuries: a prospective study. *J Trauma* 1999;47:896–902.

19 Quencer RM, Nunez D, Green BA. Controversies in imaging acute cervical spine trauma. *AJNR* 1997;18:1866–1868.

20 Hadley MN, Walters BC, Grabb PA, *et al*. Guidelines for the management of acute cervical spine and spinal cord injuries. *Neurosurgery* 2002;50(Suppl):S36–S43.

21 Chiu WC, Haan JM, Cushing BM, *et al*. Ligamentous injuries of the cervical spine in unreliable blunt trauma patients: incidence, evaluation and outcome. *J Trauma* 2001;50: 457–463.

22 Ajani AE, Cooper DJ, Scheinkestel CD, *et al*. Optimal assessment of cervical spine trauma in critically ill patients: a prospective evaluation. *Anaesth Intensive Care* 1998;26:487–491.

23 Lewis LM, Docherty M, Ruoff BE, *et al*. Flexion–extension views in the evaluation of cervical spine injuries. *Ann Emerg Med* 1991;20:117–121.

24 Geck MJ, Yoo S, Wang JC. Assessment of cervical ligamentous injury in trauma patients using MRI. *J Spinal Disord* 2001;14:371–377.

25 Benzel EC, Hart BL, Ball PA, *et al*. Magnetic resonance imaging for the evaluation of patients with occult cervical spine injury. *J Neurosurg* 1996;85:824–829.

26 Patton JH, Kralovich KA, Cuschieri J, *et al*. Clearing the cervical spine in victims of blunt to the head and neck: What is necessary? *Am Surg* 2000;66:326–330.

27 Kulkarni MV, McArdle CB, Kopanicky D, *et al*. Acute spinal cord injury: MR imaging at 1.5 T. *Radiology* 1987;164:837–843.

28 Flanders AE, Spettell CM, Tartaglino LM, *et al*. Forecasting motor recovery after cervical spinal cord injury: value of MR imaging. *Radiology* 1996;201:649–655.

29 Hall AJ, Wagle VG, Raycroft J, *et al*. Magnetic resonance imaging in cervical spine trauma. *J Trauma* 1993;34:21–26.

30 Vaccaro AR, Falatyn SP, Flanders AE, *et al*. Magnetic resonance evaluation of the intervertebral disc, spinal ligaments, and spinal cord before and after closed traction reduction of cervical spine dislocations. *Spine* 1999;24:1210–1217.

31 Katzberg RW, Benedetti PF, Drake CM, *et al*. Acute cervical spine injuries: prospective MR imaging assessment at a level 1 trauma center. *Radiology* 1999;213:203–212.

32 Hadley MN, Fitzpatrick BC, Sonntag VKH, *et al*. Facet fracture–dislocation injuries of the cervical spine. *Neurosurgery* 1992;30:661–666.

33 Vaccaro AR, Madigan L, Schweitzer ME, *et al*. Magnetic resonance imaging analysis of soft tissue disruption after flexion–distraction injuries of the subaxial cervical spine. *Spine* 2001;26:1866–1872.

34 Hadley MN, Walters BC, Grabb PA, *et al*. Guidelines for the management of acute cervical spine and spinal cord injuries. *Neurosurgery* 2002;50(Suppl):S44–S50.

35 Yashon D, Tyson G, Vise WM. Rapid closed reduction of cervical fracture dislocations. *Surg Neurol* 1975;4:513–514.

36 Brunette DD, Rockswold GL. Neurologic recovery following rapid spinal realignment for complete cervical spinal cord injury. *J Trauma* 1987;27:445–447.

37 Rizzolo SJ, Vaccaro AR, Cotler JM. Cervical spine trauma. *Spine* 1994;19:2288–2298.

38 Wolf A, Levi L, Mirvis S, *et al*. Operative management of bilateral facet dislocation. *J Neurosurg* 1991;75:883–890.

39 Marshall LF, Knowlton S, Garfin SR, *et al*. Deterioration following spinal cord injury: a multicenter study. *J Neurosurg* 1987;66:400–404.

40 Wilberger JE, Duh MS, Bracken M. The surgical treatment of spinal cord injury – the NASCIS II experience. *J Neurosurg* 1993;83:342A.

41 Mirza SK, Krengel WF, Chapman JR, *et al*. Early versus delayed surgery for acute cervical spinal cord injury. *Clin Orthop* 1999;359:104–114.

42 Hadley MN, Walters BC, Grabb PA, *et al*. Management of acute spinal cord injuries in an intensive care unit or other monitored setting. Guidelines for the management of acute cervical spine and spinal cord injuries. *Neurosurgery* 2002;50(Suppl):S51–S57.

43 Lu K, Lee TC, Chen HJ. Closed reduction of bilateral locked facets of the cervical spine under general anesthesia. *Acta Neurochir (Wien)* 1998;140:1055–1061.

44 Hadley MN, Walters BC, Grabb PA, *et al*. Blood pressure management following acute spinal cord injury. Guidelines for the management of acute cervical spine and spinal cord injuries. *Neurosurgery* 2002;50(Suppl):S58–S62.

45 Levi L, Wolf A, Belzberg H. Hemodynamic parameters in patients with acute cervical cord trauma: description, intervention and prediction of outcome. *Neurosurgery* 1993;33: 1007–1017.

46 Levi L, Wolf A, Rigamonti D, *et al*. Anterior decompression in cervical spine trauma: does the timing of surgery affect the outcome? *Neurosurgery* 1991;29:216–222.

47 Vale FL, Burns J, Jackson AB, *et al*. Combined medical and surgical treatment after acute spinal cord injury: results of a prospective pilot study to assess the merits of aggressive medical resuscitation and blood pressure management. *J Neurosurg* 1997;87:239–246.

CHAPTER 9

Surgical decision-making in spinal fracture dislocations

Robert G. Watkins

There are four basic decision-making factors in spinal fracture dislocations:
1 Neurological status.
2 Spinal stability.
3 The condition of the patient.
4 The capability of the physicians and the facilities.

Neurological status

The most important aspect of determining the patient's neurological deficit is a properly conducted series of examinations. The examination begins with a history of the mechanism of injury and is completed with physical examination of the patient. The best method of conducting serial examination involves a standardized form in which every examiner adheres to the same physical examination. Random notes made on the chart with positive findings may be helpful, but not leave the impression of a thorough examination that can be conducted with serial consistency and accuracy.

The neurological examination must include several components:
• A proper rectal examination involves anal sphincter tone at insertion and sphincter tone in response to digital motion and active voluntary rectal squeeze. Voluntary rectal squeeze is the predominant prognostic factor in ultimate bowel and bladder function. This is a different examination than the rectal examination for prostate inspection. Check the bulbocavernous reflex. Sensation to pinprick should be tested in all four quadrants. Saddle anesthesia should be documented to light touch and pinprick, testing all of the sacral dermatomes.
• The sensation examination should include pain, light touch, vibratory, hot and cold, and proprioceptive sense. Sensory sparing is not a sufficient prognostic indicator of ultimate motor function. It is important to document the completeness of the neurological deficit.
• Presence of spasticity should be evaluated by testing reflexes, strength and tone in the upper and lower extremities along with pathological signs such as the Hoffmann, Babinski, Chaddock, and Oppenheimer.

• Documentation of the sensory level is important. In cervical fractures, the nipple line is the cape-like C4 distribution and should be documented as such. Sensory level may vary in different quadrants of the body.

• A cranial nerve examination is important to rule out intracerebral, brain stem, and upper cord dysfunction.

• Motor function should be documented and graded properly. An understanding of the five levels of motor function is imperative in conducting a proper neurological evaluation. In the acute examination, loading the spine such as doing resistive shoulder abduction and adduction in a patient with a potentially unstable fracture is inappropriate. Great care should be conducted in a patient with neurological deficit as the spine is assumed to be unstable and neurological examination should not contribute to that instability.

• Frankel classification of neurological deficits is well known and should be used in simplification. Injuries are classified into complete and incomplete for upper motor neuron and lower motor neuron. The key to determining complete and incomplete deficit in upper and lower motor neuron lesions depends on an understanding of spinal shock, the transitory period of flaccid paralysis after a spinal cord injury.

• Neurological deficit as a decision-making factor depends first on accurate diagnosis. The neurological deficit must correspond to the level of the spine injury. Disparity between level of the deficit and level of the cord must be resolved to eliminate dual lesions, neurological disease and more extensive cord damage due to cephalad migration of hematoma.

• In terms of documenting the progression of a neurological deficit, a rapidly improving neurological deficit is treated differently than a deteriorating neurological deficit. Again, both depend on proper serial examinations. A complete lesion classically is not an indication for a decompressive-type operation because the ultimate chance for neurological recovery is poor. This is in contrast to an improving lesion of the cauda equina secondary to fracture where the ultimate expectation of recovery would be high.

• The extent of the neurological deficit is important, especially in incomplete lesions. A patient in which an incomplete lesion is a weak toe extensor is considerably a different situation than an incomplete lesion with impaired bowel and bladder function. Surgery would less likely be recommended with a minor deficit of no major functional consequence compared to a major lesion with extreme functional consequences.

• The severity of the neurological deficit is the chief determining prognostic factor in the ultimate functional ability of the patient. It is the prime consideration in the decision-making whether to recommend surgery to the patient versus non-operative care. Early decompressive surgery on all neurological injuries as opposed to realignment of the canal and surgery for chronic instability are two differing thoughts that have not been resolved scientifically despite numerous publications concerning this topic. Upper and lower motor neuron lesions that present with flaccid paralysis considered to be in spinal shock may, under certain circumstances, benefit from an early decompressive and stabilizing operation. This is a multifactorial decision and involves the other aspects of decision to treat rather than neurological deficit alone.

The optimum timing for spinal surgery and acute spinal cord injury is not well defined.[1] Urgent spinal stabilization can be safe and appropriate in poly-trauma patients when progressive neurological deficit, thoracoabdominal trauma or fracture instability increases the risk of delayed treatment.[2–4] While earlier surgery may improve neurological recovery and decrease hospital time in patients with cervical cord injuries treated within the first 72 h,[5] the existing body of literature fails to define the appropriate timing of surgical intervention.[1]

Spinal stability

Multiple classifications of spinal stability have been developed. Classification of spinal fractures has evolved from Holdsworth[6] in 1970 to Denis[7] in 1983 to McCormack[8] in 1994. Most classifications depend on the mechanism of injury. Holdsworth provided the classic classification for spinal injuries secondary to the biomechanics of the injury and identified the role of rotation and ligamentous injury as critical to the behavior of the fracture and its potential for neurological injury.[6] Dorr and Harvey's post-mortem evaluation of spinal injuries further demonstrate the importance of ligamentous injury by first X-raying and then directly manipulating the specimens and using body markings to demonstrate ligamentous injury based on the mechanism of the spinal injury.[9] The shear mechanism of injury demonstrated a total disruption of all ligaments without major fractures over the vertebral body.

Why use a classification of spinal injury? The predominant reason for using the classification at all is to predict the future behavior of an injury if treated non-operatively and sometimes to give insight into the best method of surgical stabilization. Any classification begins with a proper diagnosis of injury to the anatomic structures present in the fracture dislocation area. This involves a careful evaluation first of the plain X-rays, combined with additional studies such as computed tomography (CT) scan, magnetic resonance imaging (MRI) or tomography. The key is to progress anatomically in a consistent direction (e.g. posterior to anterior), naming each bone and ligament, and stating whether that bone or ligament has been injured, and the extent to which it has been injured. While this sounds basic, it is seldom emphasized. The common error is to focus too much on the classification and mechanism of injury. Often, the answer lies in thorough evaluation of the exact structures present in the injured area.

For example, on reading an X-ray of the thoracolumbar area, starting posteriorly (Figure 9.1):
• *Spinous process*: Is the spinous process splayed, spread apart, rotated, split or fractured? On evaluating the spinous processes, splaying or separation of the spinous processes may indicate disruption of the interspinous ligament. The interspinous ligament is not a major factor in decision-making and spinal stability, but splaying of the spinous processes indicates a rotatory sagittal

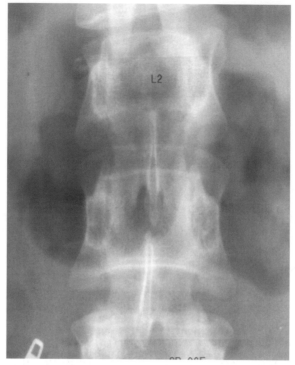

Figure 9.1 For traumatic conditions of the lumbar and thoracic spine, it is critically important to identify each structure on the AP X-ray film. The vast majority of posterior element fractures can be clearly identified with plain X-rays beginning with the more posterior structures and progressing anteriorly. This depth perception-type thinking is important in understanding spinal anatomy. We stress the beginning with the spinous process, and comment on the presence of fractures, spread, or rotation of the processes. The lamina is frequently difficult to see, superimposed on the rest of the spine, but laminar pathology should be identified. Next progress to the level of the facet joints and the pars interarticularus. Comment should be made about the spread of facet joints, integrity of articular process, and possible fractures through the pars interarticularus. The next level is the transverse process. Is it split vertically, ripped off, or damaged? Next, the pedicles; are they spread in relation to the level above and below or do they exhibit fracture lines? Next consider the posterior body wall. Spread of the pedicles indicates that there is an interruption in the posterior body wall. The lateral X-ray is often used to assess the anterior column, and oblique X-rays aid in identification of the facet and pars interarticularis area.

plane lesion that can produce disruption of the ligamentum flavum, facet joint capsules and posterior longitudinal ligament (e.g. the hidden flexion injury of McSweeney described below). Splaying of spinous processes should alert the evaluator for a disruption of posterior longitudinal ligament and a kyphotic deformity appropriate to the extent of the ligamentous injury. It is more specifically tied to the amount of angulation of the vertebrae on the lateral X-ray, with 11 degrees of kyphosis greater than adjacent level as an indication of disruption of the posterior longitudinal ligament and cervical soft tissue instability.[10]

- *Interspinous ligament*: As mentioned above.
- *Lamina*: Is the lamina fractured transversely, vertically, comminuted or a simple fracture? Transverse lamina fractures may indicate a greater potential for displacement than a vertical lamina fracture.
- *Ligamentum flavum*: The ligamentum flavum is the number one stabilizing ligament of the posterior column and its structure should be evaluated in the evaluation of the fracture. If the laminae are spread apart, the ligamentum flavum has been torn or detached. A vertical lamina fracture is in line with the fibers of the ligamentum flavum and does not disrupt the structure of the ligamentum flavum.
- *Facet joints*: Are the facet joints splayed apart or fractured? The superior facet in the cervical spine is a major impediment to rotatory injury. If fractured and displaced a major structural resistance to rotatory injury has been removed. If facet joints are dislocated or splayed apart, there is significant injury to the facet joint capsule. Each of these anatomic lesions is different in its behavior.
- *Pars interarticularis*: Identify the intact pars interarticularis to properly assess whether it has been fractured. Often facets joints would be splayed on one side and the pars fractured on the opposite side. Pars fractures may be acute or chronic. A lateral mass fracture in the cervical spine may mimic a unilateral facet dislocation. A facet dislocation that reduces with a minimal amount of weight in traction such as 10–15 pounds is classically a lateral mass fracture rather than a facet dislocation. Careful evaluation of the anterior column should be carried out with any acute pars fractures. Acute bilateral pars fractures can be completely unstable if the PLL, ALL, and annulus have been disrupted.
- *Pedicle*: Evaluation of pedicles should include the possibility of a transverse fracture indicative of a Chance-type fracture in which, instead of an oval on anteroposterior (AP) radiographs, there are two C-shaped structures facing each other. A comminuted pedicle fracture is a major destabilizing lesion whereas a vertical fracture may not be a significant destabilizing lesion. Stress fractures can occur in the pedicles as they do in the pars interarticularis.
- *Transverse process*: Each transverse process may be fractured transversely as in a Chance fracture. Avulsion fractures of the transverse process are not major destabilizing lesions. These may present with concomitant soft tissue injuries such as kidney damage and retroperitoneal hematoma. The pedicle, transverse process, and superior facet of the joint involved form a three-pronged triplane structure. Evaluation of all these structures should always be kept in mind in relationship with the others.
- *Vertebral body*: The vertebral body should be evaluated for fracture. The degree of comminution is an important factor. An anterior avulsion fracture in the cervical spine may be associated with a significant extension injury. An anterior teardrop fracture in a wedge piece of the edge of the caudal endplate of a vertebral body should always alert one to a similar wedge piece into the spinal canal in the posterior portion of that body, an indication of a compressive lesion. The degree of compression and percentage of anterior versus posterior height have commonly been used as an indication for chronic instability and progression of

kyphotic deformity. In reality, both the angulation and the percentage of the angle of compression of anterior versus posterior is more important as an indication of ligamentous disruption of the posterior column and/or posterior longitudinal ligament. A spine that is displaced enough to produce a major anterior compression may have a damaged ligament in that displacement. There is no indication that a progressive deformity will occur without the ligamentous disruption regardless of the degree of compression of vertebral body.

• *Intervertebral disk*: Disruption of the intervertebral disk may become evident on MRI, discography, careful evaluation of displacement of the vertebral body, and evaluation for intracanal obstruction not obviously attributable to bone fragment. While these disruptions are commonly considered in cases of lumbar pain and degenerative disease, it is just as important to evaluate the structural integrity of the intervertebral disk in fracture dislocations. There is a frequent incidence of disk injury at the same level and at other levels in acute cervical fracture patients. Makes sure there is no disk herniation as a secondary lesion in acute fracture dislocation patients, for example a herniated disk at L2 on evaluation for a fracture of T12. MRI evaluation is imperative in this scenario.

• *Posterior longitudinal ligament*: The posterior longitudinal ligament is the most important stabilizing ligament in the spine. Its strength is thicker and stronger in the cervical and thoracic spine than it is in the lumbar spine. In the lumbar spine, it is a very thin, inadequate-for-support ligament. Most fractures and rotatory injuries of the spine rotate around the axis of the posterior longitudinal ligament. Disruption of this one ligament indicates a major spinal displacement leading toward a chronic progressive deformity after fracture dislocation. Evaluation of the stability and integrity of the posterior longitudinal ligament is important. Displacement of the vertebral bodies may be deceptive on evaluation in that there are times when the ligament can be intact or partially intact by stripping off the back of the vertebral bodies with vertebral body displacement. Still, a diagnosis of significant posterior longitudinal ligament disruption is imperative in determining the difference between soft tissue instability or a chronically unstable spine, one that will not heal with nonoperative care and will produce a progressive deformity when external fixation is removed.

• *Anterior longitudinal ligament*: Anterior longitudinal ligaments are well developed in the lumbar spine. Rotatory injuries in the sagittal plane and kyphotic deformities normally do not disrupt the anterior longitudinal ligaments.

• *Ligamentous injuries*: Fractures and dislocation should be evaluated for ligamentous disruption. Shear injuries may disrupt all of the ligamentous structures of the spine (Figure 9.2).[9] Spinal instability means inability of the bone and ligamentous structures of the spine to prevent displacement of the spinal canal and increased neurological deficit. We classify instability as acute or chronic. Acute instability means that at the time of the injury and immediately after the injury, the spine is unable to provide stability. Every patient with neurological deficit should be considered to have an acutely unstable spine. Chronic instability is the term used for ligamentous instability of the spine, the clinical characteristic of

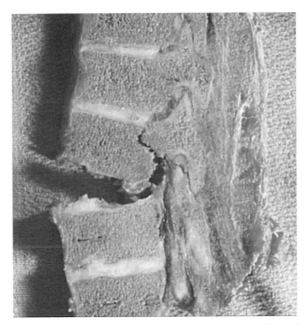

Figure 9.2 This is a demonstration of a shear injury with fracture through the endplate and vertebral body, the pedicles and the facet joints of the posterior column. This is a ligamentous injury of the posterior column, shear ligamentous injury and bony injury of the anterior column, and an unstable lesion.

which is that, even though alignment may be maintained and neurological deficit may be prevented with immediate external fixation, the ligament does not heal sufficiently. There is a much higher chance of continuing progressive deformity despite the external fixation or after the external fixation is removed. Ligamentous injuries are more likely to require surgery and permanent surgical stabilization. Ligamentous injuries may be very innocuous in appearance in the acute setting and careful diagnosis of ligamentous disruption is imperative to protect the patient's neurological status. Spinal bone fractures are more likely to heal and provide stability than ligamentous disruptions (Figure 9.3). Ligamentous disruption is important in diagnosing any fracture dislocation. There are four classic lesions frequently misdiagnosed or not diagnosed to the fullest extent of the lesion:

1 Ruptured transverse ligament (Figure 9.4). This may require flexion–extension films that are not possible in the acutely injured neck and late ligamentous instability may show up when the patient has less spasm and pain.

2 Unstable hangman's fracture (bilateral pedicle fractures and lateral mass fractures at C2, Figure 9.5). When this C2 fracture is associated with a disruption of the posterior longitudinal ligament and annulus of the disk at C2–C3, it can produce a progressive C2–C3 spondylolisthesis.

3 Hidden flexion injury of McSweeney (Figure 9.6). The classic presentation is one of a painful neck secondary to trauma. X-rays reviewed in the emergency

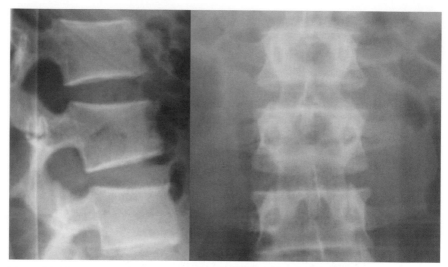

Figure 9.3 This is a bony Chance fracture. The lateral film shows the fracture extending through the pedicles into the vertebral body. The AP film demonstrates a fracture through the lamina, transverse process, and pedicle in a transverse injury. The bony Chance fracture is a chronically stable lesion.

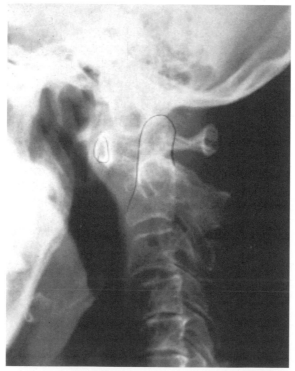

Figure 9.4 This is a demonstration of an unstable C1 ring fracture. It appears that the odontoid is in place and has anterior subluxation of the ring of C1. The transverse ligament is insufficient and ruptured.

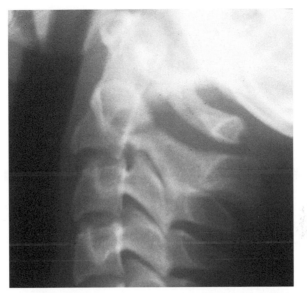

Figure 9.5 This is the extension film of the unstable hangman's fracture. Patients presenting in this fashion should have not only an evaluation of the obvious fracture of the dorsal arch at C2, but the flexion film further demonstrating the spondylolisthesis of C2 on C3 indicative of an anterior column injury.

room demonstrate no fracture or dislocation. It may be too painful for the patient to obtain adequate flexion–extension films and then the patient may not be properly followed up. The classic signs may be a small avulsion fleck of bone on the anterior vertebral body, sagittal angulation between the two vertebral endplates and some splaying of the spinous processes. The pertinent measurement is to measure the caudal vertebral endplates of adjacent vertebrae over three to four segments. If one endplate is angulated 11 degrees greater than an adjacent level, this angulation is indicative of a significant injury of the posterior longitudinal ligament that can lead to a progressive segmental kyphotic deformity. The measurement that is present on any flexion–extension films must be obtained if the standard lateral film demonstrates no instability. If the standard lateral film demonstrates instability, there is no reason to do the flexion–extension films in the acute setting; the spine is unstable. The most common errors made are not knowing how to measure caudal endplates, not doing the measurements on the lateral X-ray in patients who had trauma, and not knowing that it is 11 degrees greater than an adjacent level. The other measurement to check is for horizontal displacement of 3.5 mm of one vertebral body in relation to an adjacent vertebral body.

4. L4–L5 and L5–S1 acute spondylolytic fracture dislocation. Patients present with acute traumatic lumbar pain. There are two critical diagnostic factors: (1) Are the spondylolytic defects acute or old? Use the CT scan characteristics of old versus new spondylolytic defects, that is, formed false facets versus acute fracture lines in the pars. Always look for the intact pars in order to differentiate

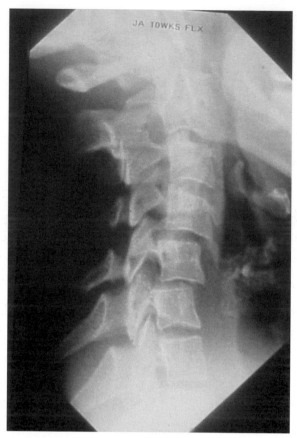

Figure 9.6 This shows a standard lateral X-ray demonstrating a reasonably aligned cervical spine, with a slight anterolisthesis at C4–C5. On the far left, the film demonstrates a hidden flexion injury of McSweeney. This is a greater than 11-degree angulation at C4–C5 with splaying of the posterior processes in the back and a small avulsion fracture anteriorly, a chronically unstable lesion that can progress without proper treatment. It may represent a unilateral facet dislocation. It looks as if these spinous processes are perched posteriorly. There is a demonstration of 25% of subluxation and significant rotation present at that segment. CT scan should demonstrate whether this is a dislocated facet rotational lateral mass fracture or a soft tissue injury.

pars fracture from facet joint. Lumbar SPECT scan maybe helpful. (2) Is there an acute ligamentous disruption of the anterior column and disk? Careful MRI assessment for acute hematoma, disk and ligament disruption, discography, and CT may be helpful. Traumatic spondylolisthesis has a different implication at L4 or L5 than it does at L2 or L3. Progressive traumatic spondylolisthesis in adults is rare. The key, just as in the hangman's fracture, is to understand the traumatic injury to the ligamentous support of the anterior column.

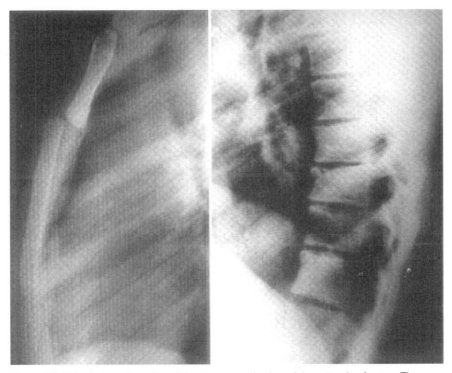

Figure 9.7 This shows a disruption of the sternum and a thoracic compression fracture. The sternum and the ribcage account for approximately 50% of the stability of the thoracic spine. Fractures in the thoracic spine can lead to a progressive deformity when the sternum displaces slowly overtime.

Additional common questions of stability are found in several other specific conditions:

• *Thoracic compression fracture with disruption of the sternum and/or ribcage* (Figure 9.7). Often patients with this injury are admitted to the coronary care unit for a cardiac contusion or to the trauma unit for pneumothorax or mediastinal injury. Traumatologists are aware of the role of unilateral scapular and clavicle fractures and its association with thoracic aortic injury, and there should be an immediate recognition that thoracic spine pain associated with a transverse sternal fracture equals an unstable thoracic fracture. The role of the ribcage has been well documented in thoracic spine instability.[11,12] The ribcage is responsible for enough thoracic spine instability that a transverse sternal fracture with what appears to be a routine compression fracture on X-ray could lead to a progressive kyphotic deformity and late neurological deficit. A classic case is a person after an automobile wreck with steering wheel impact admitted for cardiac contusion and discharged once the cardiac status is stable, presenting weeks later with a progressive kyphotic deformity of the thoracic spine.

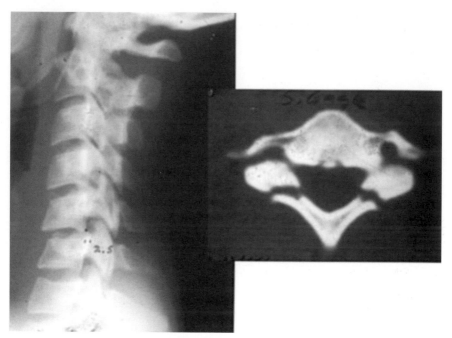

Figure 9.8 These are lateral mass fractures, a subtle subluxation at the level CAT-scanned, with some splaying of the spinous processes but not sufficient to demonstrate a soft tissue instability. A lamina fracture should be a chronically stable lesion as the bone heals to itself.

• *Lateral mass fracture versus unilateral facet dislocation* (Figure 9.8). The classic unilateral facet dislocation is a bow-tie sign when the area above or below the traumatic area or the segment above the traumatic area is rotated compared to the segment below the traumatic area. This produces an oblique view in one aspect of the spine and a lateral view in the other segment of the spine. Where CT scans are more readily available than X-ray, they should be able to distinguish between these two entities. A lateral mass fracture produces a rotation at the injured segment. As the superior facet and inferior facet joint complex rotates, it can produce a grade I spondylolisthesis as does the unilateral facet dislocation. Both are easily viewed on the plain X-ray. The difference in these two entities is that the lateral mass fracture will usually easily reduce into position with traction and extension and deformity will easily reoccur despite external mobilization of any kind, while unilateral facet dislocation is much harder to reduce and is less likely to reoccur with external mobilization.

• *Thoracolumbar junction injuries* (Figure 9.9). Certainly falls and especially motor vehicle accidents have replaced the originally described classic thoracolumbar junction injury in which the rock of a coal face falls on the upper back of a coal miner bent forward on all fours. The joints and ligaments of a thoracolumbar junction injury are amenable to diagnosis on well-read plain X-rays, but even better visualized with CT scan. It is important to diagnose every structure that is injured, name every bone, and name every ligament

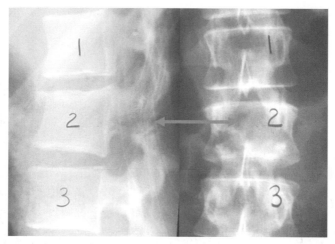

Figure 9.9 This is a thoracolumbar fracture demonstrating a gap in the spinous processes indicating posterior column ligamentous disruption. The fracture extends through the posterior ligament and the pars interarticularis of L2 into the anterior column. This anterior column may demonstrate a soft tissue discogenic disruption. This is a different type of Chance injury than that seen in Figure 9.3.

between each bone to determine the extent of injury and ultimate potential instability. Rotational injuries, common in this area, have a high propensity for ligamentous injury, instability and neurological deficit. The most significant aspect of thoracolumbar junction injury is often making the proper neurological diagnosis.

The conus medullaris, the cell bodies for the lumbar and sacral segments, is usually located at the thoracolumbar junction area. Injury of the conus medullaris produces a lower motor neuron lesion, often one with a lower motor neuron paralysis of the sacral segments, therefore affecting bowel, bladder, and sexual function. A cauda equina lesion is produced by injury to the lumbar and sacral nerve roots within the thecal sac. Ultimate functional recovery of the lumbar nerve roots has a better prognosis than injury to the conus. The cell body injury of a conus medullaris lesion may have the unfortunate result of having a walking patient with no bowel or bladder control. Lower motor neuron sacral segment injury may have a poorer functional outcome than upper motor neuron injuries involving sacral function. Recent developments in implantable electrical stimulatory devices may change this ultimate functional recovery.

• *Burst injuries.* Burst injuries that force bone into the spinal canal are classified into two categories: stable and unstable or, more precisely stated, acutely unstable or chronically unstable. Decision-making centers on two aspects:

i What neurological deficit is present? Profound incomplete neurological deficit with obstructing bone in the spinal canal often leads to spinal surgery to remove the obstructing bone. Considerations are whether the neurological deficits are truly functionally significant and whether the neurological deficit is stable. Recommendation of surgery in an attempt to improve a neurological deficit more likely will be made when the neurological deficit is functionally significant or worsening. The quantity or percentage of bone in the spinal canal is less important as a decision-making factor than is the neurological deficit.

ii Whether the burst injury is chronically unstable. Chronic instability is synonymous with ligamentous injury. A burst injury with a vertical laminar fracture but intact ligamentous structures in the posterior column can heal with a low risk of progressive neurological deficit with non-operative care. A significant ligamentous disruption of the posterior longitudinal ligament, anterior longitudinal ligament, ligamentum flavum, or facet joint capsules, such as with a rotational or shear injury component, is more likely to produce a late deformity and neurological deficit and more immediate operative fixation becomes a greater necessity (Figure 9.10).

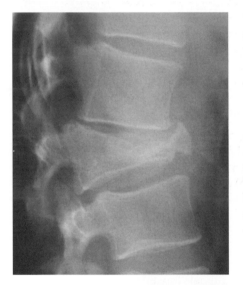
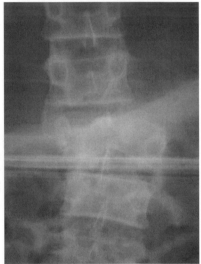
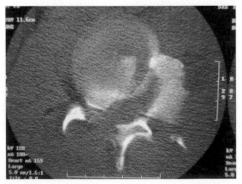

Figure 9.10 This is a burst fracture of the lumbar spine demonstrating severe splaying of the pedicles, disruption of the posterior column with fractures in the pars interarticularis and facet joint. This is a flexion–rotation injury of the upper lumbar spine.

The condition of the patient

Emergent surgery in spinal fractures is often indicated because of spinal instability and neurological deficit. The urgency of spinal surgery is greater with increase in neurological deficits and an inability to maintain acute spinal stability. In an emergency situation immediately post-injury, considerations for spinal surgery are often outweighed by the overall condition of the patient. The proper diagnosis of the patient's total medical condition is imperative in order to save the patient's life. Life-threatening conditions must be treated aggressively and take precedence over spinal instability and neurological deficit. The potential for spinal instability and proper diagnosis of neurological injury can allow protection of neurological elements in the acute setting despite continuous efforts at preventing the patient's death. From the immediate evaluation in the field at the time of a traumatic incident progressing to the hospital stay, an unconscious patient is considered to have an unstable spine until proven otherwise. Efforts must be made to determine spinal injury in massively injured patients. The converse is also true. Focusing on a patient's spinal injury must be combined with an excellent assessment of the patient's overall condition. The patient with an injured cervical spine must be assessed closely for a head, vascular and tracheoesophageal injury. The patient with a fractured thoracic spine must be assessed carefully for rupture of thoracic aorta, ruptured diaphragm, cardiac contusion, pneumothorax, spleen, and liver injuries. The patient with a lumbar spine fracture should be assessed carefully for pelvic and abdominal injuries as well as hip and pelvic injuries. Cerebral and cardiopulmonary function must be carefully evaluated in the acute traumatic patient. Patients in automobile wrecks may have heart attacks. Patients with acute traumatic injuries may have serious pre-existing conditions. The overall condition of the patient must determine the timing of the spinal surgery.

Capability of the physicians and facilities

Over the last two decades, the quality of properly trained spinal surgeons has undergone a dramatic improvement. More facilities are capable of doing excellent spinal surgery and more spinal surgeons are capable of doing excellent spinal surgery. Nevertheless, decision-making in the acutely paralyzed patient is different than the decision-making of most orthopedic surgeons and neurosurgeons practicing an elective reconstructive surgery practice. Many of the operative techniques are quite similar, if not exactly the same. The role of a spinal access surgeon is becoming more significant in daily clinical practice. A spinal access surgeon understands accessing the spine, especially anteriorly, and has the ability to deal with the potential complications of the anterior approach to the spine. Many spinal surgeons possess these abilities themselves. In the acute setting, an anterior approach to the thoracolumbar spine in an acutely injured patient requires a certain level of expertise that must be maintained in order to provide the patient the lowest potential mortality and morbidity rate.

The hospital setting, including nursing and intensive care unit (ICU) capabilities, must be able to deal with any acutely traumatized patient. Spinal and head injuries are at the top of the list of cases that require the best of facility capabilities. This is not purely distinguished as to operative versus non-operative care. Non-operative care of the paralyzed patient is complex and requires training and expertise. There are many aspects in surgical decision-making that are determined by the capability of the physicians and the facilities involved.

Summary

In summary, neurological status, spinal stability, the condition of the patient, and the capabilities of the physicians and facilities are all important decision-making factors in the care of the acutely injured spinal patient.

References

1　Fehlings MG, Tator CH. An evidence-based review of decompressive surgery in acute spinal cord injury: rationale, indications, and timing based on experimental and clinical studies. *J Neurosurg* 1999;91:1–11.

2　Tator CH, Duncan EG, Edmonds VE, *et al.* Comparison of surgical and conservative management in 208 patients with acute spinal cord injury. *Can J Neurol Sci* 1987;14:60–69.

3　Wilberger JE. Diagnosis and management of spinal cord trauma. *J Neurotrauma* 1991;8:21–30.

4　Wilmot CB, Hall KM. Evaluation of the acute management of tetraplegia: conservative versus surgical treatment. *Paraplegia* 1986;24:148–153.

5　Mirza SK, Krengel WF, Chapman JR, *et al.* Early versus delayed surgery for acute cervical spinal cord injury. *Clin Orthop Relat Res* 1999;359:104–114.

6　Holdsworth F. Fractures, dislocations, and fracture–dislocations of the spine. *J Bone Joint Surg Am* 1970;52:1534–1551.

7　Denis F. The three column spine and its significance in the classification of acute thoracolumbar spinal injuries. *Spine* 1983;8:817–831.

8　McCormack T, Karaikovic E, Gaines RW. The load sharing classification of spine fractures. *Spine* 1994;19:1741–1744.

9　Dorr LD, Harvey Jr JP. The traumatic lesions in fatal acute spinal column injuries. *Clin Orthop Relat Res* 1981;157:178–190.

10　White AA, Johnson RM, Panjabi MM, *et al.* Biomechanical analysis of cervical stability in the cervical spine. *Clin Orthop Relat Res* 1975;109:85–96.

11　Andriacchi TP, Schultz AB, Belytschko TB, *et al.* A model for studies of mechanical interactions between the human spine and rib cage. *J Biomech* 1974;7:497–507.

12　Watkins IV RG, Williams LA, Watkins III RG, *et al.* The stability of the ribcage and sternum in the thoracic spine. Presented at *North American Spine Society Annual Meeting,* October, 2004. *Spine* 2005 June 1;30(11):1283–1286.

CHAPTER 10

Spinal cord injury in pediatric patients

Philipp R. Aldana and Douglas L. Brockmeyer

Introduction

The principles of managing acute spinal cord injuries (SCIs) in children are generally similar to those in adults. These principles include recognition of the primary injury, prevention of secondary injury, timely spinal cord decompression, and spinal stabilization (Table 10.1). The controversies that surround the management of SCI in adults also apply to children. Unfortunately, well-designed studies addressing the management of SCI are much fewer in children than in adults. To date, only one prospective, nonrandomized multicenter study has been performed in children regarding the radiographic evaluation of the cervical spine in the emergency room.[1]

Table 10.1 Principles of traumatic SCI prevention and management.

1 Prevention of primary injury
  - General population education
  - Safety programs (e.g. Think First program)
  - Manufacturer improvement of safety equipment (e.g. car seat and automobile restraints improvement)

2 Prevention of acute secondary injury
  - Emergency medical transport team management at scene
  - Early spine immobilization
  - Systemic stabilization
  - Timely spinal cord decompression
    i Reduction of subluxation
    ii Operative decompression
  - Pharmacological treatment to prevent secondary molecular injury

3 Diagnosis and definitive management of SCI
  - Neurological examination
  - Radiographic studies
  - Long-term stabilization if necessary
    i External immobilization with orthoses
    ii Internal fusion with or without rigid internal fixation

4 Long-term management of chronic SCI patients
  - Physical and occupational therapy
  - Vocational rehabilitation
  - Community programs for SCI patient support and recreation
  - Management of medical complications of SCI

The specifics of SCI management in the pediatric population, however, can be quite different from the adult population. Because of a child's systemic immaturity in general and the immaturity of the spinal column and cord in particular, age-specific differences in anatomy and physiology dictate differences in SCI management as a child matures. One of these differences is a large head size relative to body ratio, which predisposes younger children to higher levels of cervical injuries (C1–3). Another difference includes increased ligament and joint capsule laxity in an infant's spine. This, coupled with immature bony anatomy (e.g. horizontally oriented facet joints, absence of the uncinate process, and wedge shaped vertebral bodies), all contribute to the propensity of the pediatric spine to become unstable if the soft tissue elements of the spine fail. A detailed description of these differences is beyond the scope of this chapter. Several reviews are available to the reader for further study.[2–4]

This chapter discusses some of the management principles of SCI in the pediatric population, both those that are controversial and those that are not. In 2002, an issue of the journal *Neurosurgery* was put forth by the American Association of Neurological Surgeons and Congress of Neurological Surgeons' Joint Section on Disorders of the Spine and Peripheral Nerves that contained comprehensive reviews of many SCI-related topics as well as evidence-based guidelines on the management of adult and pediatric SCI.[5] It is not our purpose to duplicate the material covered by these guidelines and we refer the reader to that journal to in order to review that information. We will, however, review the role of corticosteroids in the early management of pediatric SCI, the role of external immobilization in the long-term management of spinal column instability, and the problems associated with internal fixation and fusion of the growing spinal column.

Early nonsurgical management of pediatric SCI: the use of corticosteroids

We are not aware of any human studies examining the effects of corticosteroids on the outcome of SCI in children. Although corticosteroid use in pediatric SCI has been referred to by some as "standard," the data directly supporting its use in children are lacking.[6,7] Like many other treatments in the pediatric population, the use of corticosteroids for SCI was adopted based on data from studies in the adult population, which were initially encouraging.[8,9] A current analysis of the numerous adult studies evaluating the use of methylprednisolone in adult SCI classifies its use as neither a standard nor a guideline, but merely a treatment option.[10] The formulation of the guidelines by the Joint Section on Disorders of the Spine and Peripheral Nerves may have its own limitations,[11,12] but until well-designed pediatric trials on the use of corticosteroids in acute SCI are performed, we do not recommend the routine use of corticosteroids in the treatment of pediatric SCI. At best, the use of corticosteroids is an option that offers the possibility of minor motor improvement countered by an increased incidence of pulmonary and gastrointestinal complications.

Stabilization of the pediatric spinal column

One of the primary differences between pediatric and adult spinal column trauma is that children have a lower incidence of SCI. There are, however, many vertebral column injuries in children that are not usually associated with SCI but that still require careful management. Children also have a lower incidence of cervical spine fractures than adults but many still require stabilization because of ligamentous and/or soft tissue injury.

Role of external orthoses

In general, an external orthosis is preferred over operative stabilization if the orthosis provides adequate support to heal the vertebral column injury.[13] Table 10.2 lists the different types of vertebral column/SCIs, the stability typically associated with such injuries, and the preferred long-term stabilization method. Unstable injuries that have a reasonable chance of healing without internal fixation are treated first with external orthosis, then with internal fixation if this fails. Careful consideration of external orthosis placement may prevent later complications. With halo vest placement, these considerations should include the number of pins to be used, pin torque tightness, pressure ulcers, pin-site infections (both superficial and deep), and patient noncompliance. Despite attention to theses details, the use of halo vests is associated with complications and may be associated with lower fusion rates.[14,15]

Table 10.2 Pediatric spinal column injuries: stability and treatment.

Level	Type	Stability	Primary stabilization
O–C1	Occipital condyle fractures	Typically stable	Cervical collar
	Occipitoatlantal dissociation	Highly unstable	Occipitocervical fusion
C1	Jefferson fracture	Stable	Cervical collar
	C1–2 rotatory subluxation	Stable	Reduction, cervical collar
C2	Odontoid epiphysiolysis	Unstable	Halo, *possibly screw fixation and fusion*
	Type I	Typically stable	Cervical collar
	Type II	Unstable	Halo vest, *odontoid screw fixation*
	Type III	Unstable	Halo vest
	Hangman's fracture	Stable	Cervical collar
		Unstable	Halo vest
	Combination fractures	Unstable	Internal fixation
C3–7	Teardrop fractures unstable	Unstable	Halo vest or internal fixation
	Wedge-compression fracture	Stable	Cervical collar
	Burst fracture	Unstable	Halo vest if no cord compression; anterior corpectomy and fusion for cord compression
	Ligamentous injury	Stable	Cervical collar
		Unstable	Internal fixation
T & L spine	Compression fracture	Stable	TLO
	Posterior column fracture	Stable	None; TLO for comfort
	Fracture dislocation	Unstable	Reduction, Internal fixation
	Burst fracture	Unstable	TLO trial; Internal fixation

SCI without radiographic abnormality, or SCIWORA, can affect any level of the spinal cord and is managed the same way as a ligamentous spinal column injury. The vertebral column in this entity, by definition, is not unstable and therefore rigid immobilization (e.g. halo vest immobilization) is not necessary. Appropriate therapy includes a period of immobilization of the spinal segments involved (e.g. Guilford Brace for cervical lesions and thoracolumbar orthosis for thoracolumbar lesions) as well as activity limitations.[16–18] The period of time required for immobilization is controversial, and is usually decided on a case-by-case basis.

There are several indications for proceeding directly to operative stabilization of the spine rather than using external orthosis. These indications include unstable occipitoatlantal dislocation injuries, unstable burst fractures, the obvious need for spinal cord decompression, open fracture/subluxation reduction, and patient noncompliance with external orthosis. Various types of external orthoses are frequently used for additional immobilization after operative stabilization. These vary from non-rigid orthoses (such as cervical collars), thoracolumbar orthoses (TLO), cervico-thoracic orthoses (such as the Yale brace), and rigid external orthoses (such as the halo vest).

Problems of instrumentation and fusion in growing bone

Instrumentation and fusion in the pediatric spine are problematic mainly because of the immaturity of the vertebrae. In patients under the age of 6 years, the vertebral ossification centers have not matured and cartilage remains between them.[4,19] Size constraints of the involved vertebras being fused often limit the amount of purchase available for internal fixation devices. The size of these devices (e.g. C1–2 transarticular screws and anterior plate fixation) is an important consideration when performing pediatric craniocervical fixation procedures. In addition to vertebral size limitations, sources of autograft bone in a child are not abundant. The traditional autograft sources in the adult (e.g. iliac crest) may need to be supplemented by alternative sites such as rib or calvarium.[20–23] In children, allograft should only be used for anterior interbody fusions; an on-lay allograft fusion has a very high chance of failure. Another potential problem in fusing actively growing bone is the so called "creeping fusion," or the unintentional fusion of vertebral levels adjacent to the fused levels.[2,24] Because of these factors, it is not surprising that rigid *external* fixation (e.g. the halo vest) has become the traditional treatment of choice for unstable fractures in the pediatric population, especially in preadolescent children. However, external fixation, as noted above, is not without its limitations.

The limitations of external fixation, coupled with the improving techniques of modern spinal instrumentation, have made rigid internal fixation with spinal instrumentation the treatment of choice in adult spinal injury. The improvements in instrumentation hardware for the pediatric spine as well as the increasing number of surgeons skilled in these techniques will no doubt broaden the use of craniocervical instrumentation in pediatric spine surgery. The following is a discussion of our preferred treatments for stabilizing pediatric cervical spine injuries.

Occipitocervical instability

In infants up to 18 months, it is technically quite difficult to fashion any construct that will provide adequate internal stability without the need for an external orthosis. Thus, the halo vest is a reliable means of providing immediate stable fixation, coupled with bone and cable fusion for long-term stability. In post-traumatic atlanto-occipital dislocation, the patient is immobilized in a halo vest immediately after the diagnosis is made, and surgery is usually performed while the patient is immobilized in the halo, due to the significant instability of these cases.[25] As noted above, bone graft may be secured to the occiput or atlantoaxial complex with cable or suture but usually on-lay grafting suffices.[26]

In children 18 months to about 3 years of age, internal fixation techniques can be reliably used to secure bone graft to the occiput and the upper cervical spine, resulting in a fairly rigid construct. Since this still may not provide adequate internal stability, external fixation with the halo vest may be necessary for several months to allow the fusion to heal.[26]

In children 3 years and older, we prefer internal stabilization with a rigid occipital-cervical titanium loop, when anatomically feasible. This loop is pre-contoured with a flattened middle section. It is then secured to the occiput with screws; the arms of the loop are secured to the heads of transarticular screws at C1–2 via special couplers.[27,28] An iliac crest autograft is then wired between the arms of the loop and bridges the occiput and the C1–2 posterior elements (Figure 10.1). Using this method of occipitocervical fusion, there have not been any cases of non-fusion, delayed instability or fusion failures on follow-up greater than 12 months.[29] The rigidity of this construct eliminates the need for rigid external orthoses, and patients are kept in cervical collars for comfort only.

Atlantoaxial instability

The etiology of C1–2 instability as well as the child's age influences our preferences for stabilization. Congenital instability (os odontoideum, skeletal dysplasia, etc.) generally does not resolve with external fixation alone. In the child younger than 18 months, once surgical fusion is indicated, traditional C1–2 wiring techniques are used if the anatomy permits, otherwise on-lay grafting is used. The senior author (Douglas L. Brockmeyer, DLB) has described a method of atlantoaxial rib and cable fusion specifically for young children.[30] Stability may be augmented with external fixation devices, such as a halo vest or a Minerva cast. In children older than 18 months who require stabilization, we have had good success with C1–2 transarticular screw placement supplemented by a posterior iliac crest autograft bone and cable fusion.[31–33] No patients in this treatment category required postoperative rigid external immobilization.

Traumatic C1–2 instability in young children (less than 6 years) usually involves a fracture at the C1–2 synchondrosis.[34] The treatment of choice in this case is immobilization with a halo vest, since 80–100% of these cases heal with time.[24–35] If instability persists and the child is older than 12 years, then stabilization through the fracture line with an odontoid screw is usually technically possible. This might be the preferred treatment since this technique

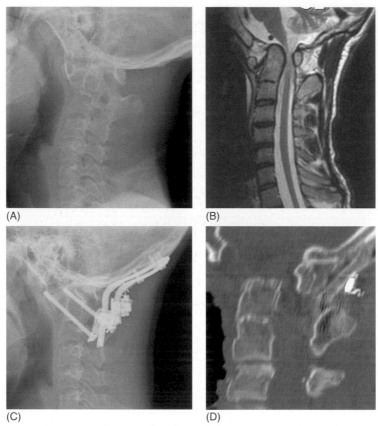

(A)   (B)

(C)   (D)

Figure 10.1 Occipitocervical instability and basilar invagination due to Morqiou's syndrome. This 8-year old boy presented with progressive neurological deficit. (A) Admission lateral cervical spine radiograph. Note basilar invagination and anterior displacement of C1. (B) Preoperative T2-weighted sagittal magnetic resonance imaging (MRI). Note canal stenosis at C1 and severe cervical cord compression. (C) Immediate postoperative lateral cervical spine radiograph showing the construct fusing the occiput to C2 with a titanium loop coupled to C1–2 transarticular screws and iliac crest autograft secured by titanium cable. (D) Computerized tomographic scan with sagittal reconstruction over area of fusion. Note that the tip of the dens has been resected and the bone graft is spanning the instrumented segments.

preserves C1–2 mobility.[28] Children who are younger than 10 years with persistent C1–2 instability despite adequate halo immobilization undergo operative stabilization with the same techniques as those described above. C1–2 instability due to transverse ligament rupture is best treated with posterior C1–2 transarticular screw fixation, if the anatomy allows (Figure 10.2). Other techniques of C1-2 instrumented fusion that have been described in recent years include the insertion of C1 lateral mass screws and C2 pars screws[36] or C2 crossing laminar screws[37], with rods connecting the C1 and C2 screws. The efficacy and safety of these techniques in the pediatric population need to be further studied on larger numbers of patients.

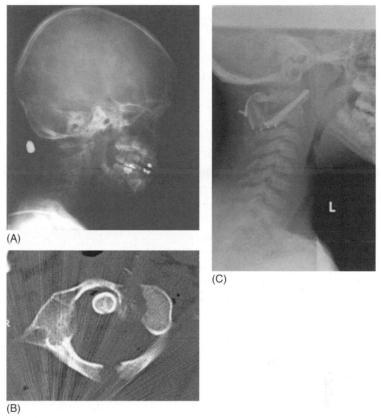

(A)

(B)

(C)

Figure 10.2 Traumatic C1–2 instability due to transverse atlantal ligament disruption and C1 arch fractures. A 9-year-old boy was playing with a blowgun loaded with a 9-mm bullet with the tip of the bullet facing him. The bullet discharged and entered his oropharynx, traveling posteriorly. (A) Admission lateral cervical spine radiograph showing the bullet lodged subcutaneously over the upper posterior cervical spine. (B) Preoperative axial computed tomographic image showing fractures of the anterior and posterior atlas arch as well as the disruption of the left tubercle of the transverse ligament. (C) Postoperative lateral cervical spine radiograph showing the C1–2 transarticular screws as well as posterior C1–2 wiring.

Subaxial instability

The determination of instability of the subaxial cervical spine is complex and beyond the scope of this discussion. The reader is directed to several references dealing with pediatric cervical spine injury for further review.[2–4,13] Once the decision to fuse the unstable subaxial spine has been made, the child's age largely determines the stabilization approach. In children younger than 4 years of age, posterior fusion techniques (e.g. simple on-lay grafting or fixation with bone and cable constructs) augmented by external rigid orthosis (e.g. halo vest) are generally our preferred methods of fusion. This is due to the size of the spine at that age, which does not allow more rigid screw constructs to be placed (e.g. lateral mass screw or anterior cervical plate constructs).[28] Anterior cervical fusion without plating supplemented by halo vest fixation has been described in a 3 years old with a severe fracture dislocation.[34]

After 5 years of age, anterior cervical fusion with plating becomes a viable option for stabilization. The vertebral body is now large enough to provide good bony purchase for the screws in the commercially available miniature plating systems (Short Stature Anterior Cervical Spine Locking Plate (Synthes); Zephyr Plate (Medtronic Sofamor Danek)). In our experience, after the age of 10 years, the lateral masses are of sufficient size to accommodate posterior screw-plating systems. Coupled with autograft fusion, these plating systems provide a rigid construct that generally does not require halo vest immobilization for long-term stability. Using both systems, we have had good success providing lasting stabilization for unstable subaxial cervical spine injuries.[31]

Effects of fusion on cervical spine growth

Although data regarding the long-term effects of cervical spine instrumentation and fusion on the growth of the pediatric cervical spine are scarce, adverse outcomes have not been noted thus far. The senior author (DLB) has previously reported 11 patients (age range 13–16 years) who underwent anterior cervical fusion with plating with at least 5 years of follow-up (abstract).[38] No kyphotic angulation or juxtafusion pathology was noted in that time period. Shacked *et al.* reported six patients (age range 3–14 years) who underwent anterior cervical fusion without plating with a mean follow-up of 4.5 years (age range 3–8 years), all of whom had normal cervical growth and alignment.[39] In our experience, young children who have undergone transarticular screw fixation of C1-C2 as well as those who have had fusion to the occiput with a rigid titanium loop have exhibited vertical growth within the fusion construct.[29]

During intersegmental cervical fusion, the vertebral end plates and disks are removed. The bone graft spans from vertebral body to vertebral body. After fusion, longitudinal growth at that level is arrested. We believe that the absence of progressive kyphosis after fusion is due to the lack of any significant growth plates in the posterior elements causing unopposed growth. In addition, continuous bony remodeling can still occur at the fused level.[19,28]

Conclusions

Little research has been conducted on the management of pediatric spinal cord or spinal column injuries compared to adults. There are no well-designed studies proving the benefit of high-dose methylprednisolone after acute SCI in children. Until further studies are conducted, its use remains an option in the pharmacological treatment of SCI. Therefore, its routine use after pediatric SCI is not recommend. The majority of unstable pediatric spinal column injuries can be treated with external orthoses, and the halo vest is the orthosis of choice for a variety of injuries. Modern spinal instrumentation techniques are not currently suited for the vertebral column of infants less than 18 months old. The increasing use of rigid spinal instrumentation techniques in older infants may provide better results than halo fixation and the initial results of these techniques are encouraging. The recent increase in the number of pediatric spine instrumentation publications likely reflects a shift toward these techniques in the treatment of pediatric spine instability. A notable text on the subject was written recently by the senior author reviews his experience and approach to pediatric craniocervical surgery and includes discussions on topics covered by this chapter.[40]

References

1 Viccellio P, Simon H, Pressman B, *et al.* A prospective multicenter study of cervical spine injury in children. *Pediatrics* 2001;108:1–6.
2 Pang D. Spinal cord injuries. In McLone DG, Marlin AE, Reigel DH, Scott RM, Walker ML, Steinbok P and Cheek WR (eds): *Pediatric Neurosurgery: Surgery of the Developing Nervous System*, 4th edn. W.B. Saunders Co, Philadelphia, PA, 2001, pp. 660–694.
3 Rauzzino MJ, Hadley MN. Pediatric spinal cord injuries. In Sonntag VKH and Menezes AH (eds): *Principles of Spinal Surgery*. McGraw-Hill, New York, 1996, pp. 817–840.
4 Heffez DS, Ducker TB. Fractures and dislocations of the pediatric spine. In Pang D (ed.): *Disorders of the Pediatric Spine*. Raven Press Ltd., New York, 1995, pp. 517–529.
5 Joint Section on Disorders of the Spine and Peripheral Nerves of the American Association of Neurological Surgeons and the Congress of Neurological Surgeons. Guidelines for the management of acute cervical spine and spinal cord injuries. *Clin Orthop Rel Res* 2002;50(Suppl).
6 Hurlbert RJ. Methylprednisolone for acute spinal cord injury: an inappropriate standard of care. *J Neurosurg (Spine)* 2000;93:1–7.
7 Pollina J, Li V. Tandem spinal cord injuries without radiographic abnormalities in a young child. *Pediatr Neurosurg* 1999;30:263–266.
8 Bracken MB, Shepard MJ, Collins WF, *et al.* A randomized, controlled trial of methylprednisolone or naloxone in the treatment of acute spinal-cord injury. Results of the Second National Acute Spinal Cord Injury Study. *New Engl J Med* 1990;322:1405–1411.
9 Bracken MB, Shepard MJ, Holford TR, *et al.* Administration of methylprednisolone for 24 or 48 hours or tirilazad mesylate for 48 hours in the treatment of acute spinal cord injury. Results of the third National Acute Spinal Cord Injury Randomized Control Trial. National Acute Spinal Cord Injury Study. *JAMA* 1997;277:1597–1604.
10 Joint Section on Disorders of the Spine and Peripheral Nerves of the American Association of Neurological Surgeons and the Congress of Neurological Surgeons. Pharmacological therapy after acute cervical spinal cord injury. *Neurosurgery* 2002;50(Suppl):S62–S72.
11 Bracken MB. Guidelines for the management of acute cervical spine and spinal cord injuries. *Neurosurgery* 2002;50(Suppl):Sxiv–Sxix (comment).
12 Bullock R, Valadka AB. Guidelines for the management of acute cervical spine and spinal cord injuries. *Neurosurgery* 2002;50(Suppl):Sv–Sviii (comment).
13 Joint Section on Disorders of the Spine and Peripheral Nerves of the American Association of Neurological Surgeons and the Congress of Neurological Surgeons. Management of pediatric cervical spine and spinal cord injuries. *Neurosurgery* 2002;50(Suppl):S85–S99.
14 Rockswold G, Bergman T, Ford S. Halo immobilization and surgical fusion: relative indications and effectiveness in the treatment of 140 cervical spine injuries. *J Trauma* 1990;30: 893–898.
15 Lowry DW, Pollack IF, Clyde B, *et al.* Upper cervical spine fusion in the pediatric population. *J Neurosurg* 1997;87:671–676.
16 Joint Section on Disorders of the Spine and Peripheral Nerves of the American Association of Neurological Surgeons and the Congress of Neurological Surgeons. Spinal cord injury without radiographic abnormality. *Neurosurgery* 2002;50(Suppl):S100–S104.
17 Pollack IF, Pang D. Spinal cord injury without radiographic abnormality. In Pang D (ed.): *Disorders of the Pediatric Spine*. Raven Press Ltd., New York, 1995, pp. 509–516.

18 Pang D, Wilberger JE. Spinal cord injury without radiographic abnormalities in children. *J Neurosurg* 1982;57:1114–1129.

19 Clark P, Letts M. Trauma to the thoracic and lumbar spine in the adolescent. *Can J Surg* 2001;44:337–344.

20 Sandhu H, Grewal H, Parvatanemi H. Bone grafting for spinal fusion. *Orthop Clin N Amer* 1999;30:685–697.

21 Boyce T, Edwards J, Scarborough N. Allograft bone: the influence of processing and safety on performance. *Orthop Clin N Amer* 1999;30:571–581.

22 Casey ATH, Hayward RD, Harkness WF, *et al.* The use of autologous skull bone grafts for posterior fusion of the upper cervical spine in children. *Spine* 1995;20:2217–2220.

23 Smith M, Phillips W, Hensinger R. Fusion of the upper cervical spine in children and adolescents: an analysis of 17 patients. *Spine* 1991;16:695–701.

24 Odent T, Langlais J, Glorion C, *et al.* Fractures of the odontoid process: a report of 15 cases in children younger than 6 years. *J Ped Orthop* 1999;19:51–54.

25 Kenter K, Worley G, Griffin T, *et al.* Pediatric traumatic atlanto-occipital dislocation: five cases and a review. *J Ped Orthop* 2001;21:585–589.

26 Schultz KD, Petronio J, Haid RW, *et al.* Pediatric occipitocervical arthrodesis: a review of current options and early evaluation of rigid internal fixation techniques. *Pediatr Neurosurg* 2000;33:169–181.

27 Brockmeyer DL, Apfelbaum RI. A new occipitocervical fusion construct in pediatric patients with occipitocervical instability: technical note. *J Neurosurg (Spine 2)* 1999; 90:271–275.

28 Brockmeyer DL. Management of cervical spine fractures in children. In Batjer H and Loftus C (eds): *Textbook of Neurosurgery*. Lippincott Williams and Wilkins, Philadelphia, 2002, pp. 1107–1114.

29 Anderson RCE, Kan P, Gluf WM, Brockmeyer DL. Long-term maintenance of cervical alignment after occipitocervical and atlantoaxial screw fixation in young children. *J Neurosurg* (1 Suppl Pediatrics) 2006;105:55–61.

30 Brockmeyer DL. A bone and cable girth-hitch technique for atlantoaxial fusion in pediatric patients. Technical note. *J Neurosurg* 2002;97(Suppl):400–402.

31 Brockmeyer DL, Apfelbaum RI, Tippets R, *et al.* Pediatric cervical spine instrumentation using screw fixation. *Pediatr Neurosurg* 1995;22:147–157.

32 Brockmeyer DL, York JE, Apfelbaum RI. Anatomical suitability of C1–2 transarticular screw placement in pediatric patients. *J Neurosurg (Spine)* 2000;92:7–11.

33 Gluf WM, Brockmeyer DL. Atlantoaxial transarticular screw fixation: a review of surgical indications, fusion rate, complications, and lessons learned in 67 pediatric patients. *J Neurosurg Spine* 2005;2:164–169.

34 Sun PP, Poffenbarger GJ, Durham S, *et al.* Spectrum of occipitoatlantoaxial injury in young children. *J Neurosurg (Spine 1)* 2000;93:28–39.

35 Mandabach M, Ruge JR, Hahn YS, *et al.* Pediatric axis fractures: early halo immobilization, management and outcome. *Pediatr Neurosurg* 1993;19:225–232.

36 Harms J, Melcher P. Posterior C1-C2 fusion with polyaxial screw and rod fixation. *Spine* 2001;26:2467–2471.

37 Leonard JR, Wright NM. Pediatric atlantoaxial fixation with bilatera, crossing C-2 translaminar screws. *J Neurosurg* 2006;104(1 Suppl Pediatrics):59–63.

38 Brockmeyer DL, York JE. Long-term follow-up of anterior cervical fusion with plating in pediatric patients. Joint section on disorders of the spine and peripheral nerves annual meeting. Rancho Mirage, CA 1998. Abstract.

39 Shacked I, Ram Z, Hadani M, *et al.* The anterior cervical approach for traumatic injuries to the cervical spine in children. *Clin Orthop Rel Res* 1993;292:144–150.

40 Brockmeyer, DL. Advanced Pediatric Craniocervical Surgery. Thieme, New York, 2006.

CHAPTER 11

Management of penetrating spinal cord injury

K. Anthony Kim, Arun Paul Amar and Michael L. Levy

Introduction: penetrating spinal cord injury is here to stay

In the United States alone, 10 to 15,000 new cases of traumatic spinal cord injury (SCI) occur each year.[1] The peak incidence of SCI occurs in adolescents and young adults.[2,3] In earlier studies, motor vehicle accidents and falls accounted for the majority of SCIs.[3,4] In urban centers, penetrating SCIs now account for one-half of all SCIs, rivaling blunt traumatic SCI (Figure 11.1).[5–7] In 1997, gunshots caused 31,636 fatal injuries and approximately 100,000 non-fatal injuries in the United States. A mean medical cost per injury of $17,000, gunshot injuries in the United States in 1994 produced $2.3 billion in lifetime medical costs, of which $1.1 billion was paid by US tax payers. Gunshot injuries due to assaults accounted for 74% of total costs.[8]

Firearm use in violent crimes is standard across the world and shows no signs of abatement. Over a thousand homicides occur in Los Angeles County alone each year, the majority involving the use of a firearm. A total of 7390 gang-related homicides have occurred in Los Angeles County from 1989 to 2000.[9] Ninety-five percent of these gang-related homicides involved firearms.[10] In Los Angeles County in 2002, there were gang-related homicides ($n = 474$), attempted homicides ($n = 726$), felony assaults ($n = 3430$), attacks on police officers ($n = 114$), random shots fired in inhabited areas ($n = 330$), and kidnappings ($n = 77$). Although the majority of these crimes involved low-velocity small-caliber or "civilian" bullet or shotgun injuries, automatic, semi-automatic rifles, submachine guns, sniper rifles, rocket launchers, and other military weapons or "artillery" are also used in urban street crimes.[9] In Los Angeles County, law enforcement officials are aware of more than 1300 street gangs with over 150,000 members. In the City of Los Angeles alone, there are approximately 407 known gangs and over 50,000 members.[11]

It is clear that penetrating SCI will continue to be an epidemic across the world.

Biomechanical principles behind traumatic spinal cord injury: $I = A + B + C + D$

Traumatic SCI is the resultant combination of (A) injury due to the initial kinetic energy (KE) of the impact, (B) the secondary injury resultant from persistent

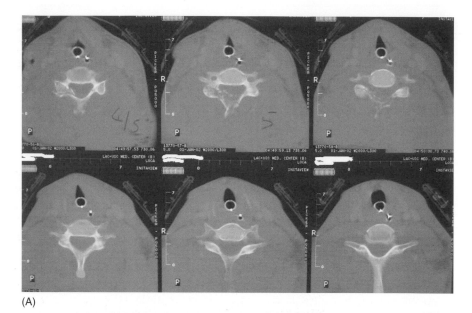

(A)

(B)

Figure 11.1 (A) (Patient A) Non-contrast axial view CT demonstrates penetrating injury to the lamina and facet of C4 and C5. This patient presented with lack of motor function and sensation below these levels. (B) (Patient B) Non-contrast axial view CT demonstrates penetrating injury to the neck and cervical spine at C6–C7 levels. Despite a relatively benign CT scan, the patient presented with paralysis below C7. There is epidural air within the spinal canal, suggesting that the bullet crossed through the neural foramenae from left to right.

compression of the spinal cord, (C) ongoing or delayed ischemic injury from vascular compromise often leading to necrosis of penumbral tissue, and (D) molecular and biochemical alterations in the environs preventing neurorestoration or healing post-injury. Whereas injury (I) is the summation of $A + B + C + D$, the portions of A, B, C, and D involved differ between blunt versus penetrating SCI.

A = Kinetic energy

Both penetrating and blunt SCI sustain initial injury via kinetic energy, KE, which is proportional to mass (m) and velocity (v): $KE = 1/2\,mv^2$. The amount of KE delivered by a missile to tissue $(totKE)$ is equivalent $totKE = \frac{1}{2}\mathrm{m}$ $(v_{initial} - v_{final})^2$, where $v_{initial}$ is the velocity of the missile on entrance into tissue and v_{final} is the velocity of the missile upon exiting the tissue. The amount of kinetic energy delivered can also be increased via the use of bullet jacket manipulation, bullet shape, use of denser missile materials, and magnum shells.

In blunt SCI, the force (F) of the impact is distributed over a wider surface area (SA) than in penetrating SCI, thereby dampening the spearhead of kinetic energy applied to the cord. Velocity (v) in blunt SCI can be considerably less than the velocity noted in penetrating SCI as well. In this regard, KE can be of less concern in blunt versus penetrating SCI. In penetrating SCI, low-velocity firearms have muzzle velocities less than 1000 ft/s whereas high-velocity firearms exceed 1050 ft/s (speed of sound). Often, magnum shells filled with extra gunpowder provide 20–60% more KE than the standard shell of the same caliber.[12–14]

Penetrating SCI and kinetic energy

In penetrating SCI, initial KE dictates the extent of tissue damage and outcome. Mass or caliber of the bullet (m), proximity of fire, type of weapon, size of the knife, velocity of the bullet (v), and extent of other organ injuries including vascular compromise contribute to the patient's eventual neurological outcome. It is unclear at this time what degree of secondary injury exists after penetrating trauma and what amount of such injury is preventable or reversible. In the absence of evidence of secondary injury in penetrating SCI, most surgeons consider penetrating SCI a *static* disease – once the missile has penetrated the spinal cord, little more is done or can be done at present to reverse or stop injury extent. Clearly, once the roles of vascular optimization (C) and molecular neurorestoration and healing (D) are better understood, penetrating SCI will be looked upon anew as a dynamic on-going process.

Most low-velocity or "civilian" bullets are designed to *increase KE* and impact. *Magnum shells* are filled with extra gunpowder to increase KE. Under the assumption that low-velocity bullets are used for gaming, civilian bullets are *partially jacketed* in such a manner that, on impact, the tip will mushroom and impart more kinetic energy, causing more tissue destruction and quick killing of game. This is not the case for military *full-metal jackets*. A partially jacketed bullet produces a cavitation and wound track three times the original diameter of the bullet.

Firearms have been optimized to transfer the highest amount of KE to its target – the resultant effect is a cavitating, shock-wave producing force capable of direct and indirect injury far beyond the limitation of a bullet's size.[12–15]

Blunt SCI $I = a + B + C + D$

Following the injury sustained after blunt trauma, one focuses on the presence of any persistent spinal cord compression or orthopedic deformity that may worsen the neurological condition. The surgeon attends to decompressing the spinal cord, optimizing blood pressure, and maintaining the vascular supply to the spinal cord in hopes to improve outcome and minimize secondary injury. Therefore, the injury from blunt SCI is $I = a + B + C + D$ where a represents a dampened version of the initial kinetic energy, A. Exceptions exist in blunt SCI management, such as SCI without radiological abnormality (SCIWORA), where secondary injury from persistent spinal cord compression is not often present.[16]

Penetrating SCI $I = A + C + D$

Unlike blunt SCI, the injury sustained from penetrating trauma is thought to be almost wholly caused by the initial KE at impact. In penetrating SCI, injury extent to the spinal cord is a direct result of the blast effect, that is, contusion of the cord from the energy imparted by the missile to adjacent tissues, the degree of cord transection, or, the disruption of spinal cord vasculature with consequent ischemia. Thus, in penetrating SCI, the injury is $I = A + C + D$.

Little is known of secondary injury C from vascular compromise or possible vasospasm post-penetrating SCI. Even less is know regarding the molecular environment at work preventing neurorestoration or healing, D. Most authors would agree that, for all intents and purposes now, penetrating SCI $I = A$.

Prudence of non-surgical intervention post-penetrating injury to the spinal cord

Current management goals of a patient post-penetrating SCI are (a) documenting the deficits on presentation, (b) ensuring the deficits do not progress over a 48-h period, and (c) treating the long-term complications that may arise during the hospital course, including cerebrospinal fluid (CSF) leak, pneumonia, urinary tract infections, and spinal instability while maintaining spinal cord perfusion.[17] Of these goals, ensuring that the deficits do not progress is the most difficult as surgical intervention is essentially limited to removal of compression or bleed.

Surgical intervention does not aid neurological outcome

The initial amount of KE received and severity of deficits, rather than the extent of medical or surgical intervention, determine ultimate neurological outcome after penetrating SCI. Numerous studies have attempted at immediate decompression of the spinal canal, retrieval of bullet, closure of dural tears with disappointing results. Neurological outcomes have been unaffected by such early operative interventions.[7,18–21] In fact, almost all patients with a complete deficit fail to improve regardless of surgical intervention. Those with incomplete deficits made similar neurological recovery regardless of surgical intervention.[19–21]

Such studies have undermined the neurosurgeon's enthusiasm to intervene early on the patient with penetrating spinal cord trauma. Operative treatment of penetrating SCI remains unusual, and, in some series, fewer than 4% of cases are explored.[6] Instead, emphasis has been placed on early orthosis, hydration, infection management, pulmonary care, and physical therapy.[22] Recovery of neurological function following several traumatic SCIs is frequently noted to be better in children than adults.[23] Little is known if this is the case as well in penetrating SCI.

Surgical intervention does not decrease infection rates

Surgical decompression and debridement after penetrating SCI seem to have no statistically significant benefit in infection control. In several large series, bullet removal and spinal debridement did not appear to diminish the incidence of infection.[7,18–21,24–26] Neurosurgical intervention in the face of associated visceral injury such as a perforated viscus was associated with a higher complication rate than with repair of the viscus and broad spectrum antibiotics alone.[1]

Surgical intervention for possible pleural fistulae should be deferred

Similarly, in penetrating SCI associated with penetrations of the pleural space, subarachnoid-pleural fistulas were rare and often self-limiting with low likelihood of parapneumonic effusions.[27–30] Hence, concern for subarachnoid-pleural or subarachnoid-peritoneal fistulas with infection is currently not a reason for early spinal cord debridement. After penetrating injury to the chest, the risk of internal CSF fistula is low. Patients are followed closely with serial chest X-rays (CXR).[28–30]

Subarachnoid-pleural fistula is the net result of a nerve root tear with CSF leak in conjunction with a pleural perforation. Alternatively, in the setting of a thoracic spine fracture, a fracture fragment may lacerate both dura and pleura and induce fistula formation. The majority of presentations are delayed with dynpnea or respiratory distress from a pleural effusion. Occasionally, headaches and nausea can occur from pneumocephalus.

In the case of subarachnoid-pleural fistulas, the initial recommendation is observation with close follow-up for headaches due to over-drainage of CSF or pulmonary compromise from CSF-pleural effusion. Daily CXR for the first week followed by once a week during the first month is recommended to look for pleural effusions, extrapleural apical densities, or a widening mediastinum. Water-soluble computed tomography (CT) myelography is the study of choice to confirm the diagnosis and define the anatomy of a fistula. False negatives occur with small fistulae. Chest tubes can be used to drain the pleural effusion while waiting for the CSF leak to seal. Lumbar drains or lumbar taps are used in conjunction to maintain low intraspinal pressure. Persistent fistulae are most often the combination of a large tear and the presence of negative intrathoracic pressure.[31,32]

Lead toxicity from the bullet is rare and serial laboratory studies are needed

Most bullets are made of lead or lead alloy. Because of its high density, lead produces less air drag and more kinetic energy at impact. In order to prevent the melting of lead in flight or from the heat of the explosive gases on firing, the bullet is shielded with copper, brass, bronze, aluminum, steel, or gold.

The risk of lead toxicity from retained bullet fragments is small and only rarely necessitates their removal.[7,24]

In a retrospective review of 12 patients post-gunshot wound to the spine with retained fragments in the intervertebral disk, one patient showed elevated lead levels and clinical evidence of plumbism after an average follow-up time of 7.8 years. This patient underwent microdiskectomy and removal of lead fragment without complications.[33]

Conservative approach to spinal stability after penetrating SCI

White and Panjabi define spinal stability as the ability to sustain physiological loads without incurring (a) structural deformation, (b) painful alterations, or (c) neurological deficit.[34] Bullet injuries to the spine commonly traverse the neural foramen, as the neurovascular bundle is a pathway of least resistance for many missiles (Figure 11.2). Because of this and other reasons, instability of the spine is uncommon after penetrating SCI.[24–27]

From a structural standpoint, Stauffer *et al.*, noted that laminectomy in patients with penetrating SCI anterior or middle column injury may lead to additional and progressive spinal instability or scoliosis requiring internal stabilization and fusion.[20] Hence, structural deformity may be paradoxically incurred with aggressive surgical management of penetrating SCI. Exceptions undoubtedly exist on a case-by-case basis. At present time, a simple spinal orthosis worn for 12 weeks or until the soft tissue and bony elements heal seems to be sufficient. The patient is followed with serial static and dynamic images.

Despite anecdotal reports of pain relief following the removal of a mobile intrathecal missile, the overall incidence of painful episodes after injury seems not to be affected by bullet removal.[24] In particular, the presence of a foreign body as a genesis point for arachnoiditis, syrinx formation, and pain generator requires further study.

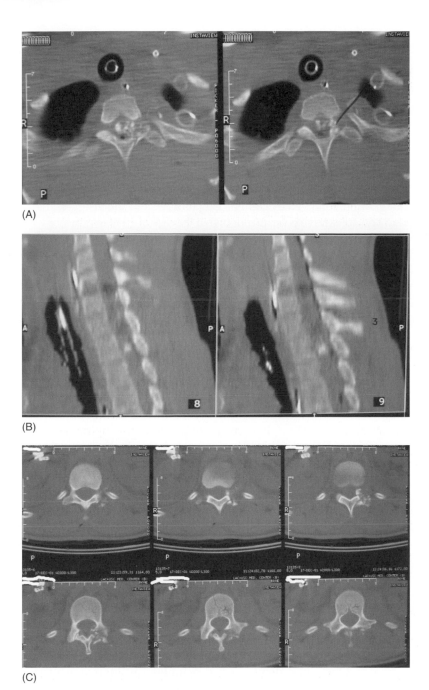

Figure 11.2 (A) (Patient C) Non-contrast axial view CT demonstrates T2 spinal canal involvement by bullet injury. The patient presented with paralysis below this level. Note involvement of the neural foramen, confirming that projectiles seem to find the neural foramen as the path of least resistance. (B) Reconstruction sagittal view CT of the same patient demonstrates three-column alignment despite spinal canal involvement by penetrating injury. Mechanical instability is uncommon after penetrating SCI. (C) (Patient D) Non-contrast axial view CT of the thoracolumbar junction demonstrates neural foraminal involvement.

Role of surgical intervention post-penetrating SCI

Early principles of surgical technique in the management of spinal cord gun-shot wound injury are derived from wartime experience and include place-ment of the skin incision distant from the missile entrance site, sharp dissection of the paraspinal muscles, debridement of all devitalized or contaminated tis-sues along the missile tract, wide bony exposure above and below the level of injury, decompressive laminectomy for removal of any compressive elements (hematomas, bony fragments, metallic fragments), and repair of dura with or without grafting, followed by copious irrigation.[19,27,35–37] Such aggressive man-agement principles have been abandoned in the case of civilian gunshot wounds as wartime high-velocity injuries seem not to correlate with the outcome of civilian low-velocity injuries.[18,20,21,25,26,36,37] Undoubtedly, new generations of powerful antibiotics have aided in promoting a more conservative management algorithm for wound care.

Although non-operative management of penetrating SCIs prevails in the majority of cases, exceptions exist. Authors agree that *persistent* external or internal CSF fistulas require repair. Vertebral dissection, occlusion with or without stroke, or the presence of an arteriovenous fistula can be managed with endovascular techniques (Figure 11.3).[38] Progressive neurological deficits due to compressive effects of a retained bullet or secondarily due to bony or disk compression should be treated as non-penetrating spinal injuries. Large epidural hematomas or epidural abscesses constitute indications for urgent surgical intervention.[19,20,27,35] In such regards, penetrating injuries cross a hazy line into non-penetrating or blunt injuries and should be treated in a case-by-case manner. The role of pharmacological agents such as steroids used in blunt SCI may be considered as well.

Injuries to the cauda equina represent a subset of penetrating SCI that may be amenable to surgical intervention. CT with or without myelography can confirm the presence of a bullet fragment impinging on or embedded in the cauda equina.[36] Studies suggest that injuries to the cauda equina are more likely to recover from the effects of blast injury or compression than cord injuries. Such patients with penetrating injuries to the cauda equina may ben-efit particularly from decompression of nerve roots, regardless of the initial severity of the patient's condition.[7,21,27,36,39,40] The theory behind the recovery presupposes that gunshot wounds below the L2 level involve the ventral and dorsal nerve roots of the cauda equina rather than tissue of the central nerv-ous system and are therefore less likely to lead to a complete deficit and more likely to heal. One study demonstrated neurological improvement in both complete and incomplete injuries after removal of bullets retained within the thoracolumbar junction, but not in those at higher vertebral levels.[21] Once again, the cauda equina represents a unique area of blending between the central nervous system and the peripheral nervous system, lending itself to differential research and management.

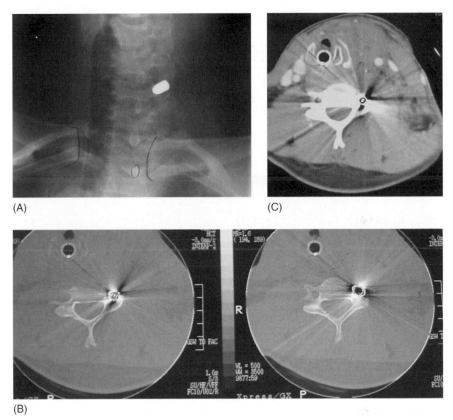

(A)   (C)

(B)

Figure 11.3 (A) (Patient E) Anteroposterior X-ray of the cervical spine demonstrates a bullet lodged in the left lateral mass of C6. Injury to the vertebral artery (dissection, occlusion, or arteriovenous fistula) should be suspected. (B) Non-contrast axial view CT of the cervical spine in the same patient demonstrates the relationship of the bullet to the transverse foramen. (C) Axial view CT angiogram of the neck in the same patient demonstrates complete occlusion of the vertebral artery at the level of injury.

Timing of surgical intervention

Non-operative management of penetrating SCIs prevails in the majority of cases. Urgent operative intervention aims at treating the compressive non-penetrating SCI segments, such as compression from hematomas, disk or bony fragments, or the bullet itself.

Rarely, an acute CSF leak or open dura communicating with the surface may necessitate urgent closure. An example is a large shotgun wound ~30 cm wide with exposure from the skin to the spinal cord. In our experience, such wounds can be closed with staged surgical procedures over the course of 1–2 months. The spinal cord and contents are debrided during the first operation. If possible, a muscle flap is used to cover the spinal cord, or, a fascial layer is closed over the spinal cord. Serial irrigation and debridements can follow, each time with closure of deeper to superficial layers as able. The use of a wound-vacuum system in-between surgeries is recommended with dressing changes each day initially and then each 3 days as needed. Heterotopic bone formation may occur and facilitate spinal stability in these cases. Otherwise, bedrest or orthosis is recommended if the wound will allow orthosis placement.

The majority of surgery is reserved for treatment of delayed complications such as abscesses or fistulae, or, in the rare occasion, for the stabilization of the spine. If possible, spinal stabilization should best be attempted after the patient's acute issues have been stabilized. Chronic spinal instability from initial missile injury is exceedingly rare.[7,24,27] In one series of 1300 cases of civilian gunshot wounds to the spine, none demonstrated instability.[24] Pneumonia, urinary tract infections, hemodynamic instability, vascular injuries should be managed first. In many cases, visceral or vascular injuries are more life threatening and must take precedence over diagnostic work-up, imaging, and management of SCIs. Alternatively, mistreated vascular or visceral lesions may aggravate SCI via sepsis, hypoxia, or hypotension.

Late manifestations of SCI such as syringohydromyelia (e.g. from arachnoiditis), migration of the missile within the thecal sac, and intractable pain can be managed surgically as well.[19,24,27,40]

Pain management should first be attempted medically as surgery has met with limited success. Surgical options include lysis of adhesions, retrieval of migratory or offending bullet or fragment, rhizotomy, cordotomy, neurolysis, neuroma excision, other ablative features, or via the use of a pain injection system. Syringohydromyelia can be treated with lysis of arachnoiditis adhesions followed by a duroplasty as needed. Syringoperitoneal or syringopleural shunting are reserved for patients who have failed adhesionolysis or at the surgeon's discretion.

Medical management of penetrating SCI

Glucocorticoids are not recommended

With the recent controversies regarding the use of glucocorticoids and the lack of efficacy noted in penetrating trauma, steroids *are not* used in penetrating SCI. The potential for a higher prevalence of wound infections at trauma and operative sites,[41–43] the theoretical potential for increased gastrointestinal hemorrhage,[44–46] and the increased risk associated with hyperglycemia and hip necrosis make the use of steroids an unnecessary risk. High-dose corticosteroids may also impede neurological recovery and neuronal regeneration.[44,47,48]

In a retrospective study of 254 patients treated post-gunshot wound to the spine between 1979 and 1994, Heary *et al.* noted no statistically significant benefits in patients who were given methylprednisone (NASCIS 2 protocol), decadron, or no steroids after 56-month follow-up.[49] Infectious, gastrointestinal complications, and pancreatitis (presumably secondary to sepsis) were higher in the steroid group.[49]

In a prospective randomized double-blinded study of 46 patients between 1993 and 1999, Takuji *et al.* noted a higher incidence of pulmonary complications in the group receiving steroids after acute cervical spinal injury than in the group receiving placebo.[50] The majority of complications were pneumonia, particularly in the elderly.

Broad spectrum antibiotics and tetanus vaccinations are recommended

All patient with penetrating SCI should be maintained on broad spectrum antibiotics with blood–brain barrier penetration, such as third-generation cephalosporins, for 10–14 days.[18–21,25–27,35,36] If meningitis is suspected, a lumbar tap is performed to rule out atypical species. As penetrating SCI will have associated visceral or vascular injury in 25–80% of patients, antibiotic use in these patients is not uncommon for other reasons.[18,39,51]

Tetanus prophylaxis should be administered in all patients who are not up to date on immunizations.[19,21]

Low-molecular-weight heparin for deep venous thrombosis (DVT) prophylaxis is currently a standard in the medical management of all SCIs. Some surgeons have opted to place an inferior vena cava Greenfield filter in patients who are immobilized.

Maintenance of systemic blood pressure and spinal cord perfusion is crucial in minimizing secondary spinal cord insult. Shock should be managed appropriately with hydration and inotropic support to render sufficient blood supply to the spinal cord.

Conclusions

Once a patient has sustained penetrating SCI, the restoration spinal cord function is limited. Current management deals with optimizing vascular supply to the cord, addressing persistent spinal cord compression, and treating sepsis, DVT, shock, pneumonia, respiratory failure, neurogenic bladder, that is, the sequelae of SCI. Until at such time a penetrating spinal cord restorative treatment modality has been established, efforts should continue at the preventive front with neurosurgeons playing a strong educational role.[1]

References

1 Amar AP, Levy ML. Surgical controversies in the management of spinal cord injury. *J Am Coll Surg* 1999;88:550–566.

2 Griffin MR, Opitz JL, Kurland LT, *et al.* Traumatic spinal cord injury in Olmsted county, Minnesota, 1935–1981. *Am J Epidemiol* 1985;121:884–895.

3 Stover SL, Fine PR. The epidemiology and economics of spinal cord injury. *Paraplegia* 1987;25:225–228.

4 DeVivo MJ, Rutt RD, Black KJ, *et al.* Trends in spinal cord injury demographics and treatment outcomes between 1973 and 1986. *Arch Phys Med Rehabil* 1992;73:424–430.

5 Kraus JF, Silberman TA, McArthur DL. Epidemiology of spinal cord injury. In Menezes AH and Sonntag VKH (eds): *Principles of Spinal Surgery*. McGraw-Hill, New York, 1996, pp. 41–58.

6 Rea GL. Subaxial injuries of the cervical spine. In Menezes AH and Sonntag VKH (eds): *Principles of Spinal Surgery*. McGraw-Hill, New York, 1996, pp. 885–898.

7 Aarabi B, Alibaii E, Taghipur M, *et al*. Comparative study of functional recovery for surgically explored and conservatively managed spinal cord missile injuries. *Neurosurgery* 1996;39:1133–1140.

8 Cook PJ, Lawrence BA, Ludwig J, *et al*. The Medical Costs of Gunshot injuries in the United States. *JAMA* 1999;282:447–454.

9 Los Angeles Police Department Website, LAPD Crime Statistics www.lapdonline.org, 2002.

10 Hutson HR, Anglin D, Kyriacou DN, *et al*. The epidemic of gang-related homicides in Los Angeles County from 1979 through 1994. *JAMA* 1995;274:1031–1036.

11 Los Angeles Almanac, www.losangelesalmanac.com, 2002.

12 Sykes LN, Champion HR, Fouty WJ. Dum-dums, hollow-points, and devastators: techniques designed to increase wound potential of bullets. *J Trauma* 1988;28:618–623.

13 Ordog GJ, Wasserberger J, Subramanian B. Wound ballistics: theory and practice. *Ann Emerg Med* 194;13:1113–1122.

14 Adams DB. Wound ballistics: a review. *Milit Med* 1982;147:832–835.

15 Bartlett CS. Clinical update: gunshot wound ballistics. *Clin Orthop* 2003;408:28–57.

16 Pang D, Wilberger Jr JE. Spinal cord injury without radiologic abnormality in children. *J Neurosurg* 1989;57:114–129.

17 Chiles BW, Cooper PR. Current concepts: acute spinal injury. *NEJM* 1996;334:514–520.

18 Venger BH, Simpson RK, Narayan RK. Neurosurgical intervention in penetrating spinal trauma with associated visceral injury. *J Neurosurg* 1989;70:514–518.

19 Heiden JS, Weiss MH, Rosenberg AW, *et al*. Penetrating gunshot wounds of the cervical spine in civilians. *J Neurosurg* 1975;42:575–579.

20 Stauffer ES, Wood RW, Kelly EG. Gunshot wounds of the spine: the effects of laminectomy. *J Bone Joint Surg* 1979;61A:389–392.

21 Yashon D, Jane JA, White RJ. Prognosis and management of spinal cord and cauda equine bullet injuries in sixty-five civilians. *J Neurosurg* 1970;32:163–170.

22 Kitchel SH. Current treatment of gunshot wounds to the spine. *Clin Orthop* 2003;408:115–119.

23 Wang MY, Hoh DJ, Leary SP, *et al*. High rates of neurological improvement following severe traumatic pediatric spinal cord injury. *Spine* 2004;13:1493–1497.

24 Yoshida GM, Garland D, Waters R. Gunshot wounds to the spine. *Orthop Clin N Amer* 1995;26:109–116.

25 Romanick PC, Smith TK, Kopaniky DR, *et al*. Infection about the spine associated with low-velocity missile injury to the abdomen. *J Bone Joint Surg* 1985;67A:1195–1201.

26 Roffi RP, Waters RL, Adkins RH. Gunshot wounds to the spine associated a perforated viscus. *Spine* 1989;14:808–811.

27 Jallo GI, Cooper PR. Penetrating injuries of spine and spinal cord. In Menezes AH and Sonntag VKH (eds): *Principles of Spinal Surgery*. McGraw-Hill, New York, 1996, pp. 807–815.

28 Beutel EW, Roberts JD, Langston HT, *et al*. Subarachnoid-pleural fistula. *J Thorac Cardiovasc Surg* 1980;80:21–24.

29 Djergaian RS, Roberts JD, Ditunno JF, Angstadt J. Subarachnoid-pleural fistula in traumatic paraplegia. *Arch Phys Med Rehabil* 1982;63:488–489.

30 Lovaas ME, Castillo RG, Deutschman CS. Traumatic subarachnoid-pleural fistula. *Neurosurgery* 1985;17:650–652.

31 Godley CD, McCabe CJ, Warren RL, *et al.* Traumatic subarachnoid-pleural fistula: case report. *J Trauma* 1995;38:808–811.

32 Lloyd C, Sahn S. Subarachnoid pleural fistula due to penetrating trauma. *Chest* 2002;122:2252–2256.

33 Scuderi GJ, Vaccaro AR, Fitzhenry LN, *et al.* Long-term clinical manifestations of retained bullet fragments within the intervertebral disk space. *J Spinal Disord Tech* 2004;17:108–111.

34 White AA, Panjabi MM. The role of stabilization in the treatment of cervical spine injuries. *Spine* 1984;9:512–522.

35 Jacobs GB, Berg RA. The treatment of acute spinal cord injuries in a war zone. *J Neurosurg* 1971;34:164–167.

36 Benzel EC, Hadden TA, Coleman JE. Civilian gunshot wounds to the spinal cord and cauda equine. *Neurosurgery* 1987;20:281–285.

37 Clark WK. Spinal cord decompression in spinal cord injury. *Clin Orthop Rel Res* 1981;154:9–13.

38 Albuquerque FC, Javedan SP, McDougall CG. Endovascular management of penetrating vertebral artery injuries. *J Trauma* 2002;53:574–580.

39 Wannamker GT. Spinal cord injuries: a review of the early treatment in 300 consecutive cases during the Korean conflict. *J Neurosurg* 1954;11:517–524.

40 Cybulski GR, Stone JL, Kant R. Outcome of laminectomy for civilian gunshot wound injuries of the terminal spinal cord and cauda equine: review of 88 cases. *Neurosurgery* 1989;24:392–397.

41 Bracken MB, Collins WF, Freeman DF, *et al.* Efficacy of methylprednisone in acute spinal cord injury. *JAMA* 1984;251:45–52.

42 Dumont RJ, Verma S, Okonkwo DO, *et al.* Acute spinal cord injury. Part II. Contemporary pharmacotherapy. *Clin Neuropharmacol* 2001;24:265–279.

43 Bracken MB. Methylprednisolone and acute spinal cord injury. *Spine* 2001;26:S47–S54.

44 Bracken MB, Shepard MJ, Collins WF, *et al.* Methylprednisolone or nalaxone treatment after acute spinal cord injury: 1-year follow up data. *J Neurosurg* 1992;76:23–31.

45 Murphy KP, Opitz JL, Cabanela ME, *et al.* Cervical fractures and spinal cord injury: outcome of surgical and nonsurgical management. *Mayo Clin Proc* 1990;65:949–959.

46 Levy ML, Gan HS, Wijesinghe HS, *et al.* Use of methylprednisolone as an adjunct in the management of patients with penetrating spinal cord injury: outcome analysis. *Neurosurgery* 1996;39:1141–1148.

47 Bracken MB, Holford TR. Effects of timing of methylprednisolone or nalaxone administration on recovery of segmental and long-tract neurological function in NASCIS-2. *J Neurosurg* 1993;79:500–507.

48 Amar AP, Levy ML. Pathogenesis and pharmacological strategies for mitigating secondary damage in acute spinal cord injury. *Neurosurgery* 1999;44:1027–1039.

49 Heary RF, Vaccaro AR, Mesa JJ, *et al.* Steroids and gunshot wounds to the spine. *Neurosurgery* 1997;41:576–584.

50 Takuji M, Tetsuya T, Mamoru K, *et al.* Early complications of high-dose methylprednisolone sodium succinate treatment in the follow-up of acute cervical spinal cord injury. *Spine* 2001;26:426–430.

51 Kumar A, Wood GW, Whittle AP. Low-velocity gunshot injuries of the spine with abdominal viscus trauma. *J Orthop Trauma* 1998;12:514–517.

CHAPTER 12

Traumatic vascular injury to the cervical spine

Michael L. DiLuna and Arun Paul Amar

Introduction

Traumatic injuries to the vasculature of the cervical spine, whether through penetrating, blunt, or iatrogenic mechanisms, are uncommon. The overall incidence of injuries to the cervical (extracranial) vessels is estimated to be between 0.2% and 0.8% depending on the institutional policies of screening aggressiveness and country of origin of the studies.[1] The result of such injuries, however, can be devastating. Published morbidity and mortality rates vary from 5% to 50%.[2–5] The cause of adverse outcomes is usually cerebral ischemia from hemodynamic or thromboembolic phenomena.

This chapter will address the epidemiology and mechanism of these various injuries, diagnostic modalities, and treatment options. Management of vascular injury may be required before, concurrent with, or after management of associated injury to the spinal cord or vertebral column, depending on the severity of each lesion. Neurological deficits in head and neck trauma patients are often attributed to cerebral cortex injuries, and vascular studies are not often performed. In many cases, the vascular injury must be suspected on the basis of traumatic mechanism or bony imaging alone.

Penetrating traumatic injury to the arteries of the neck

Injury to the carotid or vertebral arteries (VA) after penetrating trauma to the neck is a frequent finding, and the outcomes are generally poor. The first report of a penetrating injury to the carotid artery (CA), an intervention (ligation), and subsequent post-operative neurological deficit was by Ambroise Pare in 1552.[2] His patient suffered a stab wound of the left internal carotid artery (ICA) after a war-time duel; postoperatively, he was aphasic and hemiplegic.

When a penetrating injury to the anterior or lateral neck occurs, the major arteries are found to be injured in 5–10% of cases.[6] Mortality can be as high as 25%, with the majority of deaths (75%) occurring as a result of stroke.[1,2,5] It appears that the more proximal the injury (e.g. brachiocephalic artery versus carotid artery), the higher the mortality.

Two characteristics of the trauma must be recognized and diagnosed on presentation: the mechanism and the location. With respect to mechanism, the type of instrument (e.g. bullet, knife, or spear) and the interaction of said instrument with the surrounding tissues must be understood before any decision tree is implemented. Missiles and bullets vary widely with respect to velocity, mass, and kinetic energy; therefore, the potential for injury to the vessels of the neck is commensurately different. The same is true for knives, spears, swords, and other objects like screwdrivers and ice picks. Each one varies in the size (width) of tissue damaged and cutting edge characteristics. Missile and gunshot wounds are common in the developed world and during military conflict, while knives, arrows, and spear injuries are more likely to be seen in the developing world. Most of the cases reported to date of the latter are small series and the patients presented late after their injuries.[7,8] The most common complications seen, after infection, were pseudoaneurysm and fistula formation (Figures 12.1 and 12.2).[7–10]

On presentation, one should examine for characteristics of the entry site such as active hemorrhage, hematoma, or subcutaneous emphysema that would indicate the nature and extent of the injury. On physical examination, the patient might be hemodynamically unstable or present with other pertinent findings like neurological deficit (from cerebral ischemia, damage to the nearby brachial plexus, or associated spinal cord injury (SCI)), hoarseness (recurrent laryngeal nerve injury), stridor, or a bruit. Specifically, hemodynamic instability nearly triples the mortality from carotid injury.[5] It is important to note that the absence of physical examination findings does not exclude the possibility of vascular injury, as up to 20% will show no obvious sign.[11] Studies have indicated that physical examination alone carries a specificity and sensitivity of approximately 50% each.[11]

With respect to location of the injury, the trauma literature divides the neck up into three zones, each carrying a different set of potential injuries and needs for exploration:

• Zone I represents the horizontal area between the clavicle/suprasternal notch and the cricoid cartilage encompassing the thoracic outlet structures. Important vascular structures at risk include the proximal common carotid artery (CCA), VA, and subclavian arteries (ScA).
• Zone II represents the area between the cricoid cartilage and the angle of the mandible. Important vascular structures at risk include the ICA and external carotid arteries (ECA) and jugular veins (JV). The VA is somewhat protected by the bony transverse foramen.
• Zone III represents the area that lies between the angle of the mandible and the base of the skull. Important vascular structures at risk include the distal extracranial carotid (ICA, ECA) and VA and the uppermost segments of the JV.

Diagnostics

Typically, most centers favor exploration of all Zones I and III and selected Zone II injuries. In the event of hemodynamic instability, all patients should

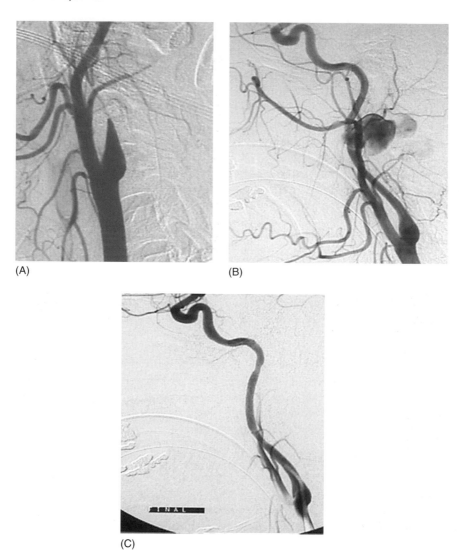

Figure 12.1 Thirty-five-year-old man who was stabbed in the left neck and subsequently developed aphasia and right hemiparesis due to an ischemic infarct of the left middle cerebral artery territory. (A) Left carotid angiogram, lateral view, arterial phase. Note occlusion of the ICA due to dissection. (B) Follow-up angiogram performed 10 days later shows recanalization of the ICA along with an enlarging, multi-lobulated pseudoaneurysm. (C) After placement of a covered stent-graft, flow through the ICA is preserved while the pseudoaneurysm is excluded (modified from Ref. [26]).

be explored with the assumption of an arterial injury.[4,12–14] Zones I and III injuries should be imaged with some vascular study, as should Zone II injuries in selected cases. Color Doppler ultrasound enjoyed brief favor in the cervical vessel trauma literature due to its non-invasive and inexpensive nature, but

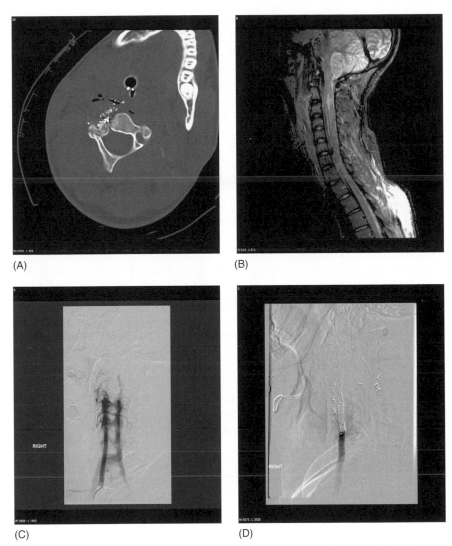

(A)

(B)

(C)

(D)

Figure 12.2 Eighteen-year-old man shot in the neck. (A) Axial computed tomography (CT) scan of the cervical spine. Note bullet shrapnel and bone fragments within the right transverse foramen, at the expected site of the VA. The spinal canal is not disrupted. (B) Sagittal magnetic resonance imaging (MRI) scan of the cervical spine. Note the abnormal signal within the spinal cord from C2 to C4 due to blast effect from the bullet, even though the bony canal was intact. The patient had an associated neurological deficit. (C) Catheter cerebral angiogram, right VA (arrow), arterial phase, lateral view. Note that antegrade flow to the brain is interrupted by an arteriovenous fistula, with rapid drainage into vertebral veins (double arrows). (D) Catheter cerebral angiogram, right VA, arterial phase, lateral view status post-endovascular embolization. The contrast column stops at the site of occlusion, proximal to the fistula. Collateral flow to the brain from the contralateral VA was sufficient.

criticism centers on operator dependency and limited sensitivity in Zones I and III.[15–17] Catheter angiography remains the gold standard,[4] but computed tomography angiography (CTA) and magnetic resonance angiography (MRA) continue to improve in their utility. Helical computed tomography angiography (HCTA) has replaced conventional angiography in many institutions. Prospective studies comparing HCTA with catheter angiography in cases of penetrating neck trauma have reported sensitivities and specificities of 90–100% in hemodynamically stable candidates.[18,19] MRA might offer improved sensitivity and specificity, however, access and speed remains an issue at most institutions, and thus its utility in penetrating injuries may be limited.

Treatment

For surgical exploration planning, it is important to understand that in true Zone I injuries, proximal control of the affected artery will be difficult, while distal control of Zone III injuries will be equally difficult. Surgical repair was long accepted as the standard treatment after injury, but this practice has recently been questioned by reports showing that some patients suffer detriment from revascularization. The primary concern is hemorrhagic conversion of ischemic injuries in the cerebral cortex. Numerous studies have compared the risks and benefits of surgical repair, and have arguments for either side have been presented.[2,20–24] Some studies suggest that younger patients who have repair or revascularization procedures do better than those who undergo ligation or "take-down" interventions.[5] Other studies confirm more favorable functional neurological outcomes (using the Carotid Neurologic Outcome Score) in patients undergoing reconstruction versus ligation.[1,5] The presence of a large stroke (by imaging or clinical criteria) must be considered in the decision to revascularize an injured vessel.

Recently, endovascular techniques have greatly improved in efficacy and are rapidly being employed to repair penetrating injuries (Figures 12.1 and 12.2). Ligation ("take-down"), repair of pseudoaneurysms, and closure of fistulae can all be performed with endovascular techniques, and indeed, the preliminary reports have been very promising.[25–31]

Blunt traumatic injury to the arteries of the neck

The incidence of blunt CA injury after trauma to the head and neck ranges from 0.08% to 0.86%,[2,32–39] and the incidence of blunt VA is up to 0.60%.[36,37,40] Even with the most aggressive of screening policies, only 1% of trauma patients with head and neck injuries have vascular injuries.[37] Mortality is estimated to be around 25% from CA injury and 10–20% (significantly less) after VA injury.[36,37,40] Motor vehicle collisions are the most common cause of these injuries, but many activities that predispose to acceleration–deceleration events, twisting, or extreme flexion/extension of the neck can also cause damage, including chiropractic manipulation, yoga, wrestling, and passive head turning.

Decades ago, blunt CA injury garnered much attention and VA injury was thought to be rare and of minimal neurological consequence. More recent studies have refuted this misconception. Though VA injuries carry an incidence of 0.4–0.6%, the associated stroke rate is as high as 25% (Figure 12.3).[36,37,40] Because

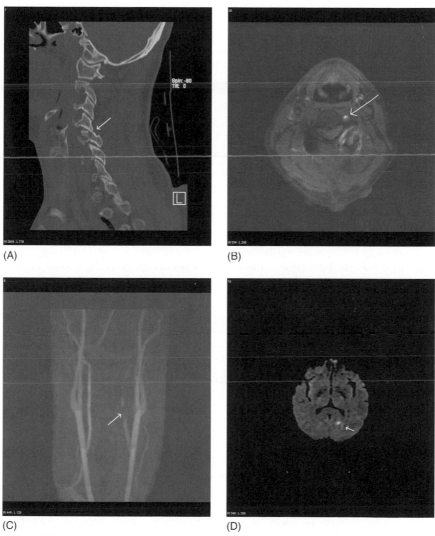

(A)   (B)
(C)   (D)

Figure 12.3 Fifty-five-year-old man involved in motor vehicle accident. (A) CT parasagittal reconstruction of the cervical spine demonstrates a fracture of the left lateral mass of C5 (arrow) resulting in a perched facet joint with slight anterolisthesis at C4–5. (B) Axial fat saturation T1 weighted MRI of the neck demonstrates dissection of left VA (arrow). (C) MRA maximal intensity projection of the neck demonstrates irregularity and focal occlusion of left VA (arrow). (D) Diffusion-weighed axial MRI of the brain demonstrates ischemic infarct of the left occipital lobe (arrow) secondary to the VA injury. The patient was anticoagulated with heparin and coumadin and had no further ischemic events.

of the potential for devastating complications and the importance of early intervention to prevent complications from cervical (extracranial) vascular injury, liberalized screening through imaging technologies is often favored.[36,37,40–42] The distribution of injuries seen in both CA and VA blunt trauma is similar with dissection (70–75%) being the most common finding, followed by occlusion (10–20%), pseudoaneurysm (3–8%), and fistula (up to 4%).[36,37,40–43]

Carotid dissections can present with any of the following features, many of which could be masked or confounded by concomitant spinal cord or vertebral column injury:
- headache or neck pain;
- ischemic features (transient ischemic attacks or completed infarcts);
  - hemiparesis, aphasia, paresthesias, amaurosis fugax, etc.
- neck swelling, bruit;
- pulsatile tinnitus;
- horner's syndrome from compression or trauma of the ascending sympathetic fibers;
- cranial nerve palsies;
- carotid bruit.

Headache and or neck pain was the most common complaint in most studies, with the incidence of neurological findings ranging from 40% to 80% and Horner's syndrome seen in up to 50%.[33,44–51]

Vertebral dissections commonly present with severe occipital headache and posterior neck pain. Additionally, one may see the following features on physical and neurological examination:
- ipsilateral facial dysesthesia or paresthesia;
- dizziness or vertigo, disequilibrium, nausea, and/or vomiting;
- diplopia;
- dysarthria, dysphagia, and/or hoarseness;
- hiccups;
- ipsilateral limb or trunk numbness;
- unilateral hearing loss.

Diagnosis of blunt vessel injury can be made through a number of means, with similar results to those seen with penetrating injuries. Conventional angiography remains the gold standard for diagnosis of blunt arterial injury and should be used when the mechanism and injuries to the spine raise suspicion of vessel injury. Furthermore, if the neurological examination findings do not correlate with non-contrast head computed tomography (CT) findings, angiography should be used to rule-out vascular injury. Duplex scanning, though operator dependent, might be useful not only as a preliminary screen for dissection, fistula, or pseudoaneurysm, but also as a means of monitoring the pathology during treatment. For example, an intimal flap can be detected and monitored with duplex ultrasound. Functional limitations include distal ICA injuries (obscuring of injury by skull base) and detection of dissections that cause minimal to no stenosis or flap. Magnetic resonance imaging (MRI) has quickly emerged as an effective, non-invasive means of detecting dissection by demonstrating mural hematomas and intimal flaps. T1 images with fat saturation will show most dissections, including some intracranial extensions. Limitations of MRI include limited ability to grade stenosis, limited ability to assess longitudinal extension, and an inability to assess flow-dynamics and velocities. MRA has improved sensitivity and can assess stenosis and flow characteristics. HCTA is also a reliable means to detect some, but not all dissections (Figure 12.4).

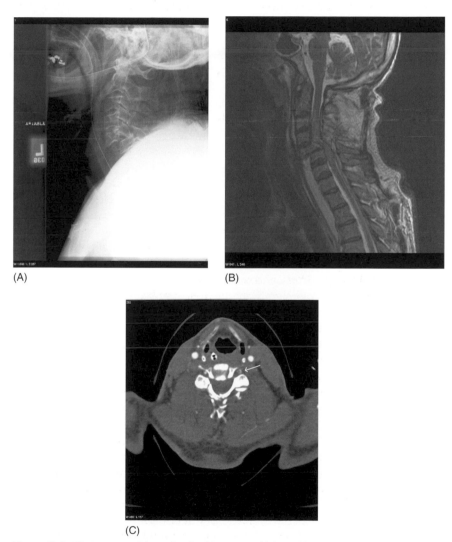

(A) (B)

(C)

Figure 12.4 Fifty-two-year-old man involved in motor vehicle accident as unrestrained driver. (A) Lateral cervical spine X-ray demonstrates grade IV subluxation of C5–6 secondary to bilateral jumped facets. (B) Sagittal MRI demonstrates associated injury to the spinal cord. The patient had complete motor and sensory loss. (C) Axial HCTA demonstrates dissection of the left VA (arrow). Note the luminal filling defect, with preservation of a crescent of contrast around the intimal flap.

Most studies have indicated that the presence of associated cervical spine fracture is the only significant predictor of injury to the VA in cervical spine trauma, and no correlation between pattern of injury to the cervical spine and injury to the VA is evident.[40,52] In one study, 33% of patients with a cervical spine injury had VA injury, and of these patients with a vascular injury, 78% had transverse foramen involvement of the fracture.[36,37] Conversely, in the same study, 48% of all patients with transverse foramen involvement (28/58) and 44% of all patients with subluxation (12/27) had arterial injury.[36,37] Despite a lack of correlation between specific fracture patterns and presence of vascular injury, the preponderance of evidence supports vascular imaging in any patient with significant cervical spine injuries (subluxation, "jumped" facets, or burst fractures), especially if the injury involves the transverse foramen (Figures 12.3–12.5).[36,37,52]

Controversy still exists with respect to optimal treatment of blunt carotid and vertebral injuries for the prevention of stroke. Anticoagulation with heparin followed by coumadin for 3–6 months is widely accepted as appropriate care (Figure 12.3). The role of intraluminal stents remains to be defined.[36,53] Some studies suggest that patients who undergo carotid stenting for blunt carotid pseudoaneurysms may have higher rates of occlusion (and thus stroke) and complication than those treated with antithrombotic therapies.[52] It is worth noting that at this time, there are no randomized trials comparing either anti-coagulants or antiplatelet drugs to control, and some argue that there is no evidence to support their routine use for the treatment of extracranial ICA dissection.[54,55] There are also no randomized trials that directly compare anticoagulants with antiplatelet drugs, and the reported non-randomized studies have not shown any evidence of a significant difference between the two. As endovascular techniques improve, stenting will likely play an increasing role in acute therapy of carotid dissection for the prevention of occlusion and stroke, but most evidence to date consists of small case series.[56–58]

Limited experience has shown that blunt vertebral occlusions frequently do not recanalize with time and conservative management.[59] Anticoagulation with heparin and coumadin[60] remains a standard option for CA and VA occlusion unless contraindicated by other elements of the trauma or intracranial extension of the vessel injury (Figure 12.5). In the latter case, many favor antiplatelet agent use (aspirin), although data remains sparse.

What we currently know about outcome after dissection from blunt cervical artery injury is extrapolated from data on all patients with dissection (including those with spontaneous dissections). The recurrence rate is reported to be between 3% and 8%,[60–62] and there is some data to suggest that two events may occur: early recurrence within the first few months to years and long-term recurrence that can happen more than a decade later.[61,62] There is no difference in recurrence rates between VA and CA dissection. The largest series in the current literature reports the annual risk of recurrence at approximately 1%.[61] Certainly underlying pathologies and risk factors such as fibromuscular dysplasia, vessel tortuosity, cystic medial necrosis, and Marfan's

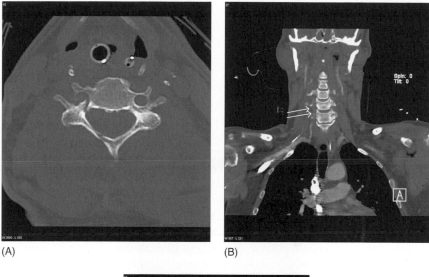

(A)   (B)

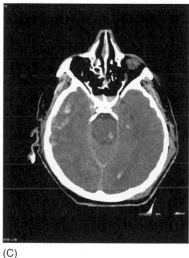

(C)

Figure 12.5 Fifty-nine-year-old male who was struck by a car as an unhelmeted cyclist. (A) Axial CT of the cervical spine shows facet fracture encroaching on the right transverse foramen. (B) Coronal CTA reconstruction demonstrates dissection and occlusion of the right VA at the level of fracture (arrows). (C) Axial head CT demonstrates diffuse intracranial injury (contusions, subarachnoid hemorrhage, and subdural hematoma) precluding the use of anticoagulation to treat the VA injury.

and Ehlers–Danlos syndromes play a large role in recurrence and complications with treatment.

Iatrogenic injury to the cervical arteries

Iatrogenic cervical artery injury is a relatively uncommon occurrence after therapeutic procedures. During surgical procedures to the anterior neck, most inadvertent injuries to the carotid arteries can be controlled with topical hemostatic agents. When they are unable to be controlled, catastrophic outcomes usually result. The incidence of carotid injury from anterior cervical procedures (e.g. anterior cervical spine decompressive procedures) is low enough to the point of being reportable.

More common is injury to the VA, with an incidence of 0.3% in the largest series.[63–65] The current literature argues that injury to the VA is most common when an anterior corpectomy is being performed and is a result of far lateral drilling. Others attribute risk of vertebral injury to tortuosity of the VA and migration toward the midline. VA injury can also occur from posterior cervical instrumentation using lateral mass screws. Care must be taken to direct the screws lateral to the transverse foramen. Although an infrequent occurrence, stroke and death is the common outcome when control of the bleeding cannot be achieved. Most advocate ligation of the artery, especially when the right VA is injured, as the left VA is typically dominant. Endovascular occlusion is often a helpful strategy when the VA is injured and direct surgical access is limited.

Carotid or vertebral injury and stroke after cervical manipulation therapy is also rare. Current estimates place the frequency at 1 in 500,000 to 1 in 3.85 million manipulations.[66–70] Fewer than 300 cases of vascular injury or stroke have been reported, and no relationship between specific factors with respect to the patient, the manipulation or the manipulator has been found.[70]

Conclusions

Injury to the cervical vessels after trauma is rare, but the complications from such injuries can be devastating. Specific characteristics of the trauma and the patient's presenting examination can often lead to sufficient clinical suspicion. Therefore, imaging or surgical exploration, depending upon the type of trauma, is paramount. Prevention of neurological sequelae is the goal of treatment. Though class 1a evidence does not exist, surgery, endovascular repair, and/or antithrombotic drugs can be effective in preventing stroke.

References

1 Martin MJ, Mullenix PS, Steele SR, *et al*. Functional outcome after blunt and penetrating carotid artery injuries: analysis of the National Trauma Data Bank. *J Trauma* 2005;59:860–864.

2 Ramadan F, Rutledge R, Oller D, *et al*. Carotid artery trauma: a review of contemporary trauma center experiences. *J Vasc Surg* 1995;21:46–55.

3 Fabian TC, George Jr SM, Croce MA, *et al*. Carotid artery trauma: management based on mechanism of injury. *J Trauma* 1990;30:953–961.

4 Demetriades D, Skalkides J, Sofianos C, *et al*. Carotid artery injuries: experience with 124 cases. *J Trauma* 1989;29:91–94.

5 du Toit DF, van Schalkwyk GD, Wadee SA, *et al*. Neurologic outcome after penetrating extracranial arterial trauma. *J Vasc Surg* 2003;38:257–262.

6 Kumar SR, Weaver FA, Yellin AE. Cervical vascular injuries: carotid and jugular venous injuries. *Surg Clin N Am* 2001;81:1331–1344.

7 Yang X, Virtaniemi J, Vuorenniemi R. Asymptomatic carotid artery occlusion from a gunshot. The role of angiography in penetrating neck trauma. *Eur Arch Otorhinolaryngol* 1995;252:440–442.

8 Jacob OJ, Rosenfeld JV, Taylor RH, *et al*. Late complications of arrow and spear wounds to the head and neck. *J Trauma* 1999;47:768–773.

9 Neal G, Downing EF. Clostridial meningitis as a result of craniocerebral arrow injury. *J Trauma* 1996;40:476–480.

10 Cogbill TH, Sullivan HG. Carotid artery pseudoaneurysm and pellet embolism to the middle cerebral artery following a shotgun wound of the neck. *J Trauma* 1995; 39:763–767.

11 Mohammed GS, Pillay WR, Barker P. The role of clinical examination in excluding vascular injury in haemodynamically stable patients with gunshot wounds to the neck. A prospective study of 59 patients. *Eur J Vasc Endovasc Surg* 2004;28:425–430.

12 Asensio JA, Valenziano CP, Falcone RE, *et al*. Management of penetrating neck injuries. The controversy surrounding zone II injuries. *Surg Clin N Am* 1991;71:267–296.

13 Kendall JL, Anglin D, Demetriades D. Penetrating neck trauma. *Emerg Med Clin N Am* 1998;16:85–105.

14 McIntyre Jr RC, Kumpe DA, Liechty RD. Reexploration and angiographic ablation for hyperparathyroidism. *Arch Surg* 1994;129:499–503.

15 Demetriades D, Theodorou D, Cornwell E, *et al*. Evaluation of penetrating injuries of the neck: prospective study of 223 patients. *World J Surg* 1997;21:41–47.

16 Gouny P, Nowak C, Smarrito S, *et al*. Bilateral thrombosis of the internal carotid arteries after a closed trauma. Advantages of magnetic resonance imaging and review of the literature. *J Cardiovasc Surg* 1998;39:417–424.

17 Friedman D, Flanders A, Thomas C, *et al*. Vertebral artery injury after acute cervical spine trauma: rate of occurrence as detected by MR angiography and assessment of clinical consequences. *AJR* 1995;164:443–447.

18 Gracias VH, Reilly PM, Philpott J, *et al*. Computed tomography in the evaluation of penetrating neck trauma: a preliminary study. *Arch Surg* 2001;136:1231–1235.

19 Munera F, Cohn S, Rivas LA. Penetrating injuries of the neck: use of helical computed tomographic angiography. *J Trauma* 2005;58:413–418.

20 Rao PM, Ivatury RR, Sharma P, *et al*. Cervical vascular injuries: a trauma center experience. *Surgery* 1993;114:527–531.

21 Cohen CA, Brief D, Mathewson Jr C. Carotid artery injuries. An analysis of eighty-five cases. *Am J Surg* 1970;120:210–214.

22 Bradley III EL. Management of penetrating carotid injuries: an alternative approach. *J Trauma* 1973;13:248–255.

23 Weaver FA, Yellin AE, Wagner WH, *et al*. The role of arterial reconstruction in penetrating carotid injuries. *Arch Surg* 1988;123:1106–1111.

24 Jebara VA, Tabet GS, Ashoush R, *et al*. Penetrating carotid injuries – a wartime experience. *J Vasc Surg* 1991;14:117–120.

25 Diaz-Daza O, Arraiza FJ, Barkley JM, *et al*. Endovascular therapy of traumatic vascular lesions of the head and neck. *Cardiovasc Intervent Radiol* 2003;26:213–221.

26 Amar AP, Teitelbaum GP, Giannotta SL, *et al*. Covered stent graft repair of the brachiocephalic vessels. *Neurosurgery* 2002;51:247–253.

27 du Toit DF, Strauss DC, Blaszczyk M, *et al*. Endovascular treatment of penetrating thoracic outlet arterial injuries. *Eur J Vasc Endovasc Surg* 2000;19:489–495.

28 Grabenwoger M, Fleck T, Czerny M, *et al.* Endovascular stent graft placement in patients with acute thoracic aortic syndromes. *Eur J Cardiothorac Surg* 2003;23:788–793.

29 McNeil JD, Chiou AC, Gunlock MG, *et al.* Successful endovascular therapy of a penetrating zone III internal carotid injury. *J Vasc Surg* 2002;36:187–190.

30 ul Haq T, Yaqoob J, Munir K, *et al.* Endovascular-covered stent treatment of posttraumatic cervical carotid artery pseudoaneurysms. *Australas Radiol* 2004;48:220–223.

31 Werre A, van der Vliet JA, Biert J, *et al.* Endovascular management of a gunshot wound injury to the innominate artery and brachiocephalic vein. *Vascular* 2005;13:58–61.

32 Sanzone AG, Torres H, Doundoulakis SH. Blunt trauma to the carotid arteries. *Am J Emerg Med* 1995;13:327–330.

33 O'Sullivan RM, Graeb DA, Nugent RA, *et al.* Carotid and vertebral artery trauma: clinical and angiographic features. *Australas Radiol* 1991;35:47–55.

34 Pearce WH, Whitehill TA. Carotid and vertebral arterial injuries. *Surg Clin N Am* 1988; 68:705–723.

35 Martin RF, Eldrup-Jorgensen J, Clark DE, *et al.* Blunt trauma to the carotid arteries. *J Vasc Surg* 1991;14:789–793.

36 Miller PR, Fabian TC, Bee TK, *et al.* Blunt cerebrovascular injuries: diagnosis and treatment. *J Trauma* 2001;51:279–285.

37 Miller PR, Fabian TC, Croce MA, *et al.* Prospective screening for blunt cerebrovascular injuries: analysis of diagnostic modalities and outcomes. *Ann Surg* 2002;236:386–393.

38 Biffl WL, Moore EE, Offner PJ, *et al.* Optimizing screening for blunt cerebrovascular injuries. *Am J Surg* 1999;178:517–522.

39 Bok AP, Peter JC. Carotid and vertebral artery occlusion after blunt cervical injury: the role of MR angiography in early diagnosis. *J Trauma* 1996;40:968–972.

40 Biffl WL, Moore EE, Elliott JP, *et al.* The devastating potential of blunt vertebral arterial injuries. *Ann Surg* 2000;231:672–681.

41 Kerwin AJ, Bynoe RP, Murray J, *et al.* Liberalized screening for blunt carotid and vertebral artery injuries is justified. *J Trauma* 2001;51:308–314.

42 Schneidereit NP, Simons R, Nicolaou S, *et al.* Utility of screening for blunt vascular neck injuries with computed tomographic angiography. *J Trauma* 2006;60:209–215.

43 Rao SK, Wasyliw C, Nunez Jr DB. Spectrum of imaging findings in hyperextension injuries of the neck. *Radiographics* 2005;25:1239–1254.

44 Anson J, Crowell RM. Cervicocranial arterial dissection. *Neurosurgery* 1991;29:89–96.

45 Biousse V, Woimant F, Amarenco P, *et al.* Pain as the only manifestation of internal carotid artery dissection. *Cephalalgia* 1992;12:314–317.

46 Sturzenegger M. Spontaneous internal carotid artery dissection: early diagnosis and management in 44 patients. *J Neurol* 1995;242:231–238.

47 Treiman GS, Treiman RL, Foran RF, *et al.* Spontaneous dissection of the internal carotid artery: a nineteen-year clinical experience. *J Vasc Surg* 1996;24:597–605.

48 Saeed AB, Shuaib A, Al-Sulaiti G, *et al.* Vertebral artery dissection: warning symptoms, clinical features and prognosis in 26 patients. *Can J Neurol Sci* 2000;27:292–296.

49 Baumgartner RW, Arnold M, Baumgartner I, *et al.* Carotid dissection with and with-out ischemic events: local symptoms and cerebral artery findings. *Neurology 11* 2001;57:827–832.

50 Bassi P, Lattuada P, Gomitoni A. Cervical cerebral artery dissection: a multicenter prospective study (preliminary report). *Neurol Sci* 2003;24(Suppl 1):S4–S7.

51 Taylor AJ, Kerry R. Neck pain and headache as a result of internal carotid artery dissection: implications for manual therapists. *Man Ther* 2005;10:73–77.

52 Cothren CC, Moore EE, Biffl WL, *et al.* Cervical spine fracture patterns predictive of blunt vertebral artery injury. *J Trauma* 2003;55:811–813.

53 Coldwell DM, Novak Z, Ryu RK, *et al*. Treatment of posttraumatic internal carotid arterial pseudoaneurysms with endovascular stents. *J Trauma* 2000;48:470–472.

54 Beletsky V, Nadareishvili Z, Lynch J, *et al*. Cervical arterial dissection: time for a therapeutic trial? *Stroke* 2003;34:2856–2860.

55 Lyrer P, Engelter S. Antithrombotic drugs for carotid artery dissection. *Cochrane Database Syst Rev* 2003:CD000255.

56 Flis CM, Jager HR, Sidhu PS. Carotid and vertebral artery dissections: clinical aspects, imaging features and endovascular treatment. *Eur Radiol* 2006;16.

57 Georgiadis D, Caso V, Baumgartner RW. Acute therapy and prevention of stroke in spontaneous carotid dissection. *Clin Exp Hypertens* 2006;28:365–370.

58 Edgell RC, Abou-Chebl A, Yadav JS. Endovascular management of spontaneous carotid artery dissection. *J Vasc Surg* 2005;42:854–860.

59 Vaccaro AR, Klein GR, Flanders AE, *et al*. Long-term evaluation of vertebral artery injuries following cervical spine trauma using magnetic resonance angiography. *Spine* 1998;23:789–794.

60 Schievink WI. Spontaneous dissection of the carotid and vertebral arteries. *New Engl J Med* 2001;344:898–906.

61 Schievink WI, Mokri B, O'Fallon WM. Recurrent spontaneous cervical-artery dissection. *New Engl J Med* 1994;330:393–397.

62 Bassetti C, Carruzzo A, Sturzenegger M, *et al*. Recurrence of cervical artery dissection. A prospective study of 81 patients. *Stroke* 1996;27:1804–1807.

63 Burke JP, Gerszten PC, Welch WC. Iatrogenic vertebral artery injury during anterior cervical spine surgery. *Spine J* 2005;5:508–514.

64 Golfinos JG, Dickman CA, Zabramski JM, *et al*. Repair of vertebral artery injury during anterior cervical decompression. *Spine* 1994;19:2552–2556.

65 Smith MD, Emery SE, Dudley A, *et al*. Vertebral artery injury during anterior decompression of the cervical spine. A retrospective review of ten patients. *J Bone Joint Surg Br* 1993;75:410–415.

66 Haldeman S, Carey P, Townsend M, *et al*. Arterial dissections following cervical manipulation: the chiropractic experience. *Can Med Assoc J* 2001;165:905–906.

67 Haldeman S, Carey P, Townsend M, *et al*. Clinical perceptions of the risk of vertebral artery dissection after cervical manipulation: the effect of referral bias. *Spine J* 2002; 2:334–342.

68 Haldeman S, Kohlbeck FJ, McGregor M. Risk factors and precipitating neck movements causing vertebrobasilar artery dissection after cervical trauma and spinal manipulation. *Spine* 1999;24:785–794.

69 Haldeman S, Kohlbeck FJ, McGregor M. Stroke, cerebral artery dissection, and cervical spine manipulation therapy. *J Neurol* 2002;249:1098–1104.

70 Haldeman S, Kohlbeck FJ, McGregor M. Unpredictability of cerebrovascular ischemia associated with cervical spine manipulation therapy: a review of sixty-four cases after cervical spine manipulation. *Spine* 2002;27:49–55.

CHAPTER 13

Intraoperative neurophysiologic monitoring during spinal surgery

Indro Chakrabarti, Jerry Larson, Gordon L. Engler and Steven L. Giannotta

Introduction

Risk of spinal cord (and spinal nerve root) injury during surgical procedures is a major concern and has led to the development of intraoperative neurophysiologic monitoring (IONM) techniques to help prevent such occurrences. Advances in surgical technology and instrumentation have expanded the aggressiveness of approaches to the spine. At the same time, this increases the likelihood of injury to nervous structures. While X-ray, computed tomography (CT), and magnetic resonance imaging (MRI) provide structural information, electrophysiologic testing provides functional assessments of the spinal column. Electrophysiologic recording has become an essential part of spine operations.

Neurophysiologic monitoring has several goals. Ideally, it must be able to detect impending or incipient injury early enough to allow for corrective measures to prevent or ameliorate it. Failing that, it provides documentation and early warning of injuries, facilitating effective postoperative treatment. IONM also allows continual verification of spinal cord and nerve root function throughout a procedure, thereby reassuring the surgeon, and permitting him or her to operate aggressively and with confidence. Mapping techniques can be used to identify and localize nervous structures, or to localize a lesion.[1,2]

Although outcome studies have demonstrated the validity and efficacy of IONM, its effectiveness depends crucially on several factors:[3–5]

1 Selection of appropriate monitoring techniques. IONM techniques are highly specific, and incorrect selection of techniques can result in false negatives.

2 Technical and clinical competence of monitoring personnel.

3 Appropriate anesthesia. Most IONM modalities are highly sensitive to volatile anesthetics, neuromuscular blockade (NMB), or both. Prompt, reliable information cannot be provided to the surgeon without the active cooperation of the skilled anesthetist.[6–8]

4 Appropriate response by the surgeon to adverse changes. The information provided by IONM can only be as valuable as the use the surgeon makes of it. It should also be noted that many efficacy studies have categorized the failure of somatosensory evoked potential (SSEP) monitoring to detect motor impairment

as a false negative. With the advent of routine motor evoked potential (MEP) monitoring, it has been argued by many investigators that since SSEP monitoring cannot be expected to detect pure motor impairment, this should not be regarded as a false negative but as deficient monitoring technique.[9]

The earliest experience with intraoperative SSEPs came from scoliosis surgery. The neurologic deficit that developed in a small percentage of patients who had undergone deformity correction could be reversed with rod removal and lessening distraction in the first few hours.[10–12] This discovery led to the search for techniques that would allow these corrective measures to be instituted intraoperatively.

Prior to the advent of neurophysiologic monitoring techniques, the gold standard for intraoperative spinal cord monitoring was the Stagnara wake-up test.[12,13] By decreasing the level of anesthesia enough to bring the patient to conscious level, the surgeon can ask the patient to move his/her extremities after the surgical correction has been completed but before surgery has been completed. This test requires cooperation between the anesthesiologist, the patient and the surgeon and should be explained and rehearsed preoperatively. Therefore, the test cannot be reliably used with patients who may be uncooperative, children, demented patients, and others. Even with "cooperative" patients there is a real risk of extubation, loss of intravenous lines, and contamination of the wound. The wake-up test is also time-consuming, and can be uncomfortable for all concerned. Its greatest drawback, however, is that it gives information only for one specific time. Injury to the spinal cord occurring after the performance of the wake-up test may go undetected, and injury occurring well before the test may be irreversible. In fairness, this test was originally developed, and worked rather well for, scoliosis surgeries, in which there is a definite moment of highest risk, namely, when the curvature is reduced. The Stagnara procedure may indeed still be useful in some circumstances, but methodologies that provide continuous monitoring throughout the procedure confer a correspondingly great advantage to the surgeon.

SSEP monitoring was the first electrophysiologic method applied to spinal IONM. The cortical or subcortical (brainstem/thalamic) SSEP response is obtained from scalp electrodes following stimulation of peripheral nerves. Spinal recording and stimulus sites have also been used. The basis for SSEP monitoring is the simple concept of stimulating caudal to the surgical site and recording rostral, so that changes in SSEP function can detect incipient injury to the intervening spinal tracts.

The SSEP is carried primarily in the dorsal columns and hence does not directly monitor motor function. In most cases of a mechanical injury to the spinal cord, SSEP is an adequate global index of spinal cord function.[3–5,12] However, SSEP monitoring is insensitive to injuries differentially affecting the motor pathways, notably in intramedullary tumors and in vascular insults to the anterior cord.[14–19] MEP monitoring techniques, especially transcranial electrical MEP (TCeMEP), have been developed for direct motor tract monitoring. Here, the concept is reversed, with rostral stimulation and recording from sites caudal to the surgery, either epidural spinal cord recordings or compound motor action potentials (CMAPs) from skeletal muscles innervated by fibers which exit the cord distal to the surgical site.

Additionally, techniques utilizing spontaneous and evoked electromyography (EMG), including pedicle screw stimulation, have been developed to assist in the avoidance of nerve root injuries.[20,21] The result is an integrated trimodal approach to spinal monitoring: SSEP for dorsal cord, TCeMEP for ventral cord, and EMG techniques for nerve roots, which is arguably the emerging standard of care. Finally, Hoffman reflex (H-reflex) recordings and other electrophysiologic reflex techniques show promise as an additional methodology for motor tract monitoring. Future directions for motor monitoring also include advanced stimulus techniques such as spatial and temporal facilitation, intraoperative collision studies, and greater integration of motor monitoring into the immediate postoperative period.[22,23]

Fundamental concepts

Evoked potentials and spontaneous activity

Electrical activity in the central nervous system (CNS) can be spontaneous or evoked. For example, electroencephalography (EEG) records spontaneous activity in the cerebral cortex. Spontaneous electromyographic activity (EMG) is recorded from muscles. Sensory evoked potentials can be elicited by electrical, auditory, or visual stimuli, and can be recorded from the peripheral or cranial nerve, spinal cord, brainstem and subcortical sites, or the cerebral cortex. MEPs can also be recorded from the spinal cord, nerves, or muscles following electrical stimulation of the motor cortex. CMAPs occurring as spontaneous EMG can indicate nerve irritation. CMAPs can also be elicited by direct electrical stimulation intraoperatively, using a hand-held probe. Thus EMG recordings can be spontaneous or evoked. The terms "free-running" and "triggered" EMG are sometimes used instead of "spontaneous" and "evoked".

Signal-to-noise ratio

Sensory evoked potentials are low in amplitude, in the range of 0.5–3 μV, compared to tens of microvolts for EEG, and up to a millivolt for EMG, evoked EMG, or electrocardiogram (EKG). Therefore, they are easily obscured by background noise and extraneous signals such as ambient electrical noise, especially from electrical equipment such as electrocautery, EEG, EMG, or EKG activity. In fact, monitoring of evoked potentials less than approximately 0.5 μV is questionable or impracticable, and even 0.5–0.9 μV is suboptimal. Signal averaging is used to improve the signal-to-noise ratio (SNR) by removing some of the noise. Most noise occurs randomly, while the evoked potential is time-locked to the stimulus, so random noise can be averaged out. The smaller the amplitude of a potential, the greater the number of responses that need to be averaged to identify non-random EPs. The SNR is proportional to the square root of the number of responses averaged. The average of as many as 1000 trials is sometimes needed to obtain a reliable SSEP recording. At a rate of 5 per second, and with some responses blocked by large artifacts, it can take as much as 5–10 min to obtain a single recording, although with modern equipment and under favorable conditions it can also take only a few seconds. Hence, whatever can be to improve the SNR is critical in allowing the neurophysiologist to provide prompt feedback with certainty.

Other methods for reducing the noise include filtering (since some noise is at frequencies outside the range of frequencies that make up the response waveform), artifact rejection (signals much larger than the expected response are presumptively rejected as being composed mainly of noise or artifact), and the common-mode rejection characteristic of differential amplifiers, which amplify the difference between two signals and cancel out that portion of the noise which is present at both electrodes.

The SNR in intraoperative recordings can be improved by:

1 Maximizing the signal by the use of appropriate anesthetic agents.

2 Decreasing the noise by means of good recording technique and troubleshooting. This includes low electrode impedances, placement of recording electrodes away from sources of electrical activity, braiding or wrapping the electrodes, and identifying offending pieces of electrical equipment and repositioning them or turning them off. Faulty grounds, microscopes and headlamps, and microprocessor-controlled infusion pumps, blood warmers, etc., are frequent offenders. Electrocautery is a source of particularly large electrical artifacts, and it is generally impossible to record during continual use of electrocautery.

Relevant properties of IONM signals

Evoked potential waveforms can be described in terms of properties such as occurrence (present versus absent); amplitude (voltage difference between peak and baseline, or most commonly between negative and positive peaks); latency (time duration from stimulus to response peak or onset); spatial distribution; characteristics of the required stimulus, such as threshold intensity, and waveform morphology.

The most relevant property of intraoperative SSEP waveforms is amplitude. Although in the past many clinicians have considered latency criteria, latency has not been found to be useful.[7] Presumably, the reason for this is that either vascular or mechanical intraoperative injuries invariably reduce amplitude by incapacitating at least some of the neurons in a tract or nerve, so that there is always an amplitude change, sometimes accompanied by a change in latency. This is the exact opposite of the situation in clinical (outpatient) evoked potentials, where amplitude is less useful, because of numerous uncontrolled factors such as head size, orientation of nervous structures, which contribute to high variability in amplitude.[24] On the other hand, clinical evoked potentials are very sensitive to latency changes caused by demyelinization, which of course does not occur during surgery. Intraoperative latency changes without significant amplitude changes generally, perhaps always, result from nonsignificant factors such as changes in anesthetic concentration.[24]

For myogenic MEP recordings, only occurrence has been shown to be reliably useful thus far. More sensitive criteria may be developed in the future. Latency and amplitude are not used in the evaluation of MEP changes due to high levels of variability in these factors. Calancie *et al.* have described a "threshold" method based on an arbitrary criterion of 100 V increase in stimulus to restore a lost response, but since in practice they do not pursue an absent response above a 50 V stimulus increase, this criterion is equivalent to an occurrence criterion.[9] Deletis and his coworkers have used amplitude criteria in the epidural MEP responses, especially in the resection of intramedullary tumors.[25] Yingling and Lyon have suggested that changes in amplitude, threshold and morphology of myogenic MEP could be used to increase the sensitivity of detection of incipient injury.[26]

For spontaneous EMG, the criterion is occurrence of excessively prolonged spontaneous activity, which indicates nerve root or spinal cord irritation. When EMG is evoked by electrical stimulation (generally using a hand-held probe applied to nerve roots), amplitude, and threshold information as well as occurrence can be used.

Baselines and significant changes

Intraoperative changes are compared not to a group norm, but to a baseline established following the induction of anesthesia. In fact, there are no normative data for anesthetized patients, who may also be hypothermic. Hence "normal" and "abnormal" are not relevant concepts in IONM. Gross abnormalities on baseline testing may be of passing interest, but as long as amplitudes are sufficiently high, monitoring can proceed.

Preoperative baseline studies are of limited value, because intraoperative results may be better (due to the patient being deeply relaxed under anesthesia and the practicability of high stimulus levels), or worse (due to anesthesia and other sources of intraoperative variability), and are generally not utilized at our institution, the University of Southern California (USC). In cases where intraoperative monitoring may or may not be possible due to the patient's pathology, the attempt is made, and if there are no monitorable data, monitoring is discontinued.

Responses that may be grossly abnormal can still be monitored as long as amplitude is adequate (generally at least $0.5 \mu V$ for SSEP). Hence, in intraoperative monitoring, the key concept is that of a significant change – significant meaning a change that is judged to represent (at least possibly) an actual physiologic change, rather than being part of the ever present variability and noise seen in intraoperative recordings. In order for a change to be considered significant, technical, anesthetic, and benign systemic factors such as hypotension, hypoperfusion, anemia, and hypothermia must be ruled out. Identification of significant changes is always accompanied by some degree of uncertainty; it is the neurophysiologist's task to reduce this uncertainty to a minimum, and to communicate accurately about it. The value of IONM depends upon correct identification of significant changes and prompt, appropriate, and effective surgical response.

Changes are invariably adverse in nature and intraoperative evoked potential "improvements" have never been documented. The second-named author has never seen a genuine case of improved responses following disk or bony decompression in over 1000 spine cases. However, even if improvements occasionally occur, they do not inform surgical decision-making. For example, decompression would not be discontinued because an improvement had not been seen.

Personnel and equipment for IONM

IONM personnel, known as surgical neurophysiologists, come from various backgrounds including neurology, neurodiagnostic technology, audiology, and neuroscience. Standardized training programs and degrees in the field do not exist at this time, and personnel learn through a mixture of on-the-job training and experience, individual study, and short-training programs such as weekend courses. Two types of certification for IONM are available: CNIM (Certified in Neurophysiologic Intraoperative Monitoring), a technologist-level certification issued by the American Board of Registered Electroneurodiagnostic Technologists (ABRET), and a professional-level board certification issued by the American Board of Neurophysiologic Monitoring (ABNM). Both credentials have experience requirements and require a written examination. The ABNM also requires a graduate degree and an oral examination.

The D. ABNM (Diplomate of the ABNM) is entitled to interpret his or her findings; in theory, the CNIM or uncertified technologist can provide technical services only, and functions under the supervision of a physician, usually a neurologist. In practice, however, it is often one person, whether CNIM, ABNM, or uncertified, who provides both the technical service and the intraoperative interpretation.

Since training, education, and competency of IONM personnel vary widely, it is important for the surgeon to be an "informed consumer" and be in close communication with the neurophysiologist. Although the surgeon cannot reasonably be expected to critique or troubleshoot the monitoring, the neurophysiologist should be able to present and explain his or her data and findings in a brief and effective way so that the surgeon can understand and evaluate them. There should also be an ongoing mutual process of education. The more the neurophysiologist understands the surgeon's concerns, and the surgeon understands the capabilities and limitations of monitoring, the more effectively IONM information can be used.

Several excellent brands of commercial IONM equipment are available. An IONM instrument for spinal monitoring should have the following:
1 At least 8 channels; 16 channels is the emerging standard, and even more may be necessary for some cases. Generally 6–8 channels are required for SSEP, the remaining channels being used for EMG and MEP. With an 8-channel machine, modalities must be alternated. Alternatively, two machines may be used, for example one for motor monitoring and one for SSEP.

2 EMG capability, including evoked EMG.

3 Interleaving (the ability to stimulate at least two sites for SSEP, for example the left and right legs, simultaneously).

4 A high-current stimulator for TCeMEP. For instruments lacking a high-current MEP stimulator, stand-alone stimulators are available for use in conjunction with the recording instrument.

5 Digital data storage and printout capabilities.

It should also have electrically isolated amplifiers and meet relevant legislative and electrical safety standards.

Anesthesia for spinal monitoring

Post-synaptic evoked potentials, including cortical SSEP and myogenic MEP, are severely affected by the volatile halogenated anesthetics such as Forane (isoflurane), Desflurane, and Sevoflurane, as well as by nitrous oxide.[6,27] Effects of halogenated agents, as far as is known, are equivalent MAC for MAC (minimum alveolar concentration, a measure of effective dosage for inhaled anesthetics), although faster-acting agents may appear more potent when first given – especially when changing from isoflurane to a faster-acting agent. It is only a slight oversimplification to say that, apart from muscle relaxants, all intravenous agents are benign with respect to SSEP and MEP recordings.

Nitrous oxide is not recommended in conjunction with halogenated agents when cortical SSEP, and particularly myogenic MEP, are to be monitored (Figure 13.1).[28] Since the MAC for nitrous oxide is slightly greater than 100%, the dosage is generally in the 50–60% range, that is approximately 0.5 MAC. Nitrous oxide by itself is therefore approximately equivalent to, a low dose of halogenated anesthetic, approximately 0.5 MAC. A regimen of nitrous oxide plus intravenous agents, such as the "nitrous/narcotic" technique, is usually reasonably compatible with IONM. However, nitrous oxide in conjunction with other inhalants can result in unpredictable synergistic effects.[8,29]

Generally, TIVA (total intravenous anesthesia) is the most favorable regimen for IONM, although low doses of volatile agents can often be tolerated (Tables 13.1 and 13.2).[27] The most popular agent for TIVA is propofol; other agents such as Droperidol, Pentothal, and Etomidate have been used. Etomidate and Ketamine actually enhance cortical evoked potentials; however, use of these agents is not a viable strategy for enhancing evoked potentials because (1) monitoring of artificially enhanced potentials may not be valid; (2) side effects of these agents generally make them unsuitable for use throughout a procedure. Opiates are also used in conjunction with other anesthetics, for their analgesic properties. Opiate dosage can be increased during the more painful parts of a procedure, thus avoiding the need to increase volatile agents.

The anesthetic protocol for IONM cases at our institution is based on a scalar concept of anesthetic effect. A 2 on the scale (minimal level of halogenated anesthetic, no nitrous oxide) is the standard dosage at USC. When SSEP or MEP responses are too low in amplitude for reliable monitoring, resorting

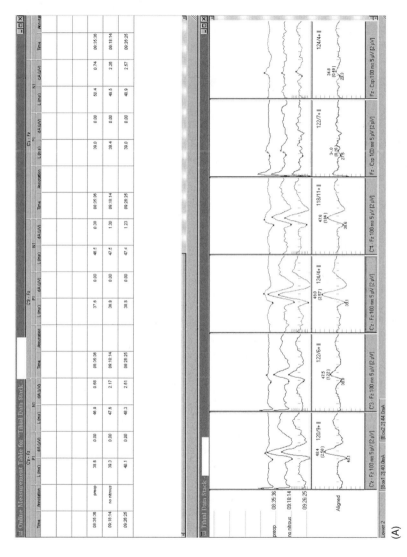

(A)

Figure 13.1 Synergistic effects of nitrous oxide with other inhaled anesthetics. (A) Top line (both of numeric amplitudes and of tracings) shows tibial nerve baseline with 50% nitrous oxide. Lower lines show the response without nitrous. Amplitudes more than tripled when nitrous was discontinued. This is not always the case; it is the result of an unpredictable synergistic drug interaction between nitrous oxide and halogenated anesthetics.

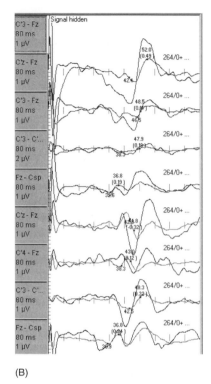

(B)

Figure 13.1 (B) Tibial nerve SSEP. Top four lines represent left leg responses, lower lines represent right leg. Baseline responses recorded without nitrous oxide are superimposed on responses after adding 50% nitrous oxide. Note the marked latency change and greater than 50% amplitude decrease. The fourth and eight lines, labeled "Fz-Csp", do not demonstrate this dramatic difference, because they show the subcortical response, which is relatively unaffected by anesthesia.

Table 13.1 Anesthetic agents' effect on IONM modalities.

Modality	Effect of halogenated anesthesia	Effect of NMB
Cortical SSEP	Moderate to severe <0.5 MAC recommended	No effect. May even be helpful in reducing muscle artifact
Subcortical SSEP	Negligible	
Transcranial MEP (epidural recordings)	Negligible	None
Transcranial MEP (myogenic recordings)	Severely affected. TIVA or <0.5 MAC recommended	NMB is incompatible with myogenic MEP. In some circumstances, MEP recording with partial blockade may be successful, but titration is difficult
EMG	None	NMB, even partial, not recommended with any type of EMG recordings
H-reflex, bulbocavernosus, and other reflex recordings	Severe. <0.5MAC recommended	NMB, even partial, not recommended
Spinal stimulation with spinal, peripheral, or subcortical (brainstem) recordings	Negligible	None

Table 13.2 The LAAFS (Los Angeles Anesthesia Friendliness Scale).

1	TIVA	*Good recording conditions.* Minimal interference with cortical SSEP. Typical response amplitudes 2–4 μV. Recommended when transcranial MEP or cortical SSEPs are to be monitored.
2	<0.5 MAC of any single inhalational agent, including nitrous oxide	*Fair-to-good recording conditions.* Some effect on cortical responses, but still *relatively favorable recording conditions.* Cortical SSEP and even transcranial MEP can usually be monitored.
3	1.0 MAC	*Fair-to-poor recording conditions.* Cortical SSEP amplitudes often less than 1 μV. In the absence of neuropathy, radiculopathy, or myelopathy, SSEPs can usually be monitored, but the reliability and promptness of monitoring feedback are significantly reduced. Myogenic MEP, H-reflex, and bulbocavernosus reflex monitoring cannot be carried out.
4	1.5 MAC	*Poor recording conditions.* Cortical SSEP amplitude 0.5 μV or less. Mixed nerve SSEPs can sometimes be monitored in the absence of pathology; single nerve root ("dermatomal") SSEPs cannot be monitored; reliability and promptness of feed back greatly reduced.
5	>1.5 MAC	*No cortical SSEPs* can be recorded.

to TIVA (1 on the scale) can often render them monitorable; conversely, when responses are very robust and the anesthesiologists require a greater anesthetic level, a slightly higher dosage, 3 on the scale, may be tolerable. Effective SSEP and MEP monitoring cannot be done at higher concentrations of inhaled anesthetic. Generally, effective SSEP monitoring cannot be done with response amplitudes of less than 0.5 μV; amplitudes of >1 μV are optimal. Myogenic MEP recordings are inherently greater in amplitude, in the tens or hundreds of microvolts; the issue there is occurrence of the response, or occurrence at practicable stimulus thresholds.

Monitoring techniques

Short latency SSEPs
Cortical and "subcortical" (brainstem/thalamus) SSEP can be recorded using scalp electrodes, following electrical stimulation of peripheral nerves. Subcortical responses generated in the brainstem and thalamus (P31/N34 lower extremity, P14/N18 for upper extremity) are recorded over frontal scalp, with a reference near one ear (or linked ears), over the cervical spine, or with another reference such as the chin. Actual cervical (spinal) potentials cannot be reliably recorded intraoperatively. The subcortical potentials can be used for spinal cord monitoring when they are sufficiently robust, and in such cases cortical response may not be required. However, the subcortical response is usually not sufficiently robust to be the sole indicator of dorsal column function – in many cases it either cannot be recorded at all, or only with prohibitively long

averaging times. Hence, cortical responses are the preferred or standard method, with subcortical responses providing a useful adjunct in some cases. A peripheral nerve response from brachial plexus or popliteal fossa, can also be helpful as a control, since it demonstrates that the stimulator is functioning properly and the peripheral nerve is not compromised by ischemia or compression (Figure 13.2).

The most convenient and effective sites for stimulation in the upper extremities are the median or ulnar nerves at wrist or elbow. The median nerve generally yields a slightly greater response, but since the root entry level of the nerve must obviously be lower than the site of surgery, the ulnar nerve, consisting primarily of C8 and T1, is generally preferred over the median (C6 and C7) for its greater coverage of the cervical spine. The median can be used when the surgery is at high cervical levels. For thoracic or lumbar surgeries, the upper extremity SSEP does not provide spinal cord monitoring because the nerves enter the cord rostral to the surgical site; however, ulnar nerve SSEP is used in these cases, as a control and also as a way to monitor for position-related nerve injury, especially to brachial plexus and ulnar nerve at the elbow. In cases of cervical instability, a baseline upper extremity SSEP should be obtained prior to positioning. If there is a significant change following positioning, corrective measures must be taken. Pre- and post-intubation recordings can also be used if desired.

The most popular stimulus sites for lower extremity SSEP are tibial nerve at the ankle or popliteal fossa, and peroneal nerve at popliteal fossa or fibular head. The sural nerve can also be used, though its amplitude is somewhat less. Lower extremity SSEP in general are lower in amplitude than upper extremity, and more susceptible to anesthesia. In thoracic cases and some cervical laminectomies, where large regions of spinal cord are exposed to air, spinal cooling can greatly reduce response amplitudes, and can compromise the effectiveness of SSEP monitoring.

Upper extremity cortical SSEP is recorded over the contralateral sensory cortex, usually with a reference either on frontal scalp or over the ipsilateral cortex (Figure 13.3). Lower extremity cortical responses are recorded over the vertex, or the ipsilateral scalp, with a frontal or contralateral scalp reference. The response is, of course, generated in the contralateral cortex, but because the leg cortex is located in the inferior mesial aspect of the cerebral hemisphere, orientation of gyri can result in a larger amplitude either at the midline, or, paradoxically, over ipsilateral scalp. Since either the longitudinal or lateral derivation may yield the larger response, and this can even change during the procedure, we routinely record multiple cortical channels. MacDonald *et al.* advocate a more elaborate procedure for maximization of cortical response amplitude.[30]

SSEP by peripheral nerve stimulation, especially in the lower extremity, can also be effected by peripheral neuropathy such as alcoholic, diabetic, or other metabolic neuropathy, and in many cases this can make SSEP monitoring impracticable. Choice of a more proximal stimulus site (e.g. knee versus ankle)

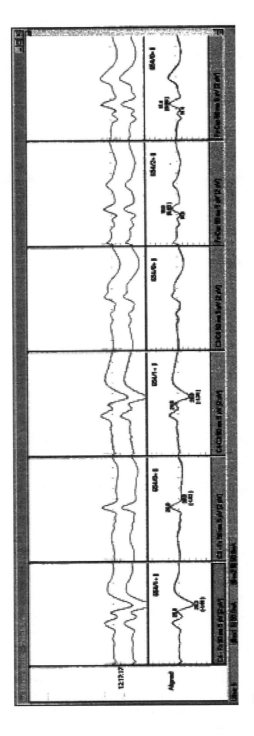

(A)

Figure 13.2 Reversible brachial plexus injury. (A) Grossly normal ulnar nerve baselines with patient in left lateral decubitus position, right arm on airplane. Neurophysiology personnel left after these tracings were taken, while general surgery opened, to return when called by neurosurgery.

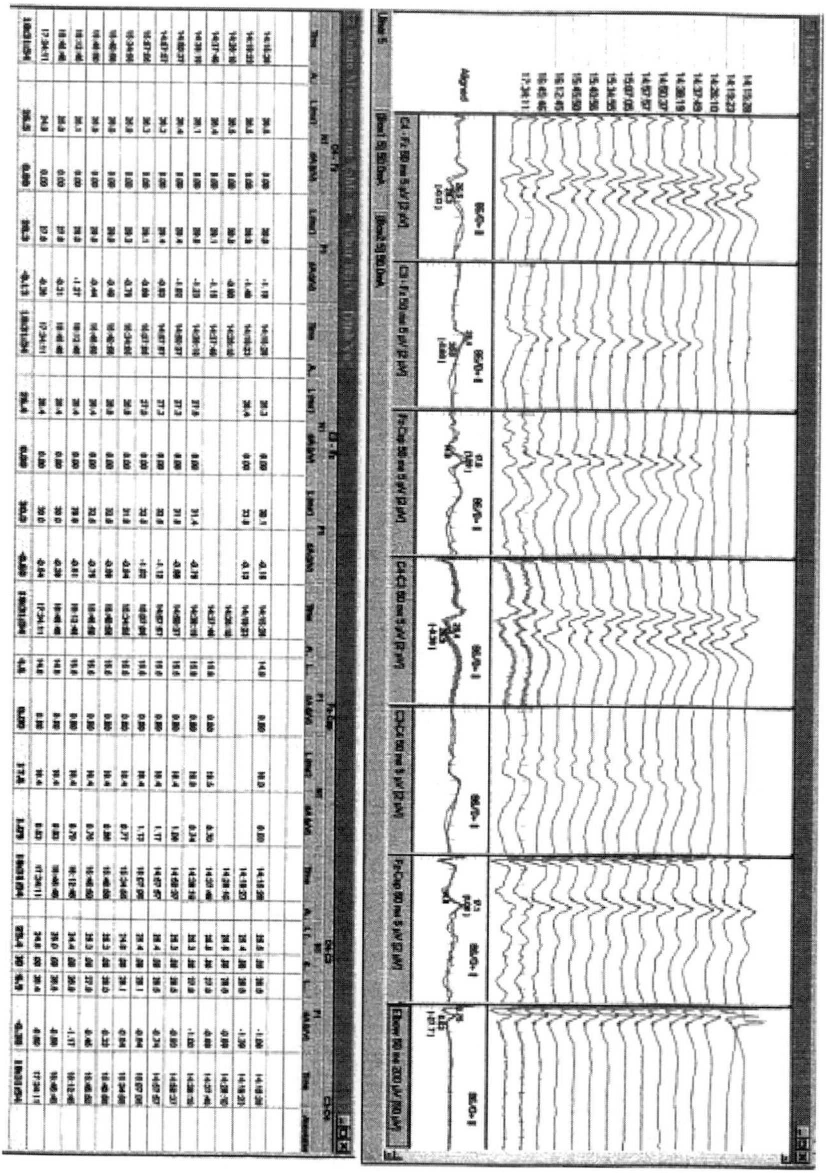

Figure 13.2 (B) Neurophysiology personnel returned to find right arm potentials (panels 2,3,5,7) absent. The arm was found to be off the airplane, hanging straight down. It was repositioned, and in approximately 20 min the response recovered.

International (10–20) electrode placement

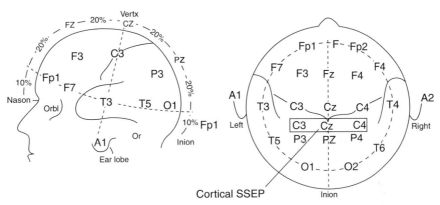

Figure 13.3 Upper extremity cortical SSEP is recorded over the contralateral sensory cortex, usually with a reference either on frontal scalp or over the ipsilateral cortex.

can sometimes ameliorate this problem. Radiculopathy should also be taken into account; for example, an L4 or L5 neuropathy may effectively abolish the peroneal or tibial nerve response, but the sural nerve response (S1 only) might still be available in such a case.

Spinal stimulation

Direct (translaminar, ligamentous, or epidural) stimulation of the spinal cord, with spinal recording offers the advantages of a large response requiring little or no averaging, and of being essentially unaffected by anesthesia. A scalp SSEP can also be recorded with spinal stimulation. The drawbacks to this method are that it is relatively invasive, and can be time consuming and inconvenient to the surgeon. It can only be used during a portion of the procedure; and it cannot differentiate left side from right. Also, once instrumentation is placed, the response may be lost because of current shunting. For these reasons, spinal stimulation has never been popular in the United States, although it is used more commonly in Japan and Europe.[31]

Spinal stimulation elicits an action potential in both directions, in all fibers (orthodromic sensory and motor, antidromic sensory and motor), so that descending potentials, including CMAPs from the extremities, can be recorded. Until the late 1990s it was thought that MEPs could be elicited by spinal stimulation – either myogenic CMAPs, or even so-called "neurogenic MEPs" recorded over a nerve (thus allowing use of muscle relaxants). However, it has been established that so-called "neurogenic motors" primarily represent antidromic sensory stimulation in the dorsal columns, expressed through reflex pathways at the root entry level as descending motor impulses in the lower motor neuron.[32] It is therefore possible that the motor tracts could be damaged, yet a "MEP" could be obtained by spinal stimulation, and in fact this does occur.[19,32] Thus spinal stimulation cannot be used for MEP monitoring.

Transcranial stimulation of the motor cortex avoids this limitation, because synapses cannot be backfired.

Motor evoked potentials

While SSEP provides an effective monitoring modality for the dorsal columns, and by extension a reasonably effective monitoring tool for mechanical injuries to the spinal cord, it cannot directly monitor the motor tracts. A way to monitor motor function directly is inherently desirable. Furthermore, in procedures where the anterior cord circulation may be compromised, such as thoracic-abdominal aortic aneurysms (TAAA) or anterior approaches, motor function can be compromised without SSEP changes, so that direct motor monitoring becomes critically important.[14–19,33] This is also true for intramedullary tumors. Although in most procedures injuries to anterior or ventral cord alone are uncommon, the use of both sensory and motor modalities allows each to confirm the other. A change in, or preservation of, both SSEP and MEP signals allows increased confidence in evaluation.

Since, as seen above, spinal stimulation cannot differentiate between motor and sensory pathways, the motor cortex must be stimulated. In spinal surgery, this means transcranial stimulation. "D" waves resulting directly from stimulation of cortical neurons can be recorded over the spinal cord using epidural electrodes and single pulse stimulation. Stimulation with multipulse trains allows the recording of centrally evoked CMAPs ("myogenic MEP") from distal musculature. Both magnetic (TCmMEP) and electrical (TCeMEP) transcranial stimulation have been successfully used, but technical limitations of magnetic stimulators, and according to some investigators greater sensitivity of magnetic stimulation to anesthetics, have prevented TCmMEP from gaining widespread popularity, although transcranial magnetic stimulation is a promising clinical tool.[34] TCeMEP, on the other hand, has proven effective, especially with the advent of high-current stimulators (Digitimer, Cadwell, Axon Systems, Medtronic Sofamor Danek). Transcranial electrical stimulation is too painful for clinical (outpatient) use, so magnetic and electrical transcranial stimulation may complement each other; the former in the clinic, the latter in the OR. Combined use of SSEP, TCeMEP, and EMG monitoring, respectively for dorsal cord, ventral cord, and nerve roots, is the emerging standard of care in spine surgery. Henceforth, "MEP" refers to MEP monitoring by transcranial electrical stimulation.

Stimulus sites and parameters for TCeMEP

Early research in transcranial stimulation used scalp-to-palate montages, large frontal electrodes, and others. More recent clinical experience has shown that simple scalp montages such as C3–C4 or C1–C2 (of the International 10–20 electrode placement system) or Cz (vertex)-to-anterior-scalp can reliably elicit epidural or myogenic MEP responses (Figure 13.4). The anode (positive electrode) stimulates more effectively than the cathode (negative electrode). The C3–C4 or C1–C2 montages are popular because the polarity of the stimulation

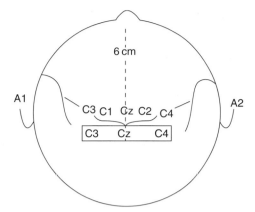

Figure 13.4 Commonly used stimulus electrode sites for TCeMEP.

can readily be reversed, allowing stimulation of each side in rapid succession. The Cz-anterior montage may be more effective in some cases for eliciting leg MEP, especially the more proximal muscles.

Early research also relied heavily on high-current levels to accomplish transcranial stimulation. The Digitimer brand stimulators still deliver up to 1000 V, with maximum current compliance of 1500 mA. Other "high-current" stimulators deliver up to 800 V or 200 mA. However, multipulse stimulation, appropriate anesthesia, and effective stimulus montages allow recording of myogenic responses at lower levels. The number of pulses in a train, length of the individual pulses, interstimulus interval (ISI), and the voltage (or current) are all relevant factors. Using the Digitimer D185, we generally use anywhere from 5 to 9 pulses (fixed at 50 µs pulse width), with an ISI usually of 3–4 ms, and obtain reliable, robust myogenic MEP responses at 200–400 V. Shorter pulse trains will require higher voltage; longer pulse width, available on other brands of stimulators, may allow lower voltage.

Recording sites for TCeMEP

Epidural recordings can be obtained caudal to the surgical site; a rostral control can also be used. Epidural MEP recordings cannot be recorded below approximately the T10 bony level. Deletis describes D-wave monitoring from epidural sites, with a 50% amplitude criterion, in intramedullary tumors, and a phenomenon of preserved D-waves in some cases where myogenic recordings are lost.[25] Lost myogenic response predicts postoperative weakness; preserved D-wave predicts recovery, whereas a lost D-wave predicts permanent loss of function.

Myogenic recording sites can be selected on either of two bases: nerve root level or ease and reliability of response recording. Generally the more distal muscles such as the hand and forearm muscles in the upper extremity, and the tibialis anterior, gastrocnemius, and intrinsic foot flexors or extensors, are more useful for spinal cord monitoring than the more proximal muscles. Also, in some cases the thenar muscles such as the abductor pollucis brevis do not respond when the hypothenar or forearm muscles do; this is presumably due to spread of current inferiorly on the lateral cranium, which reaches the trunk, arm, and fifth digit areas before reaching the thumb area.

If nerve roots are being monitored by EMG, it is generally necessary to cover all the myotomes from C5 to T1, or from L2 to S3. When recording electrodes are placed in muscles at all these levels, MEP can usually be recorded from the same sites. However, great caution must be used in the interpretation of MEP changes in surgeries below the conus medullaris, because of overlap between myotomes. It is possible, for example, that the L5 nerve root on one side could be severely injured, without abolishing the tibialis anterior MEP response, because the muscle is also innervated by L4. This objection does not apply to spontaneous or evoked EMG monitoring, where injury to a specific nerve root presumably will demonstrate spontaneous EMG activity as long as all the myotomes are covered, and where only one nerve root at a time is electrically stimulated.

Safety and practical issues with TCeMEP

Several reports have exhaustively reviewed the safety issues involved in TCeMEP and other forms of cortical stimulation, and concluded that the charge and current levels generated by TceMEP do not pose a significant threat of kindling, seizures, or brain damage, with any of the commercially available stimulators or with various pulse widths or voltages.[35,36] The most salient safety issues with transcranial stimulation for myogenic MEP (without use of NMB) are the associated contractions of head, neck and jaw muscles, and possibly also of paraspinous muscles, which pose potential risks of tongue biting or even damage to teeth or jaw, and of movement against a sharp instrument. A soft bite block must be placed to prevent injury to tongue, teeth or jaw, and the neurophysiologist and surgeon must cooperate to ensure that MEP stimulation is done only when there is no risk of movement against an instrument. However, MEP recordings must be taken frequently enough to provide continuous monitoring. Generally, movement is not an issue in thoracic and lumbar cases.

In some craniotomies and cervical procedures, where head and neck movement is especially pronounced or difficult to tolerate, myogenic MEP can be recorded under partial NMB. In our experience so far, this works well in about 50% of the cases where it is employed. However, titration of the muscle relaxants can be very difficult and time consuming. It also appears that the relationship between level of paralysis, as measured by evoked EMG amplitude or by number of twitches following train-of-four stimulation, varies from patient to patient, so that some patients have good MEP responses before they have even one twitch, while others can have four twitches (but still some weakness) before the response can be obtained. Generally, this technique is effective only when the response can be obtained at approximately one twitch paralysis level. Only short-acting agents should be used for partial blockade, preferably by intravenous infusion rather than bolus. An MEP baseline should be obtained, after positioning and before incision, before any partial blockade is attempted. If the MEP responses are lost during the procedure, it is necessary to reverse the blockade, or allow it to wear off, to verify whether or not responses are still present; this is one reason that only short-acting agents should be used.

After the MEP baseline is obtained prior to incision, it may be convenient to administer a low dose of a short-acting neuromuscular blocker, to facilitate exposure. During the first 20–30 min of most procedures, there is little need for IONM, and continual electrocautery tends to make it unfeasible in any event. In 30 min, the paralyzing agent should be worn off, and MEP monitoring can resume.

H-reflexes

The H-reflex can be recorded intraoperatively in most patients from the gastrocnemius following tibial nerve stimulation at the popliteal fossa, or from flexor carpi radialis following median nerve stimulation at the elbow (Figure 13.5). It is thought that the H-reflex is lost when afferent control, modulated by the

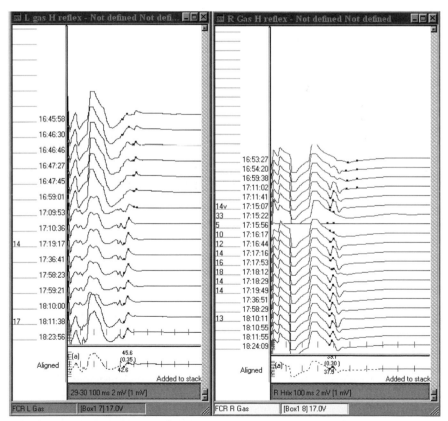

Figure 13.5 Intraoperative gastrocnemius H-reflex tracings. Note that the initial stimulus artifact is followed by the M-wave, then the H-reflex.

corticospinal tracts, is lost, so that the H-reflex offers an alternate way of monitoring corticospinal tract function intraoperatively.[37] This would provide not so much an alternative to MEP monitoring as an adjunct and confirmation, as well as another source of information about spinal cord function. From a technical standpoint, we have found it to be easy to obtain in most patients. Care must be taken to distinguish the H-reflex from the F-wave, which is non-synaptic, non-physiologic, and whose relationship to afferent control is less well understood. The H-reflex is generally found at a relatively low and narrow range of stimulus intensities, and is abolished by increased intensity. It is often abolished before the M-wave is well seen, whereas the F-wave is best seen at supramaximal intensities. Also, the H-reflex is very consistent in latency, amplitude, and morphology, whereas the F-wave is highly variable. In most institutions, the H-reflex is regarded as an investigational technique, as its significance for intraoperative spinal cord monitoring has not been established.

Spinal mapping

Approach to intramedullary spinal cord tumors is usually made through a midline dorsal myelotomy. Since the actual midline between left and right dorsal columns is not always apparent, especially when the anatomy is distorted by the underlying tumor, this myelotomy frequently results in loss of the SSEPs, which are carried in the dorsal columns, and more seriously, in a postoperative dorsal column syndrome. Krzan described a technique of dorsal column mapping by stimulation of tibial or median nerve, with recording over the spinal cord using a miniature multicontact electrode, which allows the actual midline to be located, thus avoiding damage to the dorsal columns.[1] Quinones-Hinojosa *et al.* describe an antidromic technique, stimulating the dorsal columns and recording over peripheral nerve, as well as intramedullary mapping (direct stimulation within the cord for identification of motor tracts).[2] Gardi describes antidromic mapping with myogenic recording (personal communication).[38]

Nerve root monitoring

Spontaneous and evoked EMG

In the profoundly anesthetized patient, even without the use of muscle relaxants there is generally no spontaneous EMG activity present. The patient should have full motor function for any kind of EMG testing. Therefore, NMB, even partial blockade, should be avoided. Even partial NMB can render EMG interpretation problematic.

Widespread spontaneous EMG can indicate light anesthesia and incipient movement. Single CMAPs are seen in response to mechanical stimulation of nerve roots, and generally represent no cause for concern. Prolonged bursts or "trains" of spontaneous EMG, on the other hand, and especially from a single nerve root distribution, suggest nerve root irritation (or in some cases, irritation of spinal tracts). It can be difficult to know where to draw the boundary between brief, benign bursts of activity, which are to be expected in any spinal surgery when muscle relaxants are not employed, and excessively prolonged activity that may indicate incipient injury. Rather than relying solely on the neurophysiologist to make this judgment, the surgeon should also be able to hear the audio EMG, which provides him or her with ongoing feedback (Tables 13.3 and 13.4).

Table 13.3 EMG/MEP recording montages.

Channel	Muscles employed	Myotome represented
Typical EMG/MEP recording montage for thoracic or lumbar surgery		
1	L adductors/quadriceps	L2–L4
2	L tibialis anterior/gastrocnemius	L4–S1
3	L extensor digitorum brevis/extensor hallucis longus	L5
4	L intrinsic foot flexors	S1
5	R adductors/quadriceps	L2–L4
6	R tibialis anterior/gastrocnemius	L4–S1
7	R extensor digitorum brevis/extensor hallucis longus	L5
8	R intrinsic foot flexors	S1
9	Anal sphincter	Lower sacral
Typical EMG/MEP recording montage for cervical surgery		
1	L deltoid (for potential injury to C5/brachial plexus, resulting in deltoid palsy)	C5–C6
2	L biceps/triceps	C6–C7
3	L flexor carpi radialis	C7
4	L abductor pollucis brevis/abductor digiti minimi or first dorsal interosseous/fourth dorsal interosseus	C8/T1
5	R deltoid	C5 C6
6	R biceps/triceps	C6–C7
7	R flexor carpi radialis	C7
8	R abductor pollucis brevis/abductor digiti minimi or first dorsal interosseous/fourth dorsal interosseus	C8/T1
	For MEP spinal cord monitoring, one or more lower extremity channels should also be monitored on each side. The biceps/triceps channel can be omitted to make room for this. The more distal muscles provide the most reliable response (TA, gastroc., EHL, intrinsic foot muscles).	
When nerve roots are not at issue, a simpler montage of 1 to 2 upper extremity and 1 to 2 lower extremity channels per side can be used for MEP monitoring		
1	L flexor carpi radialis/abductor digiti minimi	
2	L tibialis anterior/gastrocnemius	
3	L intrinsic foot flexors	
4	R flexor carpi radialis/abductor digiti minimi	
5	R tibialis anterior/gastrocnemius	
6	R intrinsic foot flexors	
	Here the muscles are chosen for easy elicitation of MEP, rather than for root levels. Generally the more distal muscles respond best due to their rich supply of fast corticospinal neurons.	

L: left; R: right.

Table 13.4 Selection of appropriate monitoring techniques.

Surgical site	Neural structure at risk	IONM modalities	Anesthetic requirement
Cervical	Spinal cord (cervical)	SSEP MEP EMG (optional)	• TIVA or low inhalant (<0.5 MAC, no nitrous oxide) • No NMB if EMG or myogenic MEP is used
	Sometimes cervical nerve roots	SSEP baseline prior to positioning (or prior to intubation) if C-spine is unstable	
Thoracic	Spinal cord (thoracic)	SSEP, MEP	• TIVA or low inhalant (<0.5 MAC, no nitrous oxide) • No NMB if myogenic MEP is used
Lumbar	Lumbar nerve roots (from pedicle screws)	Evoked EMG from pedicle screw stimulation	• No NMB
Thoracolumbar cauda equina	Lower extremity and sacral nerve roots	Lower extremity EMG	• TIVA or low inhalant (<0.5 MAC, no nitrous oxide) for reflex testing
Tethered cord		Anal sphincter EMG Bulbocavernosus reflex	• No NMB
Position-related injuries	Brachial plexus, ulnar nerve	SSEP ulnar nerve and optionally other nerves in upper extremity; MEP with deltoid recording	• TIVA or low inhalant (<0.5 MAC, no nitrous oxide) • No NMB if myogenic MEP is used
Anterior approaches, especially thoracic and lumbar	Ventral cord (ischemia)	MEP for ventral cord; SSEP/EMG if otherwise indicated Test occlusions before sacrificing arteries	• TIVA or low inhalant (<0.5 MAC, no nitrous oxide) for reflex testing • No NMB

One of the primary advantages of EMG monitoring over other techniques such as single nerve root SSEP (see below) is instantaneous feedback when any nerve root is affected. Hence, it is important that the recording montage provide coverage of all nerve roots at risk. Myotomes of different nerve roots vary from patient to patient, and also overlap. In any case, identification of specific nerve roots is less critical than coverage of all the involved roots. Practical limitations often dictate the ganging together of two muscles in one recording channel. MEPs can also be recorded from the same derivations.

While lower extremity EMG monitoring provides adequate coverage of nerve roots L2–S1 or S2, it does not allow monitoring of lower sacral nerve roots. Whenever the cauda equina is at risk, as in tethered cord surgery or cauda equina tumor resection, or when the conus medullaris is at risk – that is, in thoracolumbar procedures such as T12 burst fracture – some form of lower sacral nerve root monitoring must be provided. The most convenient monitoring site for this is the anal sphincter. One pair of subdermal needle electrodes, placed on the left and right sides of the sphincter, is sufficient for recording from this site, thus monitoring left and right sacral nerve roots. Evoked EMG can be obtained by direct nerve root stimulation, and transcranial MEP can also be recorded from this muscle. In addition, the bulbocavernosus reflex can be recorded from this site by stimulation of the penis, clitoris, or urethra. We use a single pair of adhesive surface electrodes in the midline dorsum of the penis. Foam vaginal sphincter electrodes can be used for clitoral/labial stimulation in females; these electrodes could also be used for vaginal sphincter recording. Finally, EMG and MEP can be recorded from a urethral ring electrode placed on the Foley catheter. This same electrode could also be used for urethral stimulation.

Recording of cortical pudendal SSEP with penile or clitoral stimulation has not proved reliable in our hands, or in those of other investigators.[39] However, anal sphincter EMG and MEP, and the bulbocavernosus reflex, have proved quite reliable and stable. According to Vodušek and Deletis, pudendal SSEP can be more effectively monitored with sacral root stimulation.[39]

We recommend a minimal sacral monitoring array of anal sphincter EMG and TCeMEP and bulbocavernosus reflex in all cases posing risk to conus medullaris or cauda equina (Figure 13.6). Where there is more specific concern about bladder control, urethral sphincter monitoring can be added. The sacral nerve roots can be mapped with direct stimulation. Since there is considerable anatomical variation here, this provides an indication as to which roots are most critical for preservation; however, it should not be assumed that a root that shows no EMG response has no function, since one cannot record from all pelvic muscles. Also, even a root with no apparent motor function may contain important sensory or autonomic fibers.

Single sensory nerve root ("dermatomal") SSEP

Mixed nerve SSEPs are insensitive to nerve root injury, because mixed nerves contain fibers from multiple nerve roots, and a single nerve root can be severely injured without greatly affecting the response. A method of single sensory nerve root evoked potential testing, usually called dermatomal somatosensory evoked potentials (DSEP) has been developed.[20,21,40] Although DSEP does provide an effective method of monitoring for nerve root injury, it is subject to severe practical limitations.[20,21] Since only one nerve root can be tested at a time, and since the responses are quite small, they are difficult to record, especially when inhaled anesthetics are used. Schwartz *et al.* ultimately concluded that DSEP monitoring is practical only under total intravenous anesthetic, and only with acute injuries.[41] EMG monitoring provides instantaneous feedback for all nerve roots covered, overcomes all the objections to DSEP monitoring, and has replaced DSEP as the standard of care.

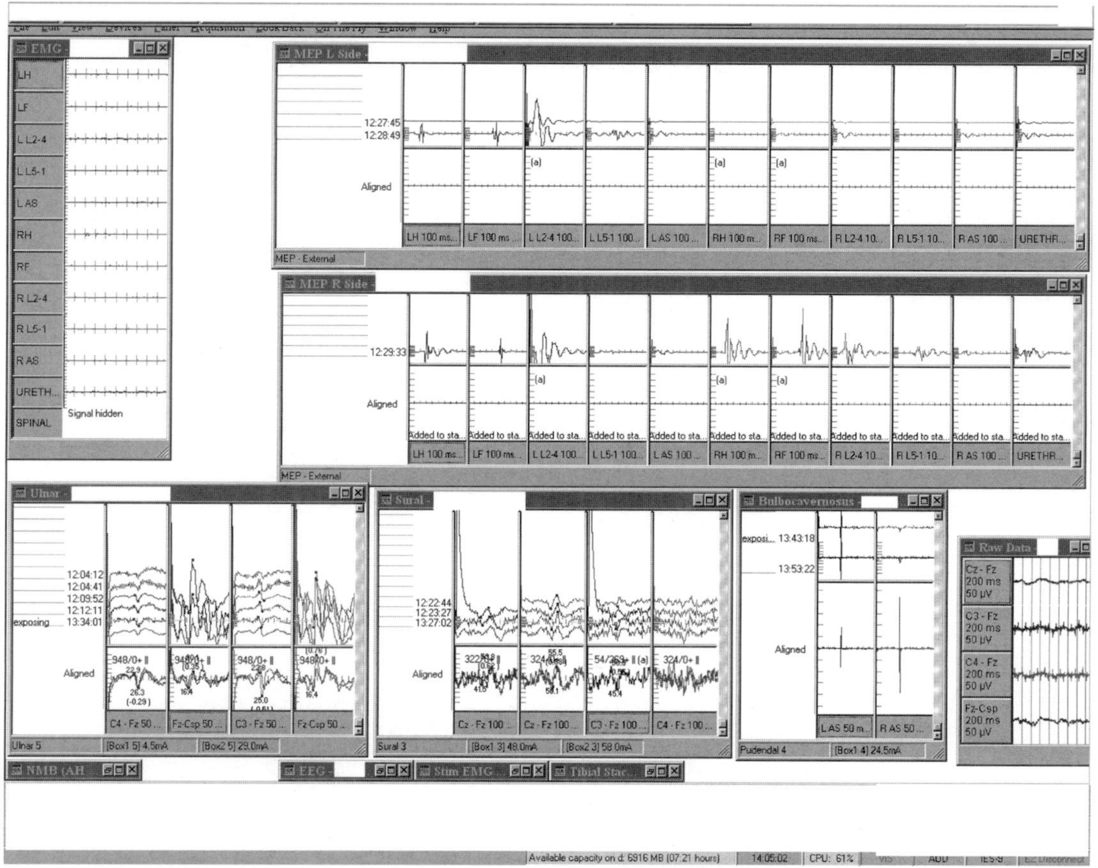

Figure 13.6 Sacral recording in a retroperitoneal approach to anterior lumbar spine in a patient with Pott's disease. Clockwise from upper left: EMG, TCeMEP (including anal and urethral sphincter responses), bulbocavernosus reflex, sural nerve SSEP, and ulnar nerve SSEP.

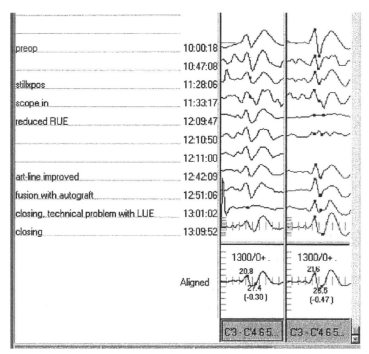

Figure 13.7 Effect of infiltrated intravenous (IV) line on SSEP. During decompression in an anterior cervical discectomy, the right ulnar nerve response was lost. Tibial nerve responses were unaffected, which rules out spinal injury as a cause for this change. The right arm was found to be swollen and blue due to obstructed venous circulation caused by an infiltrated IV. On revising the IV, the response returned. A transient change in left arm response during closing was caused by a technical problem with the stimulating electrodes; on replacing the electrodes, that response returned. The patient had no new deficits.

Monitoring for position-related injuries

Position-related brachial plexus injuries, particularly deltoid palsies, can occur, especially when the arms are in swimmer's or airplane position, or when traction is applied to the arms. Ulnar nerve SSEPs offer a convenient minimal approach to brachial plexus monitoring (Figures 13.2 and 13.7). They provide monitoring for injuries to the ulnar nerve at the elbow, and also provide a control when tibial nerve SSEPs are monitored. Ulnar nerve SSEP alone do not guarantee that there will be no brachial plexus injury, since the ulnar nerve contains only C8 and T1 fibers belonging to the lower trunk of the brachial plexus. A complete SSEP based (actually DSEP based) to brachial plexus monitoring would include median, ulnar, radial, and lateral antebrachial cutaneous nerve stimulation (C6/C7, C8/T1, C6, and C5, respectively). But this would be subject to the above-mentioned practical limitations of DSEP. EMG and MEP from cervical-innervated muscles of the arms, especially the deltoids, provide a more practical approach to brachial plexus monitoring. However, deltoid MEPs cannot always be obtained. Also, it is not feasible to monitor all upper extremity muscle groups in thoracic procedures. We recommend, at a minimum, ulnar nerve SSEP, along with EMG/MEP recordings from deltoid, wrist flexors, and intrinsic hand muscles. Biceps and triceps recordings can be added for more complete coverage of cervical nerve roots and brachial plexus.

Interpretation of IONM changes

The surgical neurophysiologist is always faced with a considerable degree of inherent variability in electrophysiologic data, due to technical factors, anesthesia, and variations in physiologic parameters including, but not limited to, blood pressure, hematocrit, perfusion, body temperature, and spinal temperature (when the cord is exposed as in laminectomies). It is his or her task to determine, with as much certainty as possible, when a genuinely significant change occurs, and to communicate this information to the surgeon promptly, succinctly, in a way that the surgeon can readily apprehend (i.e. without "neurobabble"). When possible, such a change should be correlated with surgical maneuvers. That is, it should "make sense" based on what the surgeons are doing. However, this may not always be the case; sometimes injurious events occur for other reasons such as ischemia, position-related injuries, intraoperative strokes, and drug reactions (Figure 13.8). Also, the injurious effects of surgical maneuvers may not be seen immediately.

The changes considered "critical" have been based on empiric data from large surveys of surgeon practices, rather than on neurophysiologic theory.[3–5] Many authors have proposed, for SSEP monitoring, arbitrary criteria such as a 50% drop in amplitude, or 10% increase in latency. These figures presumably are not based on any idea that a 50% loss of neurons is acceptable. That might conceivably be the case, in the sense that movement and sensation can be preserved with substantially less than 100% neuronal survival. But that does not mean that we would knowingly accept 50% neuronal death. Rather, these are attempts to allow for the above-mentioned variability – yet there is no basis for these arbitrary numeric criteria, so they do not actually improve matters.

As mentioned, latency turns out not to be useful. As for the amplitude criteria, there is no evidence on which to base the choice of a number such as 50%, rather than, for example, 30% or 70%. In fact, 50% would probably be too low; when a genuine adverse change occurs, it is usually the complete loss of the potential, or close to it. Also, in thoracic cases where a large extent of spinal cord is exposed to air, amplitudes frequently diminish by more than 50%. The problem, though, is not the choice of too low an arbitrary criterion; it is the use of arbitrary criteria to mask our uncertainty.

We recommend the following approach to the interpretation of intraoperative changes. When possible, a significant change should be sudden, definite and correlated with what is going on in the surgery. This is not to say that changes cannot be gradual, or cannot occur at unexpected times; however, when this does happen, certainty is inevitably diminished. It is the neurophysiologist's

Figure 13.8 Unexpected change during anterior cervical discectomy and fusion. The first two panels of the upper row show grossly normal baseline SSEP (first tibial nerve, then ulnar). The next two panels of the upper row show unchanged responses following exposure. The first two panels of the second row show a nearly total loss of responses from both legs and the right arm (the current traces, which are flat, are laid over the baseline responses. The difference between each pair of traces demonstrates the change). At this time anesthesia was unchanged, but blood pressure had suddenly dropped. On restoring the blood pressure, the waveforms did not recover. No surgical cause for this change was apparent. The instrumentation was performed. At closing, in the last two panels, tibial responses and right ulnar nerve cortical responses are still absent. Right ulnar subcortical responses (last trace on lower right) have recovered; this finding is inconsistent with a spinal injury, which should abolish subcortical responses. These findings, then, are inconsistent with surgical maneuvers and appear to "make no sense". The patient was taken to immediate postoperative CT scan, and found to have suffered an intraoperative stroke involving the brainstem. Intraoperative detection of this event allowed immediate treatment.

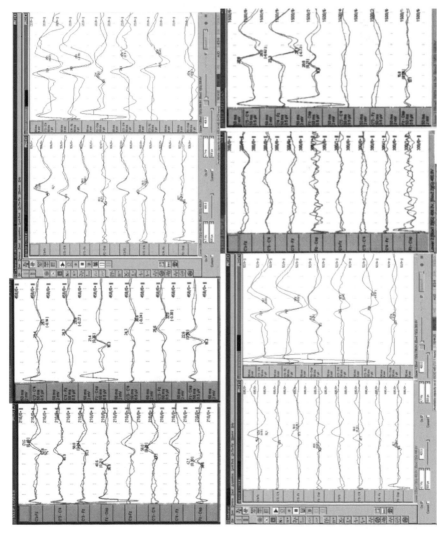

task to provide as much certainty as possible – consistent with prompt feedback. "Crying wolf" unnecessarily must be avoided, but it is equally unacceptable to take 20 min to be certain a change has occurred; it may be too late for corrective measures by that time. The surgeon must be notified, sometimes with a qualification as to the confidence level, while the process of ruling out benign causes goes forward. In some cases, the cause of the adverse neurophysiologic change may be discovered only later, may not be directly related to surgical maneuvers, or may even never be discovered.

The neurophysiologist, on suspecting that a significant change has occurred, should quickly rule out technical, anesthetic and benign causes insofar as possible, but must inform the surgeon promptly. It is acceptable, in fact sometimes necessary, to qualify one's statements: "This could be technical, but I haven't found a technical cause. I'll keep looking, and let you know". Ideally, the neurophysiologist is certain of a change, and informs the surgeon that he or she is certain; sometimes, though, it is necessary to inform the surgeon that a possibility exists, and certainty is not yet attainable.

Useful IONM data consists of:

1 The negative finding, that no significant change has occurred. No response is required, and surgery can proceed with confidence and relative aggressiveness.
2 Adverse changes, which suggest incipient injury, and which require a response.
3 In mapping and testing applications, the identification and demarcation of structures, and verification of function.

Surgeon response

Effective use of IONM requires participation by the surgeons who are making decisions based on the monitoring. The goal of IONM is to prevent incipient injury to the spinal cord or nerve roots. Therefore, IONM is a means for early detection of injury to the spinal cord, and the surgeon must respond to this warning. Otherwise, IONM merely becomes a means for documentation of injury. The initial response is to discriminate systemic and technical sources. When it is determined that incipient injury is likely, the surgeon has a few options. In a coordinated effort the surgeon must accomplish several simultaneous items. At this time the surgeon may wish to increase the blood pressure, increase the systemic oxygenation, locally hyperoxygenate the wound with peroxides, limit inhalation anesthesia, and/or administer neuroprotective agents such as mannitol, phenobarbitol, or high-dose solumedrol. At the same time the surgeon is inspecting the field. A thorough search for a hematoma or site of direct compression is undertaken. Recent placement of implants or manipulations should be undone. Deformity corrections, excessive distraction, or large grafts must be removed. After all else has been checked, he or she may choose to wait a little longer to see if the evoked potential returns spontaneously. Finally, the surgeon can order a wake-up test. This will supply the most direct evidence of spinal cord injury. When structural causes have been ruled out one must suspect inadvertent vascular injury. However, a vascular injury should differentially affect one anatomic zone of the spinal cord, sparing the other. Therefore, with multi-modal monitoring either the MEP or the SSEP only should be affected. However, classic anatomically distinct vascular territories cannot be assumed for every case. A dissipation of evoked potentials may also occur as a result of cerebral injury, as with an intraoperative cerebrovascular accident. An immediate examination of the patient's pupils may provide some cursory evidence. Ultimately, with a spinal operation the surgical team can opt to suspend the operation and allow the anesthesia to fully reverse. In this case the surgeon may wish to abort the procedure on that occasion and return to the operating room if the patient recovers and/or after appropriate diagnostic imaging is undertaken.

References

1 Kržan MJ. Intraoperative neurophysiological mapping of the spinal cord's dorsal columns. In Deletis V and Shils JL (eds): *Neurophysiology in Neurosurgery: A Modern Intraoperative Approach.* Academic Press, Burlington MA, 2002, pp.153–165.

2 Quinones-Hinojosa A, Gulati M, Lyon R, *et al.* Spinal cord mapping as an adjunct for resection of intramedullary tumors: surgical technique with case illustrations. *Neurosurgery* 2002;51:1199–1207.

3 Dawson EG, Sherman JE, Kanim LEA, *et al.* Spinal cord monitoring: results of the Scoliosis Research Society and the European Spinal Deformity Society Survey. *Spine* 1991;16:361–364.

4 Nuwer MR, Daube J, Fischer C, *et al.* Neuromonitoring during surgery: report of an IFCN committee. *Electroencephal Clin Neurophysiol* 1993;87:263–276.

5 Nuwer MR, Dawson EG, Carlson LG, *et al.* Somatosensory evoked potential spinal cord monitoring reduces neurologic deficits after scoliosis surgery: results of a large multicenter study. *Electroencephal Clin Neurophysiol* 1995;96:6–11.

6 Deletis V, Engler GL. Somatosensory evoked potentials for spinal cord monitoring. In Bridwell KH and DeWald RL (eds): *The Textbook of Spinal Surgery*, 2nd edn. Lippincott-Raven, Philadelphia, 1997, pp.85–92.

7 Schwartz DM, Wierzbowski LR, Fan D, *et al.* Surgical neurophysiologic monitoring. In Vaccaro AR, Betz RR and Zeidman SM (eds): *Principles and Practice of Spine Surgery.* Mosby, St. Louis, 2003, pp. 115–126.

8 Sloan TB, Heyer EJ. Anesthesia for intraoperative neurophysiologic monitoring of the spinal cord. *J Clin Neurophysiol* 2002;19:430–443.

9 Calancie B, Harris W, Brindle GF, *et al.* Threshold-level repetitive transcranial electrical stimulation for intraoperative monitoring of central motor conduction. *J Neurosurg* 2001; 95(Suppl):161–168.

10 MacEwan GD, Bunnel WP, Srivan K. Acute neurological complications in the treatment of scoliosis: a report of the Scoliosis Research Society. *J Bone Joint Surg* 1975;57A:404–408.

11 Spieholz NI. Intraoperative monitoring using somato-sensory evoked potentials: a brief overview. *Electromyog Clin Neurophysiol* 1994;34:29–34.

12 Engler GL, Spieholz NI, Bernard WN, *et al.* Somatosensory evoked potentials during Harrington instrumentation for scoliosis. *J Bone Joint Surg* 1978;60:528–532.

13 Vauzelle C, Stagnara P, Jouvinroux P. Functional monitoring of spinal cord activity during spinal surgery. *Clin Orthop* 1973;93:173–178.

14 Deutsch H, Arginteanu M, Manhart K, *et al.* Somatosensory evoked potentials monitoring in anterior thoracic vertebrectomy. *J Neurosurg (Spine)* 2000;92:155–161.

15 Ginsburg HH, Shetter AG, Raudzens PA. Post-operative paraplegia with preserved intraoperative somatosensory evoked potentials. *J Neurosurg* 1985;63:296–300.

16 Lesser RP, Raudzens P, Luders H, *et al.* Postoperative neurological deficits may occur despite unchanged intraoperative somatosensory evoked potentials. *Ann Neurol* 1986;19:22–25.

17 Morota N, Deletis V, Constantini S, *et al.* The role of motor evoked potentials during surgery for intramedullary spinal cord tumors. *Neurosurgery* 1997;41:1327–1336.

18 Pelosi L, Jardine A, Webb JK. Neurological complications of anterior spinal surgery for kyphosis with normal somatosensory evoked potentials (SEPs). *J Neurol Neurosurg Psych* 1994;66:662–664.

19 Zornow MH, Grafe MR, Tybor C, *et al.* Preservation of evoked potentials in a case of anterior spinal artery syndrome. *Electroencephal Clin Neurophysiol* 1990;77:137–139.

20 Toleikis RJ. Neurophysiological monitoring during pedicle screw placement. In Deletis V and Shils JL (eds): *Neurophysiology in Neurosurgery: A Modern Intraoperative Approach.* Academic Press, Burlington MA, 2002, pp. 231–264.

21 Toleikis JR, Arnold OC, Shapiro DE, *et al.* The use of dermatomal evoked responses during surgical procedures that use intrapedicular fixation of the lumbosacral spine. *Spine* 1993;18:2401–2407.

22 Journee HL, Polak HE, deKleuver M, *et al.* Improved neuromonitoring during spinal surgery using double-train transcranial electrical stimulation. Paper presented at the *IX Spinal cord Monitoring Meeting*, Rome 2004 (abstract).

23 Deletis V. MEP's monitoring. Paper presented at the *IX Spinal cord Monitoring Meeting*, Rome 2004 (abstract).

24 Chiappa KH (ed.). *Evoked Potentials in Clinical Medicine*, 3rd edn. Lippincott-Raven Press, Philadelphia, 1997.

25 Deletis V. Intraoperative neurophysiology and methodologies used to monitor the functional integrity of the motor system. In Deletis V and Shils JL (eds): *Neurophysiology in Neurosurgery: A Modern Intraoperative Approach.* Academic Press, Burlington MA, 2002, pp. 25–51.

26 Yingling CD, Lyon WR. Transcranial motor evoked potential monitoring: patterns of intraoperative changes predict postoperative deficits. Paper presented at the *IX Spinal cord Monitoring Meeting*, Rome 2004 (abstract).

27 Scheufler KM, Zentner J. Total intravenous anesthesia for intraoperative monitoring of motor pathways: an integral view combining clinical and experimental data. *J Neurosurg* 2002;96:571–579.

28 Pechstein U, Nadstand J, Zentner J, *et al.* Isoflurane plus nitrous oxide versus propofol for recording of motor evoked potentials after high frequency repetitive electric stimulation. *Electroencephal Clin Neurophysiol* 1998;108:175–181.

29 Wissel MS, Scholz M, Cunitz G. Transcranial magnetic evoked potentials under total intravenous anesthesia and nitrous oxide. *Br J Anesthesia* 2000;85:465–467.

30 MacDonald DB, Stigsby B, Al Zayed A. A comparison between derivation optimization and Cz'-Fpz for posterior tibial P37 somatosensory evoked potential intraoperative monitoring. *Clin Neurophysiol* 2004;115:1925–1930.

31 Follet KA. Intraoperative electrophysiologic spinal cord monitoring. In Loftus LM and Traynelis VC (eds): *Intraoperative Monitoring Techniques in Neurosurgery.* McGraw-Hill, 1994, pp. 231–238.

32 Minahan RE, Sepkuty JP, Lesser RP, *et al.* Anterior spinal cord injury with preserved neurogenic "motor" evoked potentials. *Clin Neurophysiol* 2001;112:1442–1450.

33 Meylaerts SAG (ed.). *Strategies to Protect the Spinal Cord during Thoracoabdominal Aortic Aneurysm Repair*. Ph.D. Thesis, 2000.

34 Padberg AM, Bridwell KH. Spinal cord monitoring: current state of the art. *Orthop Clin N Amer* 1999;30:409–433.

35 MacDonald DB. Safety of intraoperative transcranial electrical stimulation motor evoked potential monitoring. *J Clin Neurophysiol* 2002;19:416–429.

36 Agnew WF, McGeery DB. Considerations for safety in the use of extracranial stimulation for motor evoked potentials. *Neurosurgery* 1987;20:143–147.

37 Slimp JC. Electrophysiologic intraoperative monitoring for spine procedures. *Phys Med Rehabil Clin N Am* 2004;15:85–105.

38 Gardi JM. 2004. Personal communication.

39 Vodušek DB, Deletis V. Intraoperative neurophysiological monitoring of the sacral nervous system. In Deletis V and Shils JL (eds): *Neurophysiology in Neurosurgery: A Modern Intraoperative Approach*. Academic Press, Burlington MA, 2002, pp.197–217.

40 Owen JH, Toleikis JR. Nerve root monitoring. In Bridwell KH and Dewald RL (eds): *The Textbook of Spinal Surgery*, 2nd edn. Lippincott-Raven, Philadelphia, 1997, pp.61–75.

41 Schwartz DM, *et al*. Neurophysiological identification of iatrogenic neural injury during complex spine surgery. *Sem Spine Surg* 1998;10:242–251.

CHAPTER 14

Surgery after the acute phase of traumatic spinal cord injury

Michael Y. Wang and Barth A. Green

Introduction

The chronic care of spinal cord injury (SCI) victims has undergone a tremendous evolution over the past half century. Advances in emergency transport, mechanical ventilation, antimicrobial therapy, wound care, prevention of thromboembolism, and rehabilitation have drastically reduced the medical complications associated with these devastating injuries. In the contemporary era, the life expectancy for a patient who survives the acute injury phase and is not ventilator dependent approximates that of patients in the general population. This is in stark contrast to the universally lethal nature of these injuries before the development of modern medical care.[1]

Because SCI predominantly afflicts young adult men, their life expectancy following injury can span many decades. This population of patients can thus develop a myriad of unique medical problems that must be recognized and treated by physicians specializing in their care. While the focus of most neurosurgeons has been directed toward the operative treatment immediately following injury, there is a growing recognition of disorders that must be addressed operatively long after the traumatic event.

Prevention of medical complications

Any discussion of the delayed surgical care for this patient population must include some commentary on their unique medical needs. After each surgical procedure the spinal injured patient can be expected to have a more prolonged and complicated postoperative course when compared to unimpaired patients. In many ways this will recapitulate their acute hospitalization following the initial injury, and many of these patients will require a short stay at an inpatient rehabilitation center after surgery to compensate for disuse atrophy. Success in surgical intervention is thus predicated upon avoiding those disastrous medical complications associated with the loss of spinal innervation.

Cutaneous and musculoskeletal

Pressure ulcers occur after the acute injury in 25–30% of SCI patients.[2] Because of prolonged immobilization and loss of cutaneous sensation, these patients are at extremely high risk for developing skin breakdown. The most common sites of involvement are the sacrum, heels, ischium, and occiput. Immobilization in the perioperative period can result in new pressure ulcer formation.

The best treatment for pressure and decubitus ulcers remains prevention and early detection. "Log rolling" every 2 h while the patient is on bedrest is the simplest preventive measure. The use of specially cushioned beds or sequentially inflating mattresses is also useful. An alternative is the use of an electrically driven kinetic bed such as the Roto-Rest (Midmark Corporation, Versailles, Ohio).[3] Early detection is dependent upon daily inspection of the dependent areas prone to ulceration. Once skin breakdown has occurred treatment must be instituted quickly to avoid lesion growth and sepsis. Stage I lesions can be managed with aggressive mobilization and adhesive barrier dressings. However, once the dermis has been compromised daily sterile dressing changes may be needed for wound debridement. Deeper lesions may require debridement and skin grafting in the operating room. Proper management of even mild lesions will prevent devastating late sequelae such as sepsis from infected ulcers.

After prolonged immobilization progressive muscle atrophy, spasticity, and contracture formation can occur. Passive range of motioning and splinting can forestall the formation of deformities and contractures. Early involvement in a rehabilitation program incorporating both physical and occupational therapy are mandatory and allow assessment of whether a short inpatient rehabilitation stay will be necessary.

Thromboembolism

Paralyzed patients are at high risk of developing deep venous thrombosis and pulmonary embolism. The incidence of lower extremity venous thrombosis can be as high as 79% if fibrinogen scanning, impedence plethysmography, and venography are utilized.[4,5] Pulmonary embolism occurs in 2–3% of patients and is responsible for roughly 10% of all deaths after spinal cord trauma.[6] This risk of thromboembolism peaks 2–3 weeks after the acute injury, but there is a recurrence of risk with subsequent re-hospitalizations. Routine clinical screening for venous obstruction should be performed prior to surgery. A careful physical examination is utilized and even the slightest suspicion should prompt ultrasonographic investigation.

The early use of pneumatic compression devices and subcutaneous heparin can reduce the risk of thromboembolism.[7] In the absence of any medical or surgical contraindication to anticoagulation 5000 units of subcutaneous heparin should be administered twice a day starting within the first 2 days following surgery. Low molecular weight heparins can also be used for anticoagulation and may be associated with a lower incidence of hemorrhagic side effects.[8] The prophylactic use of a vena cava filter may reduce the risk of potentially fatal pulmonary embolism, and consideration should be given to placement of filters preoperatively in patients who have not had them.[9]

Genitourinary and lower gastrointestinal

The aim of bladder management is to preserve renal function and prevent urinary tract infections. Indwelling catheterization is universally employed in the immediate postoperative period. Even for incomplete patients who were not catheter dependent before surgery, operative manipulation may result in a transient loss of bladder function and urinary retention. For this reason, removal of an indwelling catheter will require meticulous attention to bladder emptying.

The liberal use of catheterization must be balanced against the risks of infection. Urinary tract infections are common and should be treated aggressively to prevent urosepsis. Urea splitting bacteria such as *Proteus* are associated with high incidence of renal calculus formation should be vigorously treated, as renal calculi are found in approximately 1% of patients.[2]

Similarly, surgery may result in transient loss of the ability to properly empty the rectum. This may be the result of surgical manipulation, anesthetic effects, or dietary changes. Constipation can easily occur if attention is not directed in this area, and frequently will be severe enough to require manual evacuation. The judicious use of rectal suppositories stimulates bowel emptying, and regular doses of stool softener should also be used. Because patients may not volunteer information about bowel movements, the physician should ensure that the patient is on a consistent bowel program prior to discharge.

Pulmonary

Respiratory diseases account for 28% of deaths and are the leading cause of mortality in the first year following SCI.[6] Spinal injury patients are at high risk for pulmonary infection for a number of reasons. Prolonged mechanical ventilation, poor pulmonary toilet, an inability to clear upper airway secretions, poor respiratory capacity, nosocomial exposure, weakened immune responses, and any accompanying chest trauma all increase the risk of pneumonia. Early mobilization can help reduce the risk of pulmonary complications. The judicious use of aggressive suctioning, chest physiotherapy, bronchodilators, positive pressure ventilation, and bronchoscopic airway clearance are also useful adjuncts.

Surgical management

The surgical management of this patient population can be broadly divided into four categories:
1 Surgery of the vertebral column.
2 Surgery for syringomyelia and cord tethering.
3 Surgery for functional restoration.
4 Surgery specifically directed at nonmechanical painful syndromes.

Delayed surgery of the vertebral column
Deformity of the spinal column
Because neurologic injuries are universally associated with failure of the musculoskeletal system, treatment of spinal instability is paramount in the acute

phase. Both surgical and nonsurgical treatment schemes share the common goal of realignment and fusion of the spinal column in a physiologic position, and failure to meet these two goals may have to be addressed with delayed surgery. This can be the result of failure to align the spine during initial treatment and fusing it in a deformed position. Alternatively, failure of the fusion can result in a pseudarthrosis which progresses to a deformity. In many cases these two etiologies will be intertwined, with spinal imbalance leading to progressively deforming forces as occurs with progressively kyphosing burst fractures.

Spinal deformity leads to a host of complications, including musculoskeletal pain, neural foraminal compression, spinal cord compression, failure of instrumentation, rib cage and respiratory compromise, functional impairment, and cosmetic abnormalities (Figure 14.1). Surgical treatment must be directed at correcting these problems by meeting three goals:

1 Neural decompression.
2 Deformity correction.
3 Successful arthrodesis.

The surgical techniques for accomplishing these goals are essentially the same as those for deformity surgery in general and outside the scope of this limited

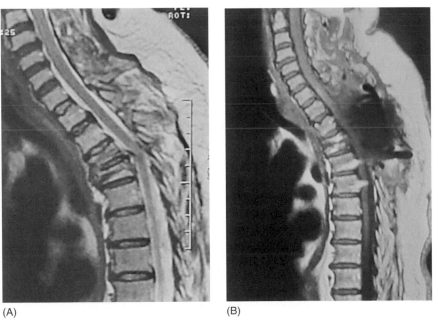

(A)   (B)

Figure 14.1 Patient who suffered a T3/4 burst fracture after a motor vehicle accident. (A) The patient was treated conservatively with bracing but developed a progressive kyphosis leading to thoracic spinal cord compression and myelopathy. (B) Decompression of the kyphus was accomplished through a T4 pedicle subtraction osteotomy to decompress the anterior spinal cord and restore sagittal balance.

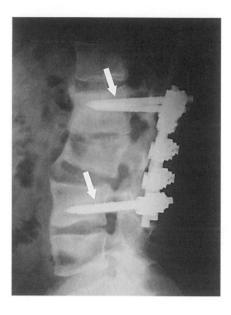

Figure 14.2 Lateral X-ray of a patient who underwent stand-alone pedicle screw fixation for a thoracolumbar burst fracture (12 months postoperative). The construct failed biomechanically with progressive kyphosis, pseudarthrosis, and "windshield wiper" effects at the bone–screw interface with progressive screw loosening (arrows).

discussion (see chapters by Roger *et al.*). However, in this particular population attention must be paid to spinal cord scarring and tethering. For patients with incomplete injuries, the correction of severe deformities can lead to traction on the spinal cord to a degree much greater than in unimpaired patients, resulting in new neurologic deficits. Intraoperative somatosensory and motor evoked potentials can help guide treatment (see chapter by Chakrabarti *et al.*).

Failure of implanted instrumentation

The development of technology for rigid internal fixation has allowed for the rapid mobilization of SCI patients. This has resulted in a reduction in associated medical complications. However, metallic implants are prone to failure over time. Implant loosening can occur at the bone–metal interface with repeated mechanical stresses (Figure 14.2). In addition, implant breakage can occurs due to fatigue from spinal motion (Figure 14.3). While frequently asymptomatic, unsecured hardware can cause a cosmetic deformity or even protrude through the skin. Motion in the soft tissue space can cause irritation and local pain, and rarely the implants may migrate to or impinge upon neural structures.

Any cases of implant failure must prompt an investigation for the cause. Because the etiologies are essentially mechanical, most cases of implant failure are due to either technical problems with the construct or a pseudarthrosis. Only rarely will a severe traumatic event will cause a metallic fracture or migration. The detection of implant problems is typically straightforward on plain X-rays. However, further investigation for a pseudarthrosis should include dynamic X-rays and bone scanning for occult cases.

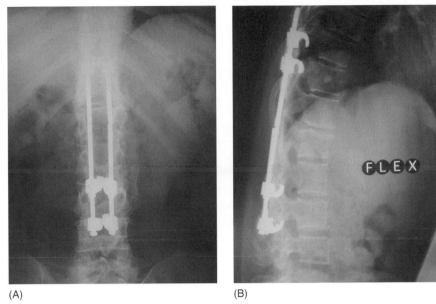

(A)   (B)

Figure 14.3 Thirty-seven-year-old patient who underwent Harrington rod fixation after suffering a thoracolumbar burst fracture from a diving accident. Ten years postoperatively the patient was continuing to experience back pain and was found to have a pseudarthrosis. AP and Lateral X-rays (A and B) demonstrate rod breakage due to continued motion and implant fatigue.

Surgical treatment is directed at removal of the hardware, and at the time of surgery direct investigation of the fusion mass can be conducted. Palpation of the fusion mass and visualization of the fused segments under mechanical stress are the gold standard for assessing fusion, far surpassing the abilities of any imaging modality. Any pseudarthrosis requires a revision of the fusion, either with or without instrumentation.

There are particular problems associated with any revision fusion surgery. The first is related to the availability of implant anchoring sites. Because the neighboring spinal segments have typically already been used for the original fusion the new constructs must frequently be extended into a long-segment fusion. The revision of pedicle screw sites requires special attention, as computed tomography (CT) imaging will have metallic artifact. Placement of larger, revision screws must be approached with care as the previously stressed pedicles are prone to blow-out fractures. The second problem is related to the availability of bone autograft. The iliac crest has typically already been harvested. This, in concert with the frequent need for a long-segment fusion, requires the surgeon to prepare adequate harvest sites and save any bone removed for decompression and exposure. Morselized bone allograft, platelet-rich concentrates, and recombinant bone morphogenetic proteins have recently become commercially available and may help to promote successful long-segment fusions.

Adjacent segment instability

The increased rigidity created by fusing spinal motion segments transfers additional mechanical stress to the adjacent disks and facet joints. This phenomenon has been well described both biomechanically[10] and in clinical series of patients fused for degenerative spine disease.[11] These factors may become accentuated in the paraplegic patient if he or she is physically active. Perturbations in normal trunk motion and stability are created by the loss in innervation of the axial musculature, and this can lead to abnormal stress risers at the level of the impairment when the patient flexes or extends.

Adjacent level degeneration typically leads to an acceleration in disk desiccation, herniation, and segmental instability. This may present as a focal radiculopathy from lateral root compression, long-tract signs from central cord compression, or pain from instability. Magnetic resonance imaging (MRI) scanning will reveal compressive lesions, but these can be obscured by metallic artifact. In such cases a myelogram is warranted. Instability can be revealed by abnormal motion on dynamic X-rays or a "hot" lesion on a radionuclide bone scan. Treatment is directed at decompressing the neural elements, and in almost all cases the fusion will have to be extended to the adjacent level.

Neural compression

Nerve root or spinal cord compression can occur for a number of reasons. In some cases, the neural impingement occurring at the time of injury was either never addressed or incompletely addressed. Adjacent segment instability can also create spinal canal or neuroforaminal impingement from disk herniations. Aggressive treatment should be undertaken in cases where the gain or loss of a single root level will have profound impact on a patient's function. In particular, compression in the lower cervical spine leading to the loss of one cephalad root level can substantially alter hand function.

Degenerative disease

The development of classic degenerative spinal disease is not limited to the uninjured population. Patients with thoracolumbar injuries can develop cervical radiculopathy or myelopathy. This can lead to the progressive loss of extremity function or trunk balance. In addition, lumbar stensosis can lead to gait deterioration in high-functioning patients. The key to the identification of degenerative disease is a high index of suspicion. Operative treatment is the same as for patients in the general population.

Surgery for syringomyelia and cord tethering

Pathologic fluid filled intramedullary spaces developing after SCI are morphologically diverse. Because not all posttraumatic cysts fit the strict definition of a syrinx, these entities are probably best categorized clinically as *progressive posttraumatic cystic myelomalacic myelopathy* (Figure 14.4). The earliest reports describing spinal cord cavitation date back to Etienne in the mid-1500's,[12] and Portal (1804) was the first to correlate the neurologic finding of motor weakness

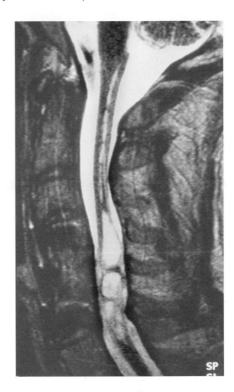

Figure 14.4 Mid-cervical multi-loculated syrinx in a patient who fell from a tree suffering incomplete quadriplegia. Ascending myelopathy prompted MRI evaluation.

as a clinical manifestation of syringomyelia.[13] Early case reports proposing a connection between cystic degeneration of the spinal cord and traumatic injury date back to the writings of Bastian and Strumpell in the late 19th century.[14] In 1890, Schmasus was able to link spinal cord trauma to cystic cavitation in a rabbit animal model, and further recognition of the connection between trauma and syringomyelia came after Charcot (1892) and Cushing (1898) reported cases of syrinx formation soon after SCI.[15–17] In 1935, Tauber and Langworthy reported the first case of delayed syringomyelia in which a patient became symptomatic 8 years after trauma.[18]

With improvements in the survival of spinal injury victims and the coincident increased availability of noninvasive imaging, posttraumatic cysts are more commonly identified. Symptomatic progressive posttraumatic cystic myelopathy occurs in up to 3.2% of SCI patients.[19] Some authors have reported a higher incidence of cysts based upon MRI studies which include asymptomatic patients.[20,21] Injuries that are more severe and that involve more intradural violation are more likely to cause cyst formation because of the increased scarring between the cord and dura. Prolonged immobility which places the spinal cord in a dependent position will also promote adhesions between the cord and dura.

The pathophysiologic mechanism that results in the formation of posttraumatic cysts is poorly understood and remains a topic of considerable controversy.

Gardner originally proposed that an obstruction to cerebrospinal fluid (CSF) flow causes pulse waves to be transmitted caudally through the spinal cord.[22] Fluid is forced into the Virchow–Robin space or central canal of the spinal cord. While this original theory was based upon studies of nontraumatic lesions it became accepted as a pathophysiologic explanation for all syrinxes. Other theories later emerged to explain the development of posttraumatic syringomyelia.[23,24] Milhorat showed that the histopathology and clinical findings seen in posttraumatic syringomyelia were different from lesions of nontraumatic origin.[25] A two-step process was proposed to explain posttraumatic cysts: cyst formation followed by cyst expansion. Cyst formation is a direct result of the injury which causes tissue edema, hemorrhage, and cell loss. Local microcystic cavitation also occurs, and these lesions may become contiguous to form a larger cyst. Cavitation may be aggravated by additional factors, such as hematoma liquefaction, cord ischemia, release of intracellular lyzosomal enzymes, and mechanical crush injury. Pathologic studies show that posttraumatic cysts become lined by flattened ependymal cells, and astrocytic gliosis forms circumferentially around the syrinx.[26]

After initial cyst formation, tethering of the spinal cord to the surrounding dura sets up abnormal CSF flow dynamics. Cyst expansion may then occur as fluid is forced into the existing cavities via transmural migration.[27] Experimental animal models of arachnoiditis in rabbits treated with intrathecal kaolin injection support these theories.[28] The "slosh" hypothesis theorizes that valsalva maneuvers such as coughing and sneezing create a rise in epidural venous pressure which cannot by dissipated when there is interference with CSF flow.[29] These forces are transmitted to the spinal cord which compresses the cystic cavity, distorting areas of structural weakness within the cord parenchyma.[13,19,27] The "suck" hypothesis proposes that increases in epidural venous pressure create a pressure gradient around a partial subarachnoid block. This causes CSF to be rapidly forced upward then sucked back down slowly around the block. Positive pressure proximal to the block leads to cephalad cyst extension. Other theories postulate that a valve-like connection between the subarachnoid space and the cyst allows CSF to enter but not the exit from the syrinx. Mechanical compression from a gibbus, kyphoscoliosis, or canal instability may also cause additional trauma to syringomyelic cavities.

The most common symptom of posttraumatic syringomyelia is pain, the quality of which can be dull, aching, sharp, or stabbing.[30,31] Milhorat reported that painful dysesthesias occur in up to 40% of patients.[32] Hyperesthesias in a dermatomal distribution are also frequently observed. Pain commonly occurs at or above the original site of injury, and cyst expansion with an ascending pain syndrome is a characteristic finding. The pain may be worsened with Valsalva maneuvers. Sensory loss is the second most common complaint and often occurs in a dissociated pattern, with proprioception being spared. Sensory loss may also be patchy, unilateral, or alternating depending on the patient's position. Progressive motor weakness is the third most common symptom but rarely occurs as an isolated phenomenon. Loss of deep tendon reflexes, changes in spasticity, hyperhidrosis, autonomic dysreflexia, Horner's syndrome, incontinence, and respiratory insufficiency are other presenting signs.

MRI is currently the most sensitive diagnostic tool for evaluating cases of possible posttraumatic cystic myelopathy and should be performed in cases of SCI with a delayed progression of symptoms. Because of the excellent soft tissue definition MRI is useful for detecting tumors and intramedullary scar. Myelomalacic cavities can also be distinguished from true syrinxes by their irregularly demarcated borders, moderate hypointensity on T1 weighted images, and non-CSF signal intensity on proton-density weighted images. The non-invasive assessment of CSF flow dynamics has more recently been made possible with CINE MRI. Spinal cord tethering can be assessed in detail using this technique, as an interruption in normal CSF flow is evident around areas where the cord is adherent to the surrounding dura. Cyst pulsatility, which occurs when the syrinx communicates with the subarachnoid space, can also be seen with CINE MRI. This finding may be predictive of future cyst expansion.

Radiographic or clinical evidence of cyst expansion is a clear indication for surgical intervention. Surgery for asymptomatic incidentally detected cysts is more controversial. Small lesions less than 1 cm in rostro-caudal extent that are not causing significant displacement of the surrounding spinal cord are managed conservatively. Narrow asymptomatic cysts spanning several spinal segment that do not expand the cord can also be followed with serial imaging studies every 3–6 months. Large cysts that expand the spinal cord and obliterate the surrounding subarachnoid space usually produce neurologic symptoms and signs and should prompt a detailed physical examination to search for missed findings. In cases followed conservatively, documentation of a detailed history and physical examination of the sensory system is essential to detect any evidence of cyst enlargement. Pain drawings may be a useful adjunct for assessing changes in symptomatology.

Contemporary sophisticated imaging techniques have led to the evolution of radiographic predictors of cyst enlargement. It is our experience that cysts having pulsatile CSF flow on CINE MRI are more frequently symptomatic and will require surgical intervention. Asano et al. used the flow-void sign on T2-weighted MR to distinguish between cases of high-versus low-pressure cysts in his report.[33] In that series cysts with high pressure showed more clinical and radiographic improvement after surgery than low-pressure cysts.

Pre-surgical evaluation should determine the exact location and extent of the syrinx, along with any associated pathology such as cord tethering, subarachnoid cysts, and fissures. Surgery should be carried out with continuous somatosensory and motor evoked potential monitoring and with the aid of the operating microscope. After laminectomy with exposure of the dura, intraoperative ultrasonography is employed to localize the cyst and to visualize any areas of cord tethering. Because cysts frequently occur at sites of previous surgery, special care must be taken in exposing the dura to free it from adhesions to surrounding soft tissue. Frequently a plane can be found using a sharp curette. If this is not possible, soft tissue may be left on the dura and opened along with it in the midline.

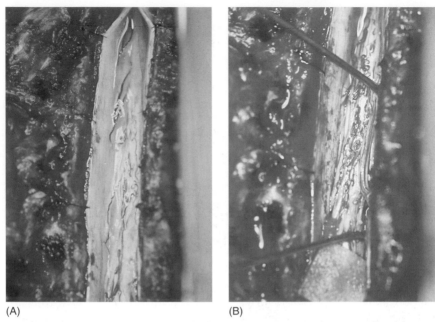

(A)   (B)

Figure 14.5 Intraoperative view: (A) of the thoracic spinal cord showing subarachnoid adhesions to the surrounding dura after trauma; (B) after adhesions have been sharply dissected, the spinal cord is untethered from the surrounding dura.

Before the dura is tacked away from the midline, care must be taken to free it from any neural tissue to prevent lateral tension on the cord. In the event of midline dorsal dural adhesions, an off-center incision can be made.

A key component of the operative intervention is spinal cord untethering with careful sharp dissection of adhesions (Figure 14.5). In our experience proper lysis of adhesions alone will lead to immediate collapse of the syrinx in greater than 50% of cases. This is accomplished primarily with sharp dissection using a No. 11 blade or microscissors. Attention must always be directed at the lateral gutters to ensure free CSF communication. Tethering to the ventral dura may be difficult to lyse and should be done only with the strictest caution to avoid neurovascular injury. It is our practice to repeat intraoperative ultrasonography after untethering to assess cyst size (Figure 14.6). If the cyst has not collapsed, shunting of the syrinx is necessary. We attempt to avoid shunts because of their associated complications. Shunt failure rates have been reported as high as 50% in some long-term studies.[34–37] Cyst overdrainage through the shunt can also be problematic, increasing the risks of arachnoiditis, cord retethering, and rarely an acquired Chiari malformation.

In the event that a shunt is needed, we prefer cyst-to-subarachnoid shunts over shunts that drain into the pleural or peritoneal cavities. The shunt entry point should be chosen at an area where the overlying neural tissue is thinnest and pial arteries are absent. In most cases the caudal end of the cyst is chosen.

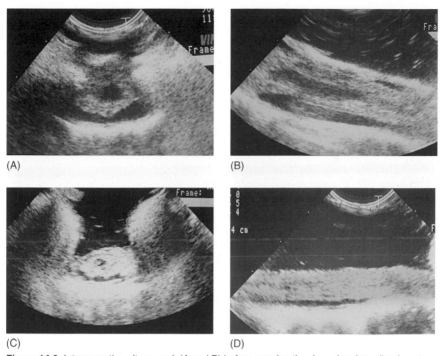

(A)   (B)

(C)   (D)

Figure 14.6 Intraoperative ultrasound: (A and B) before opening the dura showing adhesions to the dorsal surface and the intramedullary cyst; (C and D) after untethering showing cyst collapse, obviating the need for a shunt.

At this point a 2 mm section of pia is cauterized with bipolar current. A vertical myelotomy is then made using a No. 11 blade. The myelotomy can be made at the dorsal root entry zone (DREZ) for eccentrically located cysts. A thin silastic shunt catheter is then directed into the cyst in a cephalad direction. Preoperative measurement of the length of the syrinx will allow an appropriate length of tubing to be used. In the rare event that one tube will not traverse a multi-loculated or double-barreled cyst, additional myelotomies and shunt catheter placements may be necessary. After catheter placement, an X-ray is taken to ensure that it has not kinked or folded over on itself. Intraoperative ultrasound is performed to confirm that the tube is in the syrinx cavity and to evaluate the degree of cyst collapse. Several centimeters of tubing should extend from the myelotomy into the dorsal expanded subarachnoid space created by the duraplasty. Once catheter placement has been confirmed, a 6-0 prolene suture is used to secure it to the pia, preventing dislodgment. If substantial dorsal adhesions are present, the risk of distal shunt occlusion is significant; the tube may be directed between the nerve roots into the ventral subarachnoid space. Pleural or peritoneal shunting are other alternatives. Hemostasis is essential to prevent scarring or retethering and is achieved using thrombin-soaked Gelfoam and careful microbipolar coagulation.

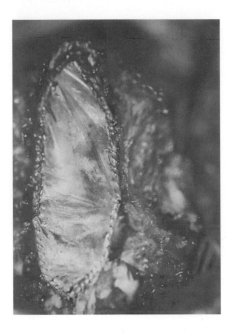

Figure 14.7 Duraplasty to expand the subarachnoid space and prevent retethering.

The prevention of retethering is critical to ensure the long-term success of the surgery. We regularly perform a duraplasty using a dural allograft to expand the dorsal subarachnoid space (Figure 14.7). The dural graft must be sewn in carefully in a watertight fashion using a 6-0 prolene running suture. Postoperatively, patients are carefully positioned in a semi-prone position to keep the spinal cord from resting in the dependent position upon the graft and suture line. Log rolling is performed religiously every 2h for the next 5 days whenever the patient is in bed.

Surgery for functional restoration
Autologous transfer and transposition techniques

It is unfortunate that the regions of the spinal column that are most frequently damaged by trauma are also areas where exiting roots for extremity function are concentrated. Because of this phenomenon, for many patients the gain or loss of a single segmental spinal level will have a profound impact on extremity function. This is particularly the case in mid-cervical injuries where, for example, the difference between a C6 and C7 injury will determine if a patient has a functional grasp.

Surgical modifications to the musculoskeletal system may be used to overcome functional impairment. In this manner, two or three muscles may be transposed to create functional movements. For C5 quadriplegics, transfer of the brachioradialis muscle to the extensor carpi radialis brevis tendon can confer wrist extension. For C6 quadriplegics, the transposition of a functional extensor carpi radialis muscle to the flexor digitorum profundis tendon combined with transposition of the brachioradialis muscle to the flexor pollicis longus tendon can create a functional grasp and pinch. Transfer of the posterior deltoid to the triceps with an interposition fascia lata graft will provide elbow extension.[38–40]

Muscular transposition has even been used to improve bladder function. Microvascular free transfer of latissimus dorsi muscle has been used to restore voluntary bladder contractions in patients with bladder atony.[41] Wrapping the bladder in innervated skeletal muscle led to long-term spontaneous bladder emptying with minimal residual urine.

In this manner substantial augmentation in function is possible, particularly when used in combination with creative dynamic splinting. Because the upper extremity and hand function as the result of complex muscular interactions, postinjury flaccidity or spasticity must be addressed in concert with these newly transposed motor unit.[42] Needless to say, the useful implementation of the transposed muscle requires extensive and lengthy retraining, and intensive work with a hand therapist both pre and postoperatively is absolutely necessary.

Neuroaugmentation for functional restoration

A second approach to restoring function after SCI is through direct control of the target organ by electrical stimulation. While this technology is in its infancy, several devices have already received Food and Drug Administration (FDA) approval. Philosophically, neuroaugmentation differs markedly from neurorestoration in that it may eventually obviate the need for spinal cord reinnervation. Given the pace with which high-technology fields have advanced in the past 50 years, "roboticized" neural control may become a reality. Research in nanotechnology, improvements in microprocessor speed, increased durability of power cells, and refinements in the electrode–neuron interface could all contribute to make life for the SCI victim near normal.

In patients with cervical injuries preliminary studies with electrical stimulation of peripheral nerves innervating the hand have added motor function that would not be possible with tendon transfers alone. With the Free-Hand System (NeuroControl Corp, Cleveland, Ohio) up to seven muscle groups can be stimulated independently. Stimulation is initiated with motions of the contralateral shoulder, and proprioceptive feedback is transmitted to sensate skin areas to assist in relearning. In many cases this has resulted in a functional grasp and improvements in activities of daily living.[43] Nevertheless, current techniques remain crude and often must be supplemented with tendon transfer procedures. In addition, muscle groups that have suffered lower motor neuron damage or prolonged denervation may not respond to electrical stimulation.[44]

Lower limb stimulation is intended to restore the ability to stand, transfer, or ambulate. Superficial transcutaneous electrical stimulation of the peroneal nerve to counteract footdrop has been available for several decades and is widely used in Europe to improve gait. Units involve separate stimulating electrodes surgically implanted intradurally on the L2–S2 rootlets. Using this technique Rushton *et al.* was able to achieve independent standing in seven out of twelve patients in the hospital and four out of twelve at home.[45] The discovery of gait generating centers within the spinal cord of animals has spurred enthusiasm for developing devices for controlled stimulation of gait centers. Clinical evidence of gait improvement with locomotion training in humans suggests that a central pattern generator may also exist in humans. Early studies with rhythmic electrical epidural stimulation of the dorsal lumbosacral spine induced stepping motions in some completely injured patients.[46] More refined microwire arrays that penetrate the ventral gray matter are currently under development.

Patients suffering high cervical injuries may become ventilator dependent as a result of denervation of the diaphragm. For these patients diaphragmatic pacing through electrical stimulation of the phrenic nerve may allow a ventilator independent existence. Since the first description of percutaneous diaphragmatic stimulation in 1948,[47] over 1000 phrenic pacers have been implanted, mostly in Europe. Quadriplegia from SCI is the most common indication for this procedure. The stimulating electrodes are sewn to the perineurium of the mediastinal portion of both phrenic nerves and the pulse generator and battery placed in the soft tissue of the abdominal wall. Thoracoscopic electrode placement is also possible. Following implantation, muscle training and adjustments in electrical amplitude, frequency, and pulse train are adjusted for successful weaning from mechanical ventilation. In most series roughly three-fourths of patients could be successfully weaned from mechanical ventilation.[48] In Mayr's series, half of the patients could have their tracheostomies closed with the patient keeping a backup ventilation mask in the event of respiratory failure.[49] In cases where the phrenic nerve has suffered severe axonal loss, intercostals to phrenic nerve anastamosis has improved the success of phrenic pacing.[50] Effective diaphragmatic pacing can improve the patient's independence and quality of life at home.

Electrical stimulation has also been used to regulate bowel and bladder evacuation.[51] The most commonly used technique is intradural stimulation of the ventral sacral roots. An electrical pulse train causes increasing intravesical pressures behind a constricted sphincter. When stimulation is discontinued the sphincter relaxes and the bladder empties. Several hundred of these devices have been implanted worldwide. A disadvantage of this procedure is the need for sacral rhizotomies to prevent reflex bladder contractions and pain. Superselective microelectrode stimulation of the parasympathetic nuclei and ventral gray matter of the spinal cord may circumvent the need for rhizotomy and improve the urodynamics of micturition.[52]

Surgery for neuropathic pain following SCI

The treatment of neuropathic pain remains difficult and is compounded by its high prevalence in SCI victims. In the study by Stormer, deafferentation pain was the most common type and was identified in 44% of respondents. This was followed by muscular pain (24%), visceral pain (6%), and pain related to spasms (9%).[53]

Neuropathic pain following SCI is also notoriously difficult to treat. It is frequently intolerable in severity and unresponsive to anti-inflammatory and opiate medications. While its etiology is unclear, neuropathic pain may in part be the result of dysfunctional neural sprouting of primary afferents.[54,55] However, even in the absence of any structural abnormality the loss of normal inhibitory processes by endogenous opiates, monoamines, gamma aminobutyric acid (GABA) and glycine may result in pathologic increases in spontaneous and evoked neural activity, and it has been suggested that this up-regulation in aberrant neuronal activity could be the cause of neuropathic pain syndromes following SCI. According to theories proposed by Melzack these pathologic processes occur above the level of injury in "suprasegmental structures." This may explain the failure of traditional ablative procedures such as cordotomy and cordectomy to produce durable pain relief. Over the long term these destructive procedures often produce even more severe neuropathic syndromes.[56]

Results with DREZ lesioning have been more encouraging. When combined with microelectrode recording of the root entry zone to localize areas of aberrant neural activity the ablation can be highly selective. Electrophysiologically guided ablation as described by Falci appears to lead to the highest success rates. However, even without microelectrode recording DREZ can be highly effective. In Gorecki's review of 56 paraplegic patients treated with DREZ, 74% experienced improvement (abstract).[57]

Nondestructive techniques such as spinal cord and deep brain stimulation have also been reported to be effective. In Tasker's recent review of spinal cord stimulation 73.9% of patients experienced greater than 50% pain reduction for 1 year.[58] Motor cortex stimulation has also been attempted in limited populations with mixed results.[59] Implantable drug delivery devices such as spinal subarachnoid and intraventricular pumps have also been used with limited success. In addition to narcotic infusions, direct administration of Baclofen into the central nervous system can decrease both spasticity-related and neuropathic pain.[60]

Conclusions

The advent of modern medical care has resulted in significant prolongation of the lifespan for SCI victims. In addition to the entire host of surgically remediable conditions in the general population at large, spinal cord injured patients have particular medical problems that should be evaluated carefully by experts well versed in this area. Future developments in stem cell as well as robotic technologies will undoubtedly lead to new vistas in the treatment of this unique patient population.

References

1 Amar A, Levy M. Surgical controversies in the management of spinal cord injury. *J Am Coll Surg* 1999;188:550–566.

2 Chen D, Apple D, Hudson L, *et al*. Medical complications during acute rehabilitation following spinal cord injury – current experience of the model systems. *Arch Phys Med Rehab* 1999;80:1397–1401.

3 Green B, Green K, Klose K. Kinetic nursing for acute spinal cord injury patients. *Paraplegia* 1980;18:181.

4 Weingarten S. Deep venous thrombosis in spinal cord injury. *Chest* 1992;102:636s–639s.

5 Harris S, Chen D, Green D. Enoxaparin for thromboembolism prophylactics in spinal injury. *Am J Phs Med Rehab* 1996;75:326–327.

6 DeVivo M, Krause J, Lammertse D. Recent trends in mortality and causes of death among persons with spinal cord injury. *Arch Phys Med Rehab* 1999;80:1411–1419.

7 Nicolasides A, Fernandez J, Pollock A. Intermittent sequential pneumatic compression of the legs in the prevention of venous stasis and deep venous thrombosis. *Surgery* 1980;87:69.

8 Deep K, Jigajinni M, McLean A, *et al*. Prophylaxis of thromboembolism in spinal injuries – results of enoxaparin used in 276 patients. *Spinal Cord* 2001;39:88–91.

9 Velmahos G, Kern J, Chan L, *et al*. Prevention of venous thromboembolism after injury: an evidence-based report. Part II. Analysis of risk factors and evaluation of the role of vena caval filters. *J Trauma* 2000;49:140–144.

10 Akamaru T, Kawahara N, Yoon ST, *et al*. Adjacent segment motion after simulated lumbar fusion in different sagittal alignments: a biomechanical analysis. *Spine* 2003;28:1560–1566.

11 Hilibrand A, Carlson G, Palumbo M, *et al*. Radiculopathy and myelopathy at segments adjacent to the site of a previous anterior cervical arthrodesis. *J Bone Joint Surg (A)* 1999; 81:519–528.

12 Finlayson A. Syringomyelia and related conditions. In Joynt R (ed.): *Neurology*, Vol. 3. JB Lippincott, Philadelphia, 1989, pp. 1–17.

13 Wilson S. Syringomyelia: syringobulbia. In Bruce A (ed.): *Neurology*, Vol. 3. Williams & Wilkins, Baltimore, 1955, pp. 1187–1202.

14 Vernon J, Silver J, Ohry A. Posttraumatic syringomyelia. *Paraplegia* 1982;20:339–364.

15 Madsen P, Falcone S, Bowen B, *et al*. Posttraumatic syringomyelia. In Levine A, Eismont F, Garfin S and Ziegle J (eds): *Spine Trauma*. Saunders, Philadelphia, 1998, pp. 608–629.

16 Cushing H. Haematomyelia from gunshot wounds of the spine. *AM J Med Sci* 1898; 115: 654–683.

17 Barnett H, Jousse A. Posttraumatic syringomyelia. In Vinken P and Bruyn G (eds): *Injuries of the Spine and Spinal Cord. Part II. Handbook of Clinical Neurology*, Vol. 26. North-Holland, Amsterdam, 1976, pp. 113–157.

18 Tauber E, Langworthy O. A study of syringomyelia and the formation of cavities in the spinal cord. *J Nervous Mental Dis* 1935;81:245–264.

19 Schwartz E, Falcone S, Quencer R, *et al*. Progressive posttraumatic cystic myelopathy: neuroradiologic evaluation. *Am J Radiol* 1999;173:487–492.

20 Hussey R, Ha C, Vijay M, *et al*. Prospective study of the occurrence rate of posttraumatic cystic degeneration of the spinal cord utilizing magnetic resonance imaging. *J Am Paraplegia Soc* 1990;13:16.

21 Backe H, Betz R, Mesgarzadeh M, *et al*. Posttraumatic spinal cord cysts evaluated by magnetic resonance imaging. *Paraplegia* 1991;29:607–612.

22 Gardner W, McMurray F. "Non-communicating" syringomyelia: a non-existent entity. *Surg Neurol* 1976;6:251–256.

23 Nurick S, Russell J, Deck M. Cystic degeneration of the spinal cord following spinal cord injury. *Brain* 1970;93:211–222.

24 Williams B, Terry A, Jones H, *et al*. Syringomyelia as a sequel to traumatic paraplegia. *Paraplegia* 1981;19:67–80.

25 Milhorat T, Capoceli A, Anzil A, *et al*. Pathological basis of spinal cord cavitation in syringomyelia: analysis of 105 autopsy cases. *J Neurosurg* 1995;82:802–812.

26 Reddy K, Bigio M, Sutherland G. Ultrastructure of the human posttraumatic syrinx. *J Neurosurg* 1989;71:239–243.

27 Biyani A, Masry WE. Posttraumatic syringomyelia: a review of the literature. *Paraplegia* 1994;32:723–731.

28 Cho K, Iwasaki Y, Imamura H, *et al*. Experimental model of posttraumatic syringomyelia: the role of adhesive arachnoiditis in syrinx formation. *J Neurosurg* 1994;80:133–139.

29 Williams B. The distending force in the production of "communicating syringomyelia". *Lancet* 1969;2:189–193.

30 Green B, Lee T, Madsen P, *et al*. Management of posttraumatic cystic myelopathy. *Top Spinal Cord Inj Rehab* 1997;2:35–46.

31 Lee T, Arias J, Andrus H, *et al*. Progressive posttraumatic cystic myelomalacic myelopathy. *J Neurosurg* 1997;86:624–628.

32 Milhorat T, Kotzen R, Mu H, *et al*. Dysesthetic pain in patients with syringomyelia. *Neurosurgery* 1996;38:940–947.

33 Asano M, Fujiwara K, Yonenobu K, *et al*. Post-traumatic syringomyelia. *Spine* 1996; 21: 1446–1453.

34 Batzdorf U, Klekamp J, Johnson J. A critical appraisal of syrinx cavity shunting procedures. *J Neurosurg* 1998;89:382–388.

35 Lee T, Alameda G, Gromelski E, *et al*. Outcome after surgical treatment of progressive posttraumatic cystic myelopathy. *J Neurosurg (Spine)* 2000;92:149–154.

36 Sgouros S, Williams B. A critical appraisal of drainage of syringomyelia. *J Neurosurg* 1995; 82:1–10.

37 Wiart L, Dautheribes M, Pointillart V, *et al*. Mean term follow-up of a series of post-traumatic syringomyelia patients after syringoperitoneal shunting. *Paraplegia* 1995;33: 241–245.

38 Lo I, Turner R, Connolly S, *et al*. The outcome of tendon transfers for C6-spared quadriplegics. *J Hand Surg* 1998;23B:156–161.

39 Freehafer A. Tendon transfers in quadriplegic patients: the Cleveland Clinic experience. *Spinal Cord* 1998;36:315–319.

40 Freehafer A. Tendon transfers in patients with cervical spinal cord injury. *J Hand Surg* 1991;16A:804–809.

41 Stenzl A, Ninkovic M, Kolle D, *et al*. Restoration of voluntary emptying of the bladder by transplantation of innervated free skeletal muscle. *Lancet* 1998;351:1483–1485.

42 McCarthy C, House J, Heest A, *et al*. Intrinsic balancing in reconstruction of the tetraplegic hand. *J Hand Surg* 1997;22A:596–604.

43 Davis S, Mulcahey M, Betz R, *et al*. Outcomes of upper-extremity tendon transfers and functional electrical stimulation in an adolescent with C-5 tetraplegia. *Am J Occupat Therap* 1997;51:307–312.

44 Keith M, Kilgore K, Peckham P, *et al*. Tendon transfers and functional electrical stimulation for restoration of hand function in spinal cord injury. *J Hand Surg* 1996;21A:89–99.

45 Rushton D, Barr F, Donaldson N, *et al*. Selecting candidates for a lower limb stimulator programme: a patient centred method. *Spinal Cord* 1998;36:303–309.

46 Pinter M, Dimitrijevic M. Gait after spinal cord injury and the central pattern generator for locomotion. *Spinal Cord* 1999;37:531–537.

47 Sarnoff S, Hardenberg E, Whittenberger J. Electrophrenic respiration. *Am J Physiol* 1948; 155:1.

48 Garrido-Garcia H, Alvarez J, Escribano P, *et al*. Treatment of chronic ventilatory failure using a diaphragmatic pacemaker. *Spinal Cord* 1998;36:310–314.

49 Mayr W, Bijak M, Girsch W, *et al*. Multichannel electrical stimulation of phrenic nerves by epineural electrodes. *ASAIO J* 1993;39:M729–M735.

50 Kreiger L, Kreiger A. The intercostal to phrenic nerve transfer: an effective means of reanimating the diaphragm in patients with high cervical spine injury. *Plast Reconstr Surg* 2000;105:1255–1261.

51 Kirkham A, Shah N, Knight S, *et al*. The acute effects of continuous and conditional neuromodulation on the bladder in spinal cord injury. *Spinal Cord* 2001;39:420–428.

52 Prochazka A, Mushahwar V, McCreery D. Neural prostheses. *J Physiol* 2001;533.1:99–109.

53 Stormer S, Gerner H, Gruninger W, *et al*. Chronic pain/dysaesthesia in spinal cord injury patients: results of a multicentre study. *Spinal Cord* 1997;35:446–455.

54 Siddal P, Taylor D, McCleland J, *et al*. Pain report and the relationship of pain to physical factors in the first 6 months following spinal cord injury. *Pain* 1999;81:187–197.

55 Siddal P, Loeser J. Pain following spinal cord injury. *Spinal Cord* 2001;39:63–73.

56 Tasker R, DeCarvalho G, Dolan E. Intractable pain of spinal cord origin: clinical features and implications for surgery. *J Neurosurg* 1992;77:373–378.

57 Gorecki J. DREZ and spinal cord injury pain. Paper presented at: *3rd IASP Research Symposium*; April 16–18, 2001; Phoenix, Arizona.

58 Seong H, Tasker R, Ol Y. Spinal cord stimulation for nonspecific limb pain versus neuropathic pain and spontaneous versus evoked pain. *Neurosurgery* 2001;48:1056–1068.

59 Nguyen J, Keravel Y, Feve A, *et al*. Treatment of deafferentation pain by chronic stimulation of the motor cortex: Report of a series of 20 cases. *Acta Neurochirurgica* 1997;(Suppl 68):54–60.

60 Broseta J, Morales F, Garcia-Marsh G, *et al*. Use of intrathecal baclofen administered by programmable infusion pumps in resistant spasticity. *Acta Neurochirurgica* 1989;(Suppl 46):39–45.

Index